TEACHING MADE EASY

The fourth edition of this highly respected book builds on the excellent reputation of its predecessors. Fully revised and updated throughout, it continues to provide essential structure, support, guidance and tips for both beginning and experienced teachers and their managers, both in the UK and internationally.

Pitched at an introductory level with an emphasis on practical tips and application of theory, rather than focussing heavily on scholarly research, its content is designed to be relevant and inclusive to all healthcare disciplines. Key points are highlighted by the inclusion of tips from experienced teachers in each chapter, while throughout chapters reflect contemporary concepts and key approaches, including teaching styles, curriculum development, e-learning, virtual learning environments, leadership and professionalism.

Teaching Made Easy, 4E will continue to benefit everyone teaching health professionals at all levels, from general practitioners and hospital doctors, nurses in primary and secondary care, and professionals allied to medicine and health service managers, and will also support the development of colleagues in new roles such as physician associates, first contact practitioners and newer nursing associates.

Teaching Made Easy
A Manual for Health Professionals

Fourth Edition

Kay Mohanna
David Wall
Elizabeth Cottrell
Ruth Chambers

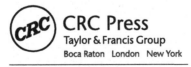

CRC Press
Taylor & Francis Group
Boca Raton London New York

CRC Press is an imprint of the
Taylor & Francis Group, an **Informa** business

Fourth edition published 2023
by CRC Press
6000 Broken Sound Parkway NW, Suite 300, Boca Raton, FL 33487–2742

and by CRC Press
4 Park Square, Milton Park, Abingdon, Oxon, OX14 4RN

CRC Press is an imprint of Taylor & Francis Group, LLC

© 2023 Kay Mohanna, David Wall, Elizabeth Cottrell and Ruth Chambers

First edition published by Radcliffe Medical Press 2000
Second edition published by Radcliffe Publishing 2004
Third edition published by Radcliffe Publishing 2011

ISBN: 978-1-032-40328-1 (hbk)
ISBN: 978-1-032-39763-4 (pbk)
ISBN: 978-1-003-35253-2 (ebk)

DOI: 10.1201/9781003352532

Typeset in Sabon
by Apex CoVantage, LLC

Contents

Section 5: For healthcare educators in relation to the management, leadership and governance of healthcare education

Foreword

I am delighted to write the foreword for the fourth edition of *Teaching Made Easy*. Past iterations have been an invaluable help to both aspiring educators and those who are more established.

This new edition is both timely and welcome during what has been a difficult period in delivering quality education amid unprecedented demands on the NHS. The COVID-19 pandemic of 2020–2022 has been a game changer not only in the delivery of services by the wider healthcare team but also the delivery of medical education and training. The explosion of online materials and the virtual learning environment are here to stay. What is now required are educators with the skills to embrace new ways of delivery and to use the new tools available appropriately. The key is to understand the educator is there to direct and facilitate the learning experience. Using the plethora of tools to engage the trainees ensures that the learning is delivered in the most appropriate way, that is, time efficient, cost effective and learner centered.

The book is not just about doctors and nurses; the authors acknowledge all health and social professionals involved in teaching and learning and the multi-professional dimension to all patient care. Including other health educators is a positive step forward in aligning the standards required of educators to deliver interprofessional education. There is no doubt that this will be the future and is likely to include all health professions going forward.

The authors (who are experts in the field and highly respected by their peers) have produced a book that gives practical tips and applications in the workplace. While they have included some references to the academic nature of the subject, they have rightly majored on the delivery. This makes it suitable to all grades and professionals to be able to dip in and out of the text using the practical tips in their day-to-day teaching. For those that seek additional reading, they have included suitable references and pointers to websites and organisations to further enhance the development of the educator.

The chapters have been updated from the last edition, and they have now included several new chapters, making this book perhaps the most up to date, go-to, adjunct for all involved in medical education.

Being an educator in the health professions does mean investing your time to update your knowledge and skills to be the educator you want to be. This book is a positive addition in helping you to achieve that goal.

Prof Derek Gallen
Emeritus Professor, University of Cardiff
President of the Association of the Study of
Medical Education (ASME)

Preface to the 4th edition

Are you a good teacher? I am not sure I am, at least not all the time. Sometimes teaching collides with clinical work and the inevitable administrative work that seems inexorably to increase year on year. I don't think I always put learners first, supervise them as well as I could or spend as much time with them outside of formal teaching. I have had several learners who struggled. Perhaps that was because of me?

But I have also had joyful experiences. Learners who transformed and flourished and flew.

In the years since our last edition of *Teaching Made Easy*, all of the authors have changed direction and focus in our teaching. We are certainly not the same as we were. What facilitates these differences both in us and in our learners?

We don't know whether the answers are to be found in this book, but we hope some will. Just about every chapter has had a make-over, some significantly so, and several new ones have been added. As I re-read our words from over a decade ago in places I am amazed by the confidence of my younger self, the assumptions I made and the certainty with which I spoke. I am much less sure of things now!

Learning will do that to you; it transforms you.

As teachers, supervisors, mentors and guides, you have picked up this book because you too are asking yourself if you are a good teacher. Like us, you are hoping to be better.

We hope this book helps.

Kay Mohanna
Worcester, UK
April 2022

About the authors

Professor Kay Mohanna FRCGP MA EdD NTF is a partner and trainer in general practice in Lichfield where she is blessed with tolerant partners who let her go off and do other things from time to time. Most recently this has included being part of the founding team for the new Three Counties Medical School at the University of Worcester where she is Professor of Values Based Healthcare Education and the programme director and admissions tutor for the MBChB. In addition, Kay is the International Development Advisor for the MRCGP in South Asia, a Professional and Linguistics Assessment Board (PLAB) examiner for the UK General Medical Council and is on the Editorial Board of Education for Primary Care. In 2020 she became the chair of the medical education sub-committee of Doctors Worldwide, an international humanitarian charity, and was part of a team delivering a Postgraduate Fellowship in Migrant and Refugee Health in the Rohingya refugee camps in Bangladesh.

Professor David Wall FRCP MMEd PhD qualified in medicine in Birmingham in 1970. He has worked in general medicine in Birmingham and in Zimbabwe in Africa for 4 years, and in general practice in Sutton Coldfield for 30 years. In addition to clinical work, he has held many roles in general practice education, and postgraduate medical education. This has included five years as regional director of general practice for the West Midlands Deanery, and then deputy postgraduate dean for the West Midlands Deanery. This included training the trainers, assessment of trainees, and latterly helping doctors and dentists in difficulty, as well as educational research as part of a team with paediatricians, physicians and intensivists. He was awarded an honorary professorship by Staffordshire University. He also served for five years on the British National Formulary for Children committee. He has over 100 peer reviewed publications, mainly on educational issues, including educational climate, workplace-based assessment, multiple mini interviews and faculty development. He retired from the West Midlands and moved to Scotland, where he served several years as a tutor in medical education at the Centre for Medical Education at the University of Dundee. He finally retired in 2016, after 46 years, but still volunteers helping individuals with their dissertations and theses at Masters and PhD level.

Dr Elizabeth Cottrell FRCGP PhD is GP Partner at a teaching and research practice in Staffordshire. She is the lead medical student tutor and a GP trainer within the practice. Lizzie has a passion for primary care and its unique value to the population and embraces the ever-widening multidisciplinary team emerging within this. Lizzie is Honorary Senior Lecturer in General Practice at Keele University, where she was awarded her PhD and worked on primary care research and implementation projects. This role allowed Lizzie to really focus on obtaining relevant evidence and educating professionals and teams to get this into practice. Now a full time GP Partner, quality improvement and maintenance is important to Lizzie, and she supports trainees and colleagues within her practice to not only learn about and deliver high quality primary care but to improve and evaluate new approaches. This has led to many national and international presentations which have been co-authored by medical students and multidisciplinary members of her team. Lizzie has undertaken evaluations to gather evidence relating to new roles in primary care such as Physician Associates, First Contact Physiotherapists and Trainee Nursing Associates. Lizzie is the topic advisor for the NICE Osteoarthritis Guidelines which are currently under national consultation.

Professor Ruth Chambers OBE FRCGP MD is an honorary professor at Staffordshire University and Keele University and has recently retired as a practising GP after 40+ years as a medic at the frontline. Ruth was a clinical lead for digital primary care transformation across Staffordshire (with focus on long-term conditions such as diagnosing and managing cardiovascular and respiratory conditions); and digital upskilling of clinicians and social workers and now social prescribers – creating 500 or so digital champions across England. Ruth has written 79 books (yes 79!!) – mainly for healthcare teams, and some for the general public on health – back pain/healthy heart/work stress; as well as carrying out research, and contributing to national guidance such as rebutting prescribing fraud and NICE guidance on weight management. Ruth has always focused on patient and public perspectives in relation to provision of care and their health and wellbeing. Recently, this has included working as a pathfinder with the Good Things Foundation, improving digital literacy of local patients (including refugees and asylum seekers), developing apps with a co-design approach, and deploying personal digital assistants such as Alexa Echo Show to those in need for their health and wellbeing. Her team have given out more than 400 devices since the COVID-19 pandemic erupted and published six articles in national journals to share the learning.

With additional contributions from:

Dr Elaine Swift BSc PhD currently Head of Digital Learning and Teaching at the University of Worcester, Elaine has twenty years' experience in leading and enabling digital organisational change for learning and teaching and professional practice. She has experience working strategically with key stakeholders in Higher Education to facilitate change in approaches to learning and teaching, digital capabilities and the adoption of digital technologies at a local, regional and national level.

Prof Janina Iwaszko PhD has nearly 50 years of experience of working in adult education and health, with over 25 years of experience using simulation in medical education. From early days studying radiation biology, she went on to get her MSc in Radiation Health and then her PhD in medical biophysics. After a few years abroad, working with barefoot doctors in the Himalayas, she went into adult education and teaching pre-medicine courses. Janina then trained in medicine but was soon involved in an educational charity training a wide spectrum of people from GPs to military personnel in specialist medical areas.

As Senior Clinical Teaching Fellow she taught a wide range of junior medical staff developing differing styles of simulation. She then entered academia as Principal Lecturer in medical education and developed the new Physician Associate MSc and is now the RCP Clinical Lead for the PA national examination. Janina has worked for the last few years integrating simulation into the curriculum of the new medical school at Worcester University. Today she works as a Professor of Clinical Education and Simulation in London promoting interprofessional, simulation and technology enhanced training for a wide range of clinical professions.

Dr Duncan Shrewsbury MRCGP MSc PhD PFHEA is a queer academic GP in Brighton and Senior Lecturer at Brighton and Sussex Medical School, where he is the deputy lead for curriculum development for the undergraduate programme. Prior to medicine, he was a biology teacher in adult education. During this time he undertook additional training (AMBDA FE/HE) to assess people for, and support people with specific learning difficulties. His Masters and PhD in medical education focused on dyslexia in doctors, and other work has focused on supporting learners with disabilities and mental ill-health.

Acknowledgements

Three new chapter authors join us in this edition, and we are grateful for the significant expertise of Dr Elaine Swift from the University of Worcester, Prof Janina Iwaszko from the University of East London, and Dr Duncan Shrewsbury from the Brighton and Sussex Medical School. Thank you also to Dr Dinusha Perera for contributing to Chapter 24. The work of all of you considerably enhances our book. We remain grateful also, for the previous contributions from Dr Mike Deighan and Prof Helen Batty, which are updated and included again here.

We would also like to thank an anonymous reviewer, whose thorough and thoughtful comments on our third edition guided this revision.

KM would like to thank colleagues at the Three Counties Medical School, discussions with whom have informed her thinking and kept her sane (-ish); notably Prof John Cookson, Prof Lisa Jones and Prof Derek Gallen.

DW would like to acknowledge two people with whom he has worked in the past, and who have each made a great contribution to his understanding of medical education over many years. These are Dr Sean McAleer – Senior Lecturer, Centre for Medical Education, University of Dundee, and Professor Alison Bullock – Professor of Medical and Dental Education, Cardiff University.

EC would like to thank her colleagues and patients at Wolstanton Medical Centre who provide a never ending supply of support and motivation as we all navigate our way through the everchanging and challenging world of primary care.

How to use this book

You will note that we have organised the chapters of this book under five headings. These are the five domains of practice identified by the UK Academy of Medical Educators.* This is a portfolio-based approach to developing and credentialling for educators (see Chapter 1).

Section 1: for healthcare educators involved in educational design and learning development processes

Section 2: for healthcare educators in relation to teaching and facilitating learning

Section 3: for healthcare educators making and reporting judgements that capture, guide and make decisions about the achievement of learners, and the feedback required

Section 4: for healthcare educators in relation to medical education research and scholarship

Section 5: for healthcare educators in relation to the management, leadership and governance of healthcare education

It may be that in your role in healthcare education you are more active in some domains than others. Or it may be that there are some areas of activity that you would like to read a bit more about. You might be looking for ways to reflect on, and demonstrate excellence in practice, in a particular domain. Either way some chapters might be of more immediate interest to you than others.

Organising it in this way, we hope the section headings will guide you and help navigate your way through the book.

You could of course sit down and read it cover to cover! Either way, we hope you find it interesting.

---

*Academy of Medical Educators (2021) *Professional standards for medical, dental and veterinary educators*. 4th edn. Cardiff: AoME. Available at www.medicaleducators.org/professional-standards (Accessed 29.3.22).

SECTION 1

For healthcare educators involved in educational design and learning development processes

CHAPTER 1

Starting out and developing as a healthcare teacher

STARTING OUT

As a healthcare professional, you have already had a lifetime of teaching and learning opportunities. You will have had both inspirational and poor educational experiences and everything in between. Reflecting on role models and mentors you have had might have encouraged you to look for ways to become involved in facilitating the learning of others. You might also have met teachers who have highlighted the sort of teacher you would never want to become! Good teaching is a bit like an elephant – hard to define in advance, but you recognise it when you see it.

As you think back over your own previous experiences as a learner, what did you find effective? Think about different teaching methods such as lectures, small group seminars or problem-based learning (PBL). Consider skills training, simulations or workshops. What characterised the teachers that you felt were effective, inspirational or 'good'? Think about previous poor or frustrating teaching experiences. Why do you think this was the case? What could have been done to change this? Compare your list with the examples in Box 1.1.

If you are interested in what effective teaching looks like, chances are you are already involved in teaching. With patients and junior colleagues in clinic perhaps, or with students or trainees or other members of the multidisciplinary team. Seeking out and offering to support the learning of junior colleagues will always be welcome since opportunities in the clinical setting can be crowded out with the hectic 'day-job' of looking after patients. Students may feel in the way, or a burden to busy healthcare professionals. Remember what it was like for you as a student or trainee and how it felt to have someone offer to talk to you about a patient, or involve you in their care. These, though informal, are important teaching moments through which you can develop your teaching and leadership skills and, as a role model, help others develop their professional identity.

DOI: 10.1201/9781003352532-2

BOX 1.1 EXAMPLES OF REFLECTIONS FROM INTERNATIONAL HEALTHCARE STUDENTS

Students' perspectives on qualities of 'good' and 'poor' teachers

Based on past experiences, learners were asked what elements resulted in a good teaching experience and/or a good teacher. They suggested the following:

- Enthusiasm, a love for the subject.
- A questioning, challenging, patient approach – ensured depth of knowledge rather than mere rote learning.
- Focussed, clear aims (outlined at the beginning of the teaching session), concentrating on the main points.
- Good knowledge of and interest in the subject, knowing what the learner needs to know, intelligent, willing to answer questions, experienced.
- Good relationship with learners: approachable; listening; interacting with learners at their level; mutual respect between teacher and learner; showing empathy, understanding and consideration in relation to learners; taking an interest in the learners and their experiences; 'understanding our feelings'; being keen to learn from learners.
- Being supportive (e.g. to those who struggle by arranging an extra tutorial, giving additional feedback on submitted work, etc.).
- High level of class participation, trying to make classes interesting, liberal use of teaching aids.
- Going back to basics – 'the teacher made us think the clinical problems through in a logical way, which made us realise that we could work answers out if we followed a logical pattern.'
- Relating the subject back to real life and/or clinical scenarios – 'we could see why each piece of information was important and where it fitted in.'
- A dynamic and adaptable style of teaching, using pictures, PowerPoint, etc. as necessary and appropriate.
- Ability to project voice across a room so that everyone can clearly hear what they are saying.
- Understanding that learners have different knowledge levels, not reacting negatively if learners do not know something, and making sure that learners have learned what they were supposed to learn.

Students' thoughts on what made teaching experiences negative

- Boring, lack of involvement of learners and/or the teacher talking all the time.
- Uncertain session objectives.
- Running out of time, poor organisation, the teacher being late for the session, the session being held at a bad time of the day, the teaching session being too long and/or without a break.
- Teaching 'bookish knowledge', repeating exactly what was available in books.

- Lack of interest in subject and/or teaching.
- Lack of guidance with assignments.
- 'Us and them' boundaries put in place between tutors and students.
- Poor communication – mumbling when addressing the class, no eye contact, reading off PowerPoint slides.
- Teaching by humiliation – 'making me feel stupid in front of my peers when I couldn't think of an answer'.
- Unnecessary emphasis on minutiae.
- Unable to test understanding or experience learners' opinions, arguments or approaches.

Effects of negative teaching experiences on the learner

- Frustration.
- Feeling as if time is being wasted and/or there is not much to gain from the teacher.
- Not looking forward to, or even not going back to, another teaching session given by the same person.
- Loss of interest, poor attention, clock watching, talking to other learners.
- Lack of respect for the teacher.
- Feeling stupid, losing confidence, and being scared of being wrong in the future.
- Missing out on the subject matter because they 'switched off', no or limited learning.
- Being 'put off' the subject.

How learners feel teaching experiences may be improved

Teacher interacting with students – for example, by using prompts to open discussion.

- Encouraging learners to participate verbally or with hands-on exercises.
- Changing the way they teach to make it more content relevant and interesting, rather than just 'bookish knowledge'.
- Using a mix of teaching styles – content rich teaching when necessary, group work, class participation, discussing theory.
- Having a clear structure, being organised, clarifying what the aims and objectives of the session and/or programme are.
- Sometimes asking learners what their expectations of the session are causes those who are not clear to understand, and enables the teacher to direct the learners to the actual point of the session if they have this wrong.
- Relating the teaching to clinical scenarios, telling the learners what they need to know both for exams and for clinical practice.
- Ensuring that there is enough time for the planned content of the teaching session to be delivered.

Maybe you now want to move on and 'formalise' your role or undertake some further training; where would you start? You could start by seeking out the views and advice of local educationalists about careers options. If you are in a training role yourself, speak to your own preceptor or educational supervisor about how they started and what the steps are. Perhaps approach current or previous tutors or seek out relevant people from staff lists on university websites to obtain discipline-specific information. A good source of advice and guidance can be found in Donnelly and Gallen (2017) who have included vignettes and case studies from current teachers describing their route into teaching.

General information is also available from educational associations and organisations (see Box 1.2).

BOX 1.2 EXAMPLES OF EDUCATIONAL ASSOCIATIONS AND ORGANISATIONS

- The Academy of Medical Educators is a multi-professional body which is the standard setting body for clinical teachers in the United Kingdom www.medicaleducators.org
- Health Care Education Association (HCEA) www.hcea-info.org
- MedEdWorld www.mededworld.org (The international community developed by the International Association for Medical Education in Europe) https://amee.org/home

Dentists and/or dental students

- American Dental Education Association (ADEA) www.adea.org
- Association for Dental Education in Europe (ADEE) www.adee.org
- International Federation of Dental Educators and Associations (IFDEA) www.ifdea.org

Doctors and/or medical students

- Association for the Study of Medical Education (ASME) www.asme.org.uk
- American Society of Teachers of Family Medicine (STFM) www.stfm.org

Physiotherapists and/or physiotherapy students

- Chartered Society of Physiotherapists (CSP) www.csp.org.uk/careers-jobs/career-development/becoming-educator

Nurses and/or student nurses

- American National League for Nursing (NLN) www.nln.org
- American Professional Nurse Educators Group (PNEG) www.pneg.org
- Royal College of Nurses (RCN) Educator forum, www.rcn.org.uk/get-involved/forums/education-forum

Midwives

- Association for Midwifery Educators www.associationofmidwiferyeducators.org

The Academy of Medical Educators in the UK has a portfolio-based approach to developing and credentialing for educators (AoME 2021). The framework is built around standards in five domains of practice (see Figure 1.1) and focuses on four core values of the effective educator:

1. Demonstrates professional identity and integrity.
2. Is committed to scholarship and reflection in medical education.
3. Demonstrates respect for others.
4. Promotes quality and safety of care.

Undergraduates who already have an interest in medical education can apply for student membership of the Academy and with advancing expertise aspire to membership, fellowship and principal fellowship recognising increasing experience and commitment as an educator. This can be a good way to start networking with educators and advancing your competence and career.

You might have noticed that the section headings in this book are taken from the AoME standards. We hope that this means this book will become a source of guidance for you as you seek to reflect on your practice for your appraisal and revalidation as a teacher.

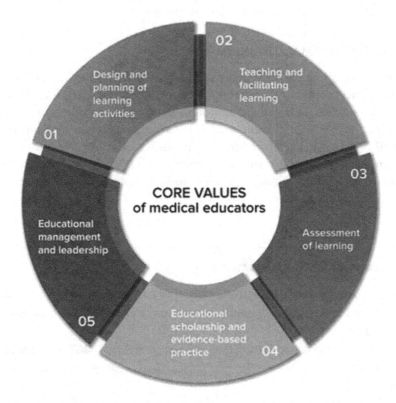

FIGURE 1.1 AoME standards: five domains of practice.

For those who are still students, many healthcare courses now include peer-assisted learning (PAL) initiatives that provide experience of teaching, experience of being role models for juniors and improved success in studies and exams. PAL initiatives may exist within your university/college, so find out from your tutors. If such initiatives do not exist, consider starting one, as medical students in Sheffield, UK, did when they founded a 'Peer Teaching Society' to facilitate those with an interest in education to develop their skills (MacKinnon et al. 2009). National PAL initiatives also exist. For example, Sexpression:UK (www.sexpression.org.uk) is a near-peer initiative involving UK medical students teaching sex education to local secondary school children.

Increasingly healthcare programmes involve students in interviewing applicants or assessments. You can seek opportunities to understand assessments 'from the other side' by assisting with a station in a practical clinical examination or an objective, structured, clinical examination (OSCE), for example. You will see how learners are marked and the limitations of such examination methods.

Speak with senior faculty staff, express your interest in teaching and they may direct you to, or create opportunities for you to become involved in undergraduate course development, management or delivery. Certain opportunities may only be available to postgraduates, but expressing your interest early on may invite opportunities such as facilitating problem-based learning (PBL) groups, teaching anatomy, running special interest groups or committees or journal clubs.

UNDERTAKING FORMAL TRAINING

If you are serious about teaching and would like to formalise this, you should gain a theoretical background and undertake a course or recognised educational qualification in the subject. This will enable you to improve your skills, and will provide good evidence of your commitment and level of attainment when applying for future educational posts. Multiple accredited qualifications exist (see Box 1.3). The right one for you will depend upon your discipline/specialty, where you live and/or work and your current level of training. Specific information can be found on the relevant awarding institution's website.

BOX 1.3 EDUCATIONAL QUALIFICATIONS

Introductory courses: Teaching the Teachers basic skills courses. (Individual higher education institutions, royal colleges and postgraduate deaneries run these courses differently, so consult local information.)

Consider the introductory Academy of Medical Educators in Europe (AMEE) Essential Skills in Medical Education (ESME) Online course https://amee.org/courses/amee-esme-online-courses/esme-online.

Higher degrees (Certificate/Diploma/Masters/PhD) in medical education. The Foundation for Advancement of International Medical Education and Research (FAIMER) has collated details of institutions that host Masters programmes in medical education (www.faimer.org/resources/mastersmeded.html).

For blended, distance learning consider online programmes such as the medical education iHEED programme, delivered by faculty around the world for international students, validated by the University of Warwick in the UK www.iheed.org.

LOOKING FOR FORMAL ROLES

Depending on your discipline, the country in which you work and your level of experience and qualifications, a large range of formal educational posts are available (see Box 1.4). Further details can be from the appropriate professional organisation websites.

BOX 1.4 FORMAL EDUCATIONAL POSTS

Integrated academic and clinical training schemes: When the importance of streamlining academic and clinical training was recognised, integrated training schemes were developed. For example, the UK National Institute for Health Research (NIHR) Integrated Academic Training scheme funds posts for trainee doctors that enable them to continue training in their chosen specialty while undertaking basic training in the academic field. A few of these schemes are education and educational research based. See https://research.ncl.ac.uk/clinical-education-research-incubator

Clinical and/or educational supervisory roles:

- Doctors – educational/clinical supervisors, trainers or faculty for junior doctors
- Physiotherapists – clinical educators
- Nurses – practice educators, preceptors, clinical supervisor
- Midwives – supervisor of midwives (UK), midwife preceptor (Canada, USA, New Zealand)

Within training and/or postgraduate continuing professional development organisations, deaneries and/or universities: Examples of teaching posts are Teaching Fellow, Lecturer, Lecturer Practitioner, Lead Midwife for Education, Clinical Nurse Educator, Professor, Dean and Programme Director. Such roles may involve the following responsibilities to varying extents: developing courses and curricula, teaching students/postgraduate trainees/fully qualified professionals, evaluating teaching and learning and devising assessments. Some posts may also require you to undertake formal research, including writing grant proposals.

Within professional organisations: Specialty-specific professional bodies and/or educational organisations offer formal posts that enable you to develop your field of education using a top-down approach (e.g. committee positions, being an appraiser or quality assessor).

REVIEWING PERFORMANCE

In order to achieve and maintain good teaching practice, you must review your performance. Good quality preparation of supervisors and ongoing assessment of their performance is essential for effective supervision. This can be particularly true with the identification of your strengths, especially the areas of 'unconscious competence' where your strengths might not be clear or obvious to you.

So how do you do this? Your performance can be reviewed through the following:

- Self-evaluation
- Peer observation of teaching
- Learner feedback
- Multi-source feedback

Certain evaluations in some formal posts are compulsory. However, if they are not, you should still seek feedback to facilitate your development. Review of your performance will highlight areas that are in need of improvement and those in which you excel. This knowledge can be developed into a personal development plan (PDP) and reviewed in your annual appraisal as evidence both for career progression and development as a teacher.

Reflecting on your skills and progress and undertaking a realistic assessment of your teaching are crucial for ongoing development. By gathering evidence and reflecting on why your teaching sessions have gone exceptionally well (or were a disaster), you can use this information, along with the advice in the rest of this book, to address your personal development areas and to refine your teaching techniques and styles.

CREATING A PERSONAL DEVELOPMENT PLAN (PDP)

Once you are armed with your strengths, weaknesses and areas for further development, you can plan how you will address these. PDPs allow for variations in learning style, personality, experience, interests and job requirements. An effective PDP consists of the following:

- Identification of your areas for improvement in knowledge, skills or attitudes
- Specification of topics for learning as a result of changes in your role, your responsibilities and the organisation
- A description of how you identified your learning needs
- Prioritisation and setting of your learning needs and associated goals
- Justification of your selection of learning goals:
  - A description of how you will achieve your goals and over what time period
  - A description of how you will evaluate learning outcomes

Many healthcare professionals are required to maintain PDPs for managing their personal learning, often in the form of an electronic portfolio. This often starts in undergraduate years where the habit of self-assessment for life-long learning can be developed. Many medical schools require students to organise and evidence their learning in a portfolio, usually electronic. Although not universally appreciated by students, some of whom find difficulties with the necessary organisational skills and skills of reflective practice, such portfolios do allow evidence for progression to be presented. If electronic portfolios are unfamiliar you to, you could ask your student or trainee to talk you through theirs – adopting and modelling the role of the novice is a good way to start building a learning environment where your learner also feels confident to share things they don't know.

Otherwise, examples of what such portfolios can look like might be found here:

1. The UK Foundation Programme for postgraduate doctors in training: https:// foundationprogramme.nhs.uk/curriculum/e-portfolio/
2. Medical Royal College portfolios, such as www.fourteenfish.com for GP trainees and GP appraisal

Some of the elements in such a portfolio will be mandatory or statutory training requirements. However, these should not be completed in isolation. Teachers should guide learners through an educational conversation, or formative appraisal, to ensure careful and accurate review and well-defined, realistic, achievable and necessary goals. This will make demonstrating your competence as a healthcare teacher much easier.

To assist in the development of a clinical and/or educational PDP, learning objectives must be appropriate (see Box 1.5).

BOX 1.5 HOW TO ENSURE THAT PDP LEARNING OBJECTIVES ARE APPROPRIATE

Be SMART

Learning objectives should be:
- **Specific**
- **Measurable**
- **Achievable**
- **Relevant**
- **Time-bounded**

A PDP is a dynamic document, and ideally it should be regularly reviewed and updated, at least annually, as you achieve the agreed objectives and identify new learning needs. Early in your clinical and educational career you should review your PDP more than once a year, as your needs change rapidly. While undertaking your PDP objectives, gather evidence that each of the objectives has been met, reflect on how you have achieved them, and make a note of further learning objectives that have arisen and how each has changed your practice. Your organisational appraisal will very likely be organised to facilitate this.

GATHERING SUPPORTING INFORMATION AND DEMONSTRATING ACHIEVEMENTS AND COMPETENCE

Competence is a person's ability to perform, and their competences are their total capability (what they can do – which might not necessarily be the same as what they actually do). A helpful definition of 'competence' is: 'the state of having the knowledge, judgement, skills, energy, experience and motivation required to respond adequately to the demands of one's professional responsibilities' (Roach 1992). The measurement of competence may be based on three levels of expertise – aware, competent, expert (Benner 1984) – and you might use these concepts to organise and reflect on your practice and areas for improvement.

Your portfolio is a compendium of evidence of your learning, practice and maintenance of standards. How you present this evidence depends upon the purpose of your portfolio. All teachers and learners should maintain a portfolio to demonstrate learning that has occurred. Often the PDP is a good starting point for a portfolio, as it highlights the ongoing development of learning objectives and your plans for improvement. A portfolio can be used to obtain credits for prior learning with higher degree courses, or to prove experience and competence in the future. Finally, your portfolio might form the basis of professional revalidation (see Section 1.7).

Portfolio-based learning involves the following steps:

- Identifying significant experiences to serve as important sources of learning
- Reflecting on the learning that arose from those experiences
- Demonstrating that learning has been put into practice
- Analysing the portfolio and identifying further learning needs and ways in which these needs can be met

As a personal document, a portfolio will have a varied content, which may include some or all of the following:

- An outline of your current post, responsibilities, aspirations and goals
- Workload logs
- Case descriptions
- Evidence of continuing professional development (certificates of attendance can be useful but are not as powerful as reflections on what has been learned and how your practice will change as a result of learning)
- Audiovisual examples of your practice (e.g. teaching/presentations given)
- Patient and/or learner satisfaction surveys
- Research or service evaluations
- Audit projects
- Publications

- Report of a change or innovation (e.g. in curricula/course design, assessment)
- Commentaries on published literature or books
- Records of critical incidents, complaints and learning points
- An outline of formal teaching sessions with reference to clinical work or other supporting information (e.g. self-, peer and/or learner evaluations, reflections on teaching experiences, whether the style/methods were appropriate for the learners/content/situation)
- A summary of your learners' outcomes compared with those of others

Analysis of experiences and learning opportunities should show demonstrable learning outcomes and resulting educational or developmental needs. Learners may be guided by a mentor as they compile and analyse the material in their portfolio to obtain another perspective that challenges them to think more deeply about their own attitudes, knowledge or beliefs. Much of the learning emanating from a portfolio comes from individual reflection and self-critique.

To ensure that your portfolio demonstrates the standards to which you must work, you must explicitly link the expected standards and your achievement of, or work towards, them. For example, as we saw previously, the Academy of Medical Educators (AoME) has produced a framework to assist with the demonstration of expertise and achievements in medical education, organised under five domains, which are mirrored in the sections of this book. Table 1.1 shows a simplified version of how expected standards can be mapped to evidence, and this can be generalised across specialties and educational posts.

TABLE 1.1 Mapping Evidence to Standards

	Domain	Evidence	TME chapters
1	*Designing & planning learning: outlining standards for medical educators involved in educational design and learning development processes.*	*Examples of needs assessments, curriculum design, lesson plans, feedback gathering measures, strategies for evaluation and quality assurance of teaching.*	*1,2,3,4,5,6*
2	*Teaching and facilitating learning: standards in relation to the practice of teaching and supporting learning.*	*Peer observation and feedback on teaching, videos of teaching with self-assessment and critique, student feedback, examples of environmental or instructional media design including virtual learning environments.*	*7,8,9,10,11,12, 13,14*

(continued)

TABLE 1.1 (Continued)

	Domain	Evidence	TME chapters
3	*Assessment of learning: the expected standards in making and reporting judgements that capture, guide and make decisions about the achievement of learners, and the feedback required.*	*Examples of blueprinting and standard setting activities, knowledge of different methodologies of assessment, involvement in selection and admission of learners, participation in equality and diversity activities.*	*15,16,17,18,19,20*
4	*Educational scholarship and evidence-based practice: outlines the expected standards for medical educators involved in medical educational research.*	*Examples of audit and service evaluation of teaching practice, scholarly articles or publications such as books and papers, research funding or participation.*	*21*
5	*Educational management and leadership: for medical educators in relation to the management, leadership and governance of medical education.*	*Examples of public speaking, conferences etc, leadership of risk management activities, or strategic governance, refereeing for peer-referenced journals, reflection on external examinerships.*	*22,23,24*

(See the AoME Framework Standards document for details of the standards themselves and an illustration of how achieving the standards can be an iterative and developmental process. The Framework standards document highlights each domain and the hierarchy of evidence that might be presented.)

Expectations of teachers across different healthcare disciplines are similar (see Box 1.6) (CSP 2004).

BOX 1.6 THE CHARTERED SOCIETY OF PHYSIOTHERAPY'S EXPECTATIONS OF PHYSIOTHERAPY CLINICAL EDUCATORS

The clinical educator should provide evidence that they are able to:
- Describe the role and identify the attributes of the effective clinical educator
- Apply learning theories that are appropriate for adult and professional learners
- Plan, implement and facilitate learning in the clinical setting
- Apply sound principles and judgement in the assessment of performance in the clinical setting
- Evaluate the learning experience
- Reflect on experience and formulate action plans to improve future practice

---

REVALIDATION

Revalidation is part of a system that is designed to demonstrate to the public and other stakeholders – such as funders and commissioners of services – the competence of health professionals and the maintenance of standards. This applies as much to healthcare educators as it does to those in clinical roles.

Revalidation with the General Medical Council for UK doctors was implemented in 2012, and requires doctors to collect information about all of their professional work, including teaching and training and supported by annual workplace-based appraisal. This is informed by evidence of involvement in continuing professional development (CPD) or continuing medical education (CME) as a teacher and includes audit, learner, patient and colleague feedback as well as other quality measures of performance. Developing the habit of creating an active personal development plan and building a portfolio as you complete that plan enables you to fulfil that requirement.

THE CHANGING LANDSCAPE OF HEALTH PROFESSIONS LEARNING

The 2020/2022 COVID-19 pandemic brought into sharp relief changes that were already starting to occur in instructional media design and organisation of teaching and learning. Asynchronous, at-a-distance, 'just-in-time' learning is replacing group attendance in the same place at the same time. Online learning is well established with blended delivery and virtual learning environments (see Chapter 11).

As we increasingly move to teaching over the internet, with learners who we might rarely if ever meet, healthcare teachers will need to develop innovative, creative and imaginative ways to ensure their teaching is effective. How will we know if students are actively engaging with (or even present during) teaching if their cameras are off or their internet crashes? Similarly, reliance on interpersonal skills to enabling role modelling of professional requirements and the development of communities of practice to foster professional identity becomes more challenging. Tried and tested modalities of teaching that work well in face-to-face learning environments might not work so well online. Access and barriers to learning for differently-abled learners and those in low resource settings need to be thought through carefully. As you progress as a teacher, reflection on your experiences as a learner in changing times can be very valuable to inform and strengthen your practice.

The principal challenges of staying up to date and maintaining your performance as a healthcare teacher remains the same, even as the environment changes around us. But we will all need to develop new modalities of evaluation and self-assessment and enhanced skills of reflexivity and criticality if we are to continue to meet the challenge of excellence as teachers.

REFERENCES

Academy of Medical Educators (2021) *Professional standards for medical, dental and veterinary educators.* 4th edn. Cardiff: AoME. Available at www.medicaleducators.org/professional-standards (Accessed 29.3.22).

Benner P. (1984) *From novice to expert: Excellence and power in clinical nursing practice.* Menlo Park, CA: Addison-Wesley.

Chartered Society of Physiotherapy (2004) *Accreditation of clinical educators scheme guidance.* London: Chartered Society of Physiotherapy.

Donnelly P. and Gallen D. (2017) *Becoming a medical educator.* London: BPP Learning Media Ltd.

Mackinnon R., Haque A. and Stark P. (2009) Peer teaching: By students for students. A student-led initiative. *Clin Teacher,* 6: 245–248.

Roach S. (1992) *The human act of caring: A blueprint for health professions.* Ottawa, ON: Canadian Hospital Association Press.

CHAPTER 2

Healthcare professionals as teachers

....

FORMAL AND INFORMAL TEACHING ROLES AMONG HEALTHCARE PROFESSIONALS

Informal teaching by role modelling, observation and apprenticeship has a long and distinguished history in the perpetuation of clinical skills, professional roles and responsibilities. Teaching is an integral aspect of the healthcare provider's role. Indeed the Hippocratic Oath includes reference to teaching:

> I swear by Apollo the physician . . . to teach others this art, without fee and covenant; to give a share of precepts and oral instruction and all the other learning to those who have taken this oath under medical law.
>
> *(Translation in Beauchamp and Walters 1978)*

In modern times, this part of the oath is still in practice worldwide:

> As Scholars, physicians demonstrate a lifelong commitment to excellence in practice through continuous learning and by teaching others, evaluating evidence, and contributing to scholarship.
>
> *(CanMEDS 2015)*

Similar responsibilities exist in the curricula of other healthcare professionals around the world. There is an accepted obligation that all members of the multi-professional healthcare team should be prepared to teach and to learn from each other and to support and teach junior colleagues. There is also recognition of the teaching role with patients and the public. A note of caution is added by the World Medical Association (WMA) as stated in the *International Code of Medical Ethics*:

DOI: 10.1201/9781003352532-3

A physician shall recognise his/her important role in educating the public but should use due caution in divulging discoveries or new techniques or treatment through non-professional channels.

(WMA 2006)

This obligation to teach sits well with the fact that the good communication skills of the effective clinician show considerable overlap with the skills needed to be an effective teacher – shown in Box 2.1.

BOX 2.1 SKILLS NEEDED TO BE AN EFFECTIVE TEACHER

- Listen with genuine interest.
- Create a conducive environment.
- Be encouraging.
- Show understanding and empathy.
- Check current understanding.
- Reflect/summarise and paraphrase answers.
- Use closed questions for exploration.
- Use open questions for clarification.
- Adopt a similar language and avoid jargon.
- Use plural pronouns to indicate partnership.
- Be provisional rather than dogmatic.
- Be descriptive not judgemental.
- Comment on behaviours and issues rather than personalities or appearances.
- Encourage eye contact.
- Give information in clear, simple terms and use repetition.
- Check understanding.
- Use silence.

Source: Adapted from Tate (2000).

POSSESSING SUCH SKILLS HOWEVER, ALTHOUGH NECESSARY, IS NOT SUFFICIENT TO BE A GOOD TEACHER

Traditionally (in the education of junior doctors), formal healthcare teaching qualifications or roles were not the norm. Clinical teachers may have ended up in that role as a result of their seniority and clinical experience, rather than by training and educational experience. Teachers in higher education similarly may have entered their roles as a result of their research experience, and not until the Dearing Report in 1997 was it a requirement that all teachers in higher education institutes had training in teaching (Dearing 1997). Hospital consultants frequently act as educational supervisors of junior doctors, and previously may have had little or no formal training in that role. The buddy or assistant-operator pairing is much more formal, but still a version of the 'sitting with Nelly' observational form of teaching, and was used in the training and assessment of dentists.

Medical teaching has changed significantly in the UK however since the General Medical Council (GMC) made it a requirement that all those involved in supervision should be trained and recognised as teachers. There is now an entry in the GMC generalist and specialist registers to recognise teacher status alongside a concomitant responsibility to stay up to date and be revalidated in that domain (see also Chapter 1).

This followed on from the already established and more rigorous approach to preparation of teachers in UK general practice and the therapies. For nurses and midwives, educational roles with specific definitions and standards for teaching practice had been formalised in 2001/2 by the English National Board (ENB 2001) and the Nursing and Midwifery Council (NMC 2002). Teaching is expected of nurses and midwives as part of their contract of employment.

In these formal roles, a distinction is drawn between mentors, assessors, practice educators and lecturers. Slightly different competences are expected within these different roles (see Box 2.2). These definitions are shared here because, although initially and primarily defined for nursing, midwifery and health visiting, the competences defined can be generalised to other health professions.

BOX 2.2 TEACHING ROLE DEFINITIONS OF THE ENGLISH NATIONAL BOARD FOR NURSING, MIDWIFERY AND HEALTH VISITING

1. Mentor denotes the role of the nurse, midwife or health visitor who facilitates learning and supervises and assesses students in the practice setting. (In nursing, the term 'assessor' is often used to denote a role similar to that of the mentor.)

2. Practice educator denotes the role of the teacher of nursing, midwifery or health visitor, who:
    Makes a significant contribution to education in the practice setting, coordinating student experiences and assessment of learning.
    Leads the development of practice.
    Provides support and guidance to mentors and others who contribute to the students' experience in practice, enabling students to meet learning outcomes and develop appropriate competencies.

3. Lecturer denotes the role of the teacher of nursing, midwifery or health visitor employed in an educational institution, who has responsibility for the development and delivery of educational programmes in nursing, midwifery or health visiting.

Please note that the definitions are different for other healthcare disciplines.

The UK Nursing and Midwifery Council advisory standards for nursing mentors are listed in Box 2.3.

BOX 2.3 UK NURSING AND MIDWIFERY COUNCIL ADVISORY STANDARDS FOR NURSING MENTORS

Effective [nursing] mentors will develop the following skills:

Communication and working relationships that enable:

1. The development of effective relationships based on mutual trust and respect.
2. An understanding of how learners integrate into practice settings and assist with this process.
3. The provision of ongoing and constructive support for learners.

Facilitation of learning in order to:

1. Demonstrate sufficient knowledge of the learner's programme to identify current learning needs.
2. Demonstrate strategies that will assist with the integration of learning from practice and educational settings.
3. Create and develop opportunities for learners to identify and undertake experiences to meet their learning needs.

Assessment in order to:

1. Demonstrate a good understanding of assessment and ability to assess and implement approved assessment procedures.

Role modelling in order to:

1. Demonstrate effective relationships with patients and clients.
2. Contribute to the development of an environment in which effective practice is fostered, implemented, evaluated and disseminated.
3. Assess and manage clinical developments to ensure safe and effective care.

An environment for learning in order to:

1. Ensure effective learning experiences and the opportunity to achieve learning outcomes for students.
2. Implement strategies for quality assurance and quality audit.

Improvement of practice in order to:

1. Contribute to the creation of an environment in which change can be initiated and supported.

A knowledge base in order to:

1. Identify, apply and disseminate research findings within the area of practice.

Course development which:

1. Contributes to the development and/or review of courses.

Please note that the definition of mentor for UK nurses is different to that for other healthcare disciplines.

As we have seen, both formal and informal, recognised and unrecognised teaching roles exist within healthcare and, as healthcare demand increases for an aging population living with multiple co-morbidities, and increased technological advances stimulates healthcare activity, the need and opportunity for such roles are increasing. The role of the healthcare professional as teacher is 'a core professional activity . . . that cannot be left to chance, aptitude or inclination' (Purcell and Lloyd-Jones 2003).

RESPONDING TO CHANGING HEALTHCARE SYSTEMS AND EDUCATIONAL INFRASTRUCTURES

The impact of continuing changes in and modernisation of healthcare systems is felt in training and education through changes in patient care patterns and working arrangements. For example, there is recognition of the detrimental effect on high-quality graduate medical education of the long hours worked, reduced length of inpatient stays and the often increased acuity of the average inpatient that place additional demands on juniors' time and energy.

Changes in the environmental aspects of healthcare delivery however can have unintended consequences for teaching and learning. The introduction of the European Working Time Directive (EWTD) aimed to improve the work–life balance of doctors, and subsequently improve patient care (Legislation.Gov.uk 2003). However, this has resulted in less time being available for teaching and training, due to a direct reduction in clinical exposure and changes to rotas, with subsequent staff shortages. More frequent handovers and reduced exposure to each patient prevent follow-up throughout a patient's admission, and this risks training jobs becoming focused on service provision rather than training.

Other changes in healthcare and teaching capacity also have impact. In 2008 a review of the UK postgraduate medical education and training system recognised an 'erosion' of the 'traditional clinical academic departments' and the existence of fewer clinical academic posts in medical schools, resulting in increased reliance on clinical staff to deliver undergraduate teaching and postgraduate supervision. Integrated educational and clinical training pathways were suggested to facilitate formal training, development and qualification in educational skills (Tooke 2008).

A significant problem was identified in 2010 of faculty shortages at nursing schools in the USA due to budget constraints that have made salaries for teachers lower compared with those for clinical or private-sector workers. Furthermore, the ageing population of faculty staff was thought to predict a wave of faculty retirements. Multiple initiatives have been introduced to improve funding for individuals who are entering a career in education, and to provide funding for increased numbers of faculty staff in schools of nursing (AACN 2010).

Funding for education is dynamic and vulnerable to changes in healthcare system and political priorities. We see for example the recurrent impact of medical school student numbers on the UK Foundation Programme where a mismatch in workforce planning leads every year to challenges finding employment for all graduating doctors and the creation of a reserve list of qualified doctors, at the same time as clinical settings are significantly understaffed (Lok 2022). Preventing such a bottleneck due to a shortage of Foundation Programme places numbers is given as one of the reasons for funding for medical student places to remain capped – again when according to the Royal College of Physicians, the number of medical school places should be doubled to meet workforce needs (Wilkinson 2022).

Funding overhauls can either be beneficial or detrimental to various groups of healthcare professionals, and significant changes can be implemented at relatively short notice. Therefore teachers must be equipped, adequately represented and supported to provide good-quality education in a flexible and changing environment.

GLOBAL ASPECTS IMPACTING ON TRAINING AND EDUCATION IN HEALTHCARE: SOCIAL ACCOUNTABILITY AND SUSTAINABILITY

The World Health Organization has defined social accountability of medical schools as the 'obligation to direct their education, research, and service activities toward addressing the priority health concerns of the community' (Boelen et al. 1995). At the time of writing, it is nearly 30 years since Boelen defined a triad of social responsibility, social responsiveness, and social accountability.

> Countries worldwide increasingly demand more value for money in healthcare. [Health professions educational institutions] which both shape the health care system and are shaped by it, must continue to be [responsive to need, and] socially responsible on their own initiative. In addition they must accept and acknowledge being held to account by society: being socially accountable . . . is a balance between relevance, quality, cost effectiveness and equity, through their activities in education, research and service delivery. . . . Social accountability addresses the priority health concerns of the community, region and/or nation they have a mandate to serve.
>
> *(Boelen et al. 1995, p. i)*

Despite being unable to define or recall the 'obligation triad' of responsibility, responsiveness and accountability, faculty members were nonetheless sensitive to their responsibilities towards students and the community in research in an Indian medical school (Dandekar et al. 2021). Four major themes were described in this qualitative research: (1) perceptions of the importance of the social obligation owed by faculty and others, (2) the importance of an awareness of social and cultural values, (3) the role and value of community partnerships and (4) the structural requirements of building a socially accountable model of healthcare education.

There are many stakeholders sharing a reciprocal relationship in healthcare education: policymakers, tax-payers, healthcare professionals, patients, communities and academic institutions. Medical schools and the community share a symbiotic association where the school responds to societal needs by collaborating in identifying priority health needs – both clinical and research orientated needs – and also learns from clinical encounters. Insight into the role of all the stakeholders is paramount to the understanding of social obligation. If healthcare education is to become more socially responsive, it will also be important to sensitise students towards community needs and the impact of a patient's cultural and socio-economic backgrounds on their own health and the health infrastructure that the community can afford. Faculty members need to imbed this understanding of the importance of a contextual curriculum. Health professionals involved in teaching play important roles as change agents and role models in healthcare education.

Case study

The establishment of a new medical school not only triggers the development of an infrastructure which is conducive to learning for the medical students but also leads to 'handshaking' with the community. Healthcare settings are not primarily designed for teaching but as the site for delivery of healthcare, yet those same environments are vitally important as the site of educational transformation of students into healthcare professionals. Patients, tax-payers and healthcare providers sign an invisible 'social contract' (Dandekar et al. 2021). Educators, researchers and clinicians are drawn in higher numbers to the area which enhances patient care, but the system needs then to accommodate teaching and training obligations.

The Three Counties Medical School, University of Worcester, was established in a largely rural and under-doctored area. The aim was to become part of the workforce solution in the area but also to widen the participation of students from backgrounds that have hitherto not been well represented in medical careers. The mission statement of the school is: 'To enhance the health and wellbeing of communities, through challenge and transformation; leading to integrity and compassion in the care of patients'. Approval by the General Medical Council in 2021 was however not followed by government funding for student places. A funding model was instead developed that drew on local NHS financial support to enable the intake of 20 students. For four years NHS money was used to support placement, education and training costs, including faculty time, premises and infrastructure.

The 'social compact' thus formed means that the NHS will become both the recipient and funder of the environmental support for the educational development of newly graduated doctors.

Sustainability

In a survey across more than 100 countries, only 15% of medical schools were found to have included the health effects of climate change in the curriculum. Even fewer schools have included air pollution in the curriculum, despite 91% of the world's population living in places where air quality exceeds the WHO safety levels (Omrani et al. 2020). In some ways this is not surprising because of the pressures on space in the curriculum caused by the tendency for new subjects to be included without older topics giving way.

However, the medical student authors who took on the challenge of reviewing 2817 medical school curricula around the world for this paper said:

> With deteriorating ecosystems, the health of mankind is at risk. Future health care professionals must be trained to recognize the interdependence of health and ecosystems to address the needs of their patients and communities.
>
> *(Omrani et al. 2020, p. 1107)*

They point to statistics that suggest 'the healthcare sector, which aims to protect and promote health, is a significant global producer of greenhouse gases, contributing approximately 4.4% of global net emissions, the equivalent to two gigatons of carbon dioxide' (Healthcare Without Harm 2019).

The views of these authors build on notions of social accountability as described previously. The student, as a future healthcare provider, is seen to have an obligation not only to patients but to communities and future populations. The role of healthcare professionals in promoting public health is not new, but the potential interaction of health and climate change is three-fold: first, health is a contributing site for greenhouse gas production; next, healthcare workers will be at the forefront of dealing with the social and health challenges which have variously been described to include respiratory and cardiac problems due to air pollution, as well as 'poverty, starvation, the resurgence of previously managed infectious diseases, mass dispossession of populations, and increasing cancers due to carcinogenic pollutants' (McLean et al. 2020); finally, health systems themselves risk disruption by extreme events that might be provoked by a climate crisis or environmental disaster, challenging their capacity to deliver services at critical times.

The Academy of Medical Educators of Europe issued a consensus statement on planetary health and education for sustainable healthcare and laid out a shared purpose by and for healthcare educators. The aim was:

> to provide . . . an inclusive vision for educating an interprofessional healthcare workforce that can deliver sustainable healthcare and promote planetary health. It is intended to inform national and global accreditation standards, planning and action at the institutional level as well as highlight the role of individuals in transforming health professions education.
>
> *(Shaw et al. 2021)*

Widening participation

There is currently high, and increasing, interest in widening access and participation to ensure that the healthcare professions mirror the make-up of society. All UK Medical Schools are required to run an outreach scheme that widens access to courses. The NHS Long Term Plan and NHS Interim People Plan laid out an aspiration for the NHS to 'train more people domestically [and] recruit people from the widest possible range of backgrounds' (NHS 2019).

However, as the BMA points out, 'Despite efforts to increase gender parity and ethnic diversity among UK doctors, the lack of people from lower socio-economic backgrounds entering the profession is still a reality' (BMA 2021).

The General Medical Council highlighted that:

> there remains limited representation from those from lower socio-economic backgrounds within medicine . . . [we] found that over one-third of trainee doctors attended private school compared with 7% of the general popula-tion and just 8% of trainee doctors received free school meals at any point during their schooling, compared with one quarter of the general population while 6% of participants grew up in a socio-economically deprived area within the UK.
>
> *(GMC 2013)*

The barriers are multifactorial but include self-belief and aspiration in some students, their parents and their schools, but also lack of access to resources and preparation to enable all students to meet admission criteria. This latter includes some of the soft criteria, such as access to work experience opportunities to develop an understand-ing of what daily life is like for different types of healthcare professionals.

A current student expressing interest in medicine recently illustrated this when she emailed:

> I cannot afford to pay for a graduate entry medicine course as the current po-sition is that [even with a Bursary] I would have to put almost £4000 a year towards the studies which is money that I don't have. I am state school edu-cated and from a working class background and due to my background I never thought that medicine was a possibility for me.

The BMA Aspiring Doctors scheme is a network of doctors and medical students who can help schools whose students are interested in applying to medical school, in the following ways:

- Offer insight into the application process and a doctor's career path
- Provide work experience
- Help with personal statements and interview practice
- Help to prepare for admission tests

Medical schools also run outreach schemes such as the following:

- School programmes to inspire children at a young age to consider medicine
- Summer schools to assist with medical school applications and gaining work experience

- MBChB programmes with dedicated places for disadvantaged backgrounds
- Individual medical school programmes, such as the one at Edge Hill University offering programmes of talks and practical sessions, contact with students and clinicians and access to learning materials (www.edgehill.ac.uk/medicalschool/widening-participation/widening-access-to-medicine)
- Some universities run programmes not just for medicine but to encourage applications to university, for example, the Bright Minds in Birmingham initiative for supporting disadvantaged students (www.birmingham.ac.uk/birmingham-in-action/about-the-campaign/support-students.aspx)

This chapter has looked at how healthcare professionals bring all their skills from clinical care into teaching but are also influenced by and can influence socio-economic and political changes in the environment of healthcare education delivery. Healthcare settings impact aspects of social accountability which can be seen in initiatives around community engagement and faculty development, but also in curriculum developments such as inclusion of issues of sustainability and climate change. Thinking about widening access or participation in health professions education pulls together some of these roles, responsibilities and structural aspects of designing effective and equitable learning environments in healthcare.

REFERENCES

American Association of Colleges of Nursing (2010) *Nursing faculty shortage fact sheet.* Washington, DC: American Association of Colleges of Nursing.

Beauchamp T. and Walters L. (1978) The hippocratic oath. In *Contemporary issues in bioethics.* Encino, CA: Dickenson.

Boelen C., Heck J.E. and WHO (1995) *Defining and measuring the social accountability of medical schools.* Geneva: World Health Organisation. Available at https://apps.who.int/iris/handle/10665/59441 (Accessed 30.3.22).

British Medical Association (2021) Available at www.bma.org.uk/advice-and-support/studying-medicine/becoming-a-doctor/widening-participation-in-medicine.

Dandekar S.P., Mhatre R. and Mohanna K. (2021) Perceptions of faculty toward "social obligation" at an Indian medical school. *Education Health*, 34: 48–54.

The Dearing Report (1997) *Higher education in the learning society.* London: Her Majesty's Stationery Office. Available at www.educationengland.org.uk/documents/dearing1997/dearing1997.html (Accessed 30.3.22).

English National Board for Nursing, Midwifery and Health Visiting (ENB) and Department of Health (2001) *Preparation of mentors and teachers.* London: English National Board and Department of Health.

General Medical Council (2013) *State of medical education and practice in the UK 2013.* London: GMC.

Healthcare Without Harm (2019) Health care's climate footprint: How the health sector contributes to the global climate crisis and opportunities for action. Available at https://noharm-global.org/sites/default/files/documents-files/5961/HealthCaresClimate Footprint_090619.pdf (Accessed 3.12.22).

Legislation.Gov.uk (2003) The working time regulations (1998): European working time directive. Available at https://www.legislation.gov.uk/uksi/1998/1833/contents/made (Accessed 3.12.22).

Lok P. (2022) The UK's foundation training programme for 2022 oversubscribed by almost 800 places. *BMJ*, 376: 650.

McLean M., Gibbs T. and McKimm J. (2020) Educating for planetary health and environmentally sustainable health care: Responding with urgency. *Medical Teacher*, 42(10): 1082–1084. DOI: 10.1080/0142159X.2020.1795107.

National Health Service (2019) *Interim NHS people plan*. London: NHS. Available at www.longtermplan.nhs.uk/wp-content/uploads/2019/05/Interim-NHS-People-Plan_June2019.pdf (Accessed 21.3.22).

Nursing and Midwifery Council (NMC) (2002) *Standards for the preparation of teachers of nursing and midwifery*. London: Nursing and Midwifery Council.

Omrani O., Dafallah A., Castillo B.P., Amaro B.Q.R.C., Taneja S., Amzil M., Sajib M.R.U. and Ezzine T. (2020) Envisioning planetary health in every medical curriculum: An international medical student organization's perspective. *Medical Teacher*, 42(10): 1107–1111. DOI: 10.1080/0142159X.2020.1796949.

Purcell N. and Lloyd-Jones G. (2003) Standards for medical educators. *Medical Education*, 37: 149–154.

Royal College of Physicians and Surgeons of Canada (2015) The CanMEDS Physician competency framework. Available at www.royalcollege.ca/rcsite/canmeds/framework/canmeds-role-scholar-e (Accessed 30.3.22).

Shaw E., Walpole S., McLean M., Alvarez-Nieto C., et al. (2021) AMEE consensus statement: Planetary health and education for sustainable healthcare. *Medical Teacher*, 43(3): 272–286. DOI: 10.1080/0142159X.2020.1860207.

Tate P. (2000) *The doctor's communication handbook*. 3rd edn. Oxford: Radcliffe Medical Press.

Tooke J. (2008) *Aspiring to excellence: Findings and final recommendations of the Independent inquiry into modernising medical careers*. London: MMC Inquiry.

Wilkinson E. (2022) The real reason that new UK medical schools are focusing on international students. *BMJ*. DOI: 10.1136/bmj.o421.

World Medical Association (2006) International code of medical ethics. Available at www.wma.net/wp-content/uploads/2006/09/International-Code-of-Medical-Ethics-2006.pdf (Accessed 30.3.22).

CHAPTER 3

Healthcare teaching in context

....

Following the Mid-Staffordshire NHS Foundation Trust public inquiry into poor standards of care (The Frances Report 2010), a report by the Commission on Education and Training for Patient Safety made 12 recommendations about education and training (CETPS 2016). These recommendations emphasise the importance of learning in context:

1. Ensure learning from patient safety data and good practice.
2. Develop and use a common language to describe all elements of quality improvement science and human factors with respect to patient safety.
3. Ensure robust evaluation of education and training for patient safety.
4. Engage patients, family members, carers and the public in the design and delivery of education and training for patient safety.
5. Supporting the duty of candour is vital, and there must be high quality educational training packages available.
6. The learning environment must support all learners and staff to raise and respond to concerns about patient safety.
7. The content of mandatory training for patient safety needs to be coherent across the NHS.
8. All NHS leaders need patient safety training so they can have the knowledge and tools to drive change and improvement.
9. Education and training must support the delivery of more integrated 'joined up' care.
10. Ensure increased opportunities for inter-professional learning.
11. Principles of human factors and professionalism must be embedded across education and training.
12. Ensure staff have the skills to identify and manage potential risks.

DOI: 10.1201/9781003352532-4

CHANGING HEALTHCARE SERVICES CHANGES LEARNING NEEDS

Changes in the focus of healthcare delivery create new educational and training needs for healthcare professionals, managers and other non-clinical staff. As we will see in Chapter 4, the healthcare setting is the site of frequent changes in traditional health professionals' roles and a growing emphasis on emerging models of care delivery. Basing clinical care, management or health policy on evidence, when available, or being able to justify performance where it diverts from the norm or best practice, continue to be learning needs for many healthcare professionals. These complex areas require as great an understanding of the context of the topics as the subject areas themselves. For example, changing approaches to developing healthcare services involves learning more about 'health needs assessment' and requires knowledge about the differences and interrelationships between 'need' (the potential to benefit from care), 'demand' (expressed desire for services) and 'supply' (services that are actually provided in relation to need or demand).

Public health has adopted a population-based perspective, whereas clinicians traditionally focus on the needs of individual patients. Now, healthcare workers and managers must take both 'macro' *and* 'micro' perspectives on health, rather than just considering individual patients. They must also develop the skills to manage the conflict that results from using both approaches.

The educational requirements and learning needs of people working in healthcare services are diverse (see Box 3.1).

BOX 3.1 EDUCATIONAL REQUIREMENTS OF TODAY'S HEALTHCARE SERVICES

- Education and training plans should complement those of the individual unit or practice, healthcare organisations and central priorities.
- Implementation of clinical governance, quality assurance and safety measures: knowledge, positive attitudes, new skills and learning culture.
- Adoption of evidence-based practice: where and how to get information, how to apply evidence and monitor changes.
- Needs assessments: how to conduct them, who to work with, linking needs assessment with commissioning and providing care, finding ways to reduce health inequalities.
- Working in partnerships: with other disciplines, clinicians and managers, clinicians and patients or the public, others from non-health organisations.
- Involving the public and patients in planning and delivering healthcare.
- Health service management developments: understanding and working with new models of delivery of care; as work-based teams and across primary/secondary care interfaces.
- Delivering tangible outcomes: thinking and planning in terms of 'health gains' rather than improvements in structures and systems.
- Research and development: encouraging a culture whereby the two are inextricably linked.

The involvement of patients and the public in healthcare decision making is now common but to be done effectively requires healthcare professionals to develop new attitudes and beliefs, and not just to update their knowledge and skills (see also Chapter 13). Such cultural changes will only be achieved if traditional boundaries between healthcare professionals and patients, or between the healthcare service and the voluntary sector, are eradicated. Achieving quality improvements and establishing a clinical governance culture requires everyone's willing cooperation. Similarly, there was a time when the approach to health professions' learning kept individual professions isolated, and individuals opted for postgraduate courses based on personal preferences rather than service needs. Increasingly we now see inter-professional learning opportunities recognising the strength in the multidisciplinary team. Working in partnerships with a wide range of healthcare disciplines requires learning about the roles, responsibilities and capabilities of other professionals which can lead to greater understanding and improvement in the way that multi-professional teams work together.

In the UK, the Centre for the Advancement of Interprofessional Education (CAIPE) is a leading organisation for interdisciplinary education. CAIPE defines interprofessional education as 'occasions when members or students of two or more professions learn with, from and about each other to improve collaboration and the quality of care and services' (CAIPE 2016).

CAIPE identifies the following values for effective interprofessional education and collaborative practice:

- Focus on the needs of individuals, families and communities to improve their quality of care, health outcomes and wellbeing.
- Apply equal opportunities within and between the professions and all with whom they learn and work.
- Respect individuality, difference and diversity within and between the professions and all with whom they learn and work.
- Sustain the identity and expertise of each profession.
- Promote parity between professions in the learning environment.
- Instil interprofessional values and perspectives throughout uniprofessional and multi-professional learning.

Common priorities for education and training from local, district and national perspectives can overlap. Education and training needs should be assessed against all of these development priorities so that educational programmes are relevant to service needs. Ever changing educational and training needs cannot be met by sending individuals on various ad hoc courses. Service changes affect everyone, so a coordinated and integrated approach to educational provision is needed at local levels if the healthcare service is to deliver new models of care that better target the needs of the community. Teachers should support individual learners to follow programmes of activities that are matched to their own predetermined educational plans, but they must also help individuals to design plans to complement the overall business and development plans of their local healthcare service to deliver central and district priorities.

You may need to acquire new knowledge and skills to become more aware of, and expert in, reconciling the needs of individual healthcare professionals and organisations, or recommendations from external sources such as providers of national guidelines and service frameworks. The learning culture for the modern healthcare systems cannot be delivered simply through lectures or seminars, but requires a partnership between educationalists, managers and healthcare professionals, and imaginative educational programmes.

BENEFITS OF INTER-PROFESSIONAL EDUCATION

The benefits of inter-professional education can include the following:

- Reduced isolation of different professionals
- Enhancement of the collaborative approach necessary for cost-effective delivery of quality and safe care and for meeting the needs of local communities, including the development of competences in group decision making:
  - Teamwork
  - Leadership
  - Conflict resolution
- Increasing learners' understanding of others' roles and responsibilities, skills and knowledge, powers and duties, value systems and codes of conduct, opportunities and constraints
- Developing a more appropriate skill-mix of healthcare professionals, resulting in more efficient and effective employment
- Improving patient and healthcare professional satisfaction
- Improving access to healthcare

However, a systematic review looked at the evidence for inter-professional learning and concluded that although there is some evidence for the above list and that interprofessional learning is generally well received, it is not accepted consistently by all learners from similar professional backgrounds. The authors found it is reliant on teachers being adequately competent and confident as facilitators in this mode of teaching and has the potential to worsen perceptions and attitudes towards other professional groups among some learners. This must be sought, monitored and addressed by teachers (Hammick et al. 2007).

The proposed mechanisms through which the benefits of inter-professional working and learning may occur are outlined in Box 3.2.

BOX 3.2 BENEFITS OF INTER-PROFESSIONAL WORKING AND LEARNING

- Development of new roles
- Respect for other professions
- Professionals working together in an atmosphere of openness and trust
- Real communication between professionals
- An appreciation of the strengths of the diversity of other professionals and the complex nature of professional judgement and ways of working
- A common set of values and attitudes
- An understanding of the contribution that other professionals can make and how different professions work best together

---

POTENTIAL BARRIERS TO INTER-PROFESSIONAL EDUCATION

Inter-professional education is not always appropriate and, as we have seen, is not always well received. Some subjects are so specialised that they apply to only one particular discipline or subspecialty. Participants from one discipline may not be comfortable being taught alongside other learners from a traditionally more dominant discipline, or where their learning needs are more basic than those of participants from other disciplines. This challenges the basic principle of inter-professional learning, where all learners should feel equal, regardless of their workplace status. The evidence suggests that undergraduate inter-professional learning may not be as well received as such learning delivered at the postgraduate level. Perhaps because learners do not appreciate the relevance of inter-professional learning if they have yet to work in a multi-professional environment.

Practical barriers include inequalities in study budgets and study leave arrangements between professions, and different working arrangements. These differences may prevent certain groups from attending education or training events, or they may alter the perceived priority of such events. Issues such as space within learning environments may prevent or limit participation.

Inter-professional education can be invaluable. However, the benefits are dependent upon the topic being taught. It appears most useful for professionals to learn about the roles of other disciplines, and least useful for them to learn about knowledge or content, as different healthcare professionals have different priorities, training and knowledge bases.

TEACHING ABOUT WORKING IN PARTNERSHIPS IN THE HEALTHCARE SYSTEM

People are more likely to learn about the benefits of working in partnerships and develop new and meaningful partnerships by observing successful role models.

Teaching should focus on encouraging a common understanding of people's roles, responsibilities and capabilities.

You can help people to understand more about how they perform in a certain role within a team by using psychometric or psychological measurements or interpersonal assessment, such as the Belbin Self-Perception Inventory (Belbin 1981). Such tools have significant limitations and are best not thought of as 'diagnostic tools' but can stimulate a debate about difference, and the importance of a well-balanced team with distinct areas of responsibility playing to individual members' characteristics or strengths.

Teams consist of individuals, with each member fulfilling a different role. Different situations dictate the role that an individual will adopt. Roles may be duplicated, or one person may play a combination of roles. All roles will be evident in any effective social or work group, although groups may survive and achieve some of their objectives with one or more of the roles unfilled.

Belbin described eight roles within a 'winning team':

1. Chairman or Coordinator: coordinates leadership, clarifies goals and priorities
2. Plant: generator of ideas, solves difficult problems
3. Monitor or evaluator: 'sifts' ideas, sees all the options, analyses, judges the likely outcomes
4. Team worker: looks after internal relationships, listens, handles difficult people
5. Resource investigator: looks after external relationships, engages in networking, explores new possibilities
6. Company worker: loyal to the group, organises, turns ideas and plans into practical forms of action
7. Shaper: challenges, pressurises, finds ways round obstacles
8. Completer finisher: ensures that tasks and projects are completed, keeps others to schedules and targets

The move to establish integrated team models of delivery requires more understanding of the capabilities and range of skills of the different disciplines participating, rather than just team roles.

The following list includes the positive features of partnerships that are most likely to be successful. Good partnerships between different disciplines within the healthcare system, the voluntary sector and social care depend on creating trust, mutual respect and joint working for common goals.

Tips on establishing successful working partnerships

Make sure that you establish the following:

*   A written memorandum of partnership
*   A joint strategy with agreed goals and outcomes
*   Widespread support from individuals working within the partnership and their organisations

- Clear roles and responsibilities with regard to joint working
- Shared decision making on partnership matters
- That each partner has different attributes that fit well with the other partner
- Partnership benefits for all organisations
- A partnership where the whole is greater than the sum of the components
- An environment where each partner makes a 'fair' investment in the partnership – and the risk-benefit balance is fair between partners
- Partners who trust each other and are honest about partnership matters
- Partners who appreciate, respect and tolerate each others' differences
- A common understanding about language and communication

As an educational facilitator you can set a learning environment that emphasises and supports the principles of partnerships through project working. Consider the following:

- Set a task that requires the learner to work in partnership with others, and then analyse how that partnership was created and sustained.
- Establish inter-professional learning events to promote understanding of others' roles and responsibilities while undertaking an educational event.
- Ask the learner to gather information that is only available within other sectors, including both healthcare settings and non-healthcare settings (e.g. housing or transport).
- Write case vignettes that describe situations which cross healthcare sectors and settings and involve several health disciplines. By debating who will do what, when and how, the participants will gain further understanding of other colleagues' capabilities and expertise.

CONTINUING PROFESSIONAL DEVELOPMENT (CPD)

Perhaps the most obvious example of learning in context is CPD or continuing medical education (CME). This is usually seen as a process of 'lifelong learning' which enables professionals to enhance their practice and fulfil their potential as well as stay up to date as their role changes or develops.

CPD includes the following:

- Pursuing personal and professional growth by widening, developing and changing your own roles and responsibilities
- Keeping abreast of, and accommodating, clinical, organisational and social changes that affect professional roles in general
- Acquiring and refining the knowledge and skills that are needed for new or current roles or responsibilities or career development
- Putting individual development and learning needs into a team, organisational and multi-professional context

Box 3.3 highlights the criteria for successful CPD learning. The minimum amount of CPD that should be undertaken is often defined by an individual's professional organisation. This can be increased if additional roles are taken on.

To make the most of CPD activities, however, it is not enough to attend learning events; you must reflect on what you have learned, and often this is encouraged through the requirements of an appraisal portfolio. However, in reality, the process of reflection also arises through formal and informal discussions with colleagues. Capturing these thoughts and conversations, and the application of learning in practice and demonstrating change, is of much more value than collecting the traditional certificates of attendance.

BOX 3.3 THE MOST SUCCESSFUL CPD INVOLVES LEARNING WHICH:

- Has a clear need or reason for the particular CPD to be undertaken
- Is led by the learner's own identified needs
- Is based on what is already known by the learner
- Appropriately uses a variety of learning modalities
- Involves active participation by the learner
- Uses the learner's own resources
- Includes relevant and timely feedback
- Includes follow-up to reinforce learning (e.g. self-assessment, reflection)

Note: as a healthcare teacher you should make any education or training relevant to the service needs of your healthcare system, while remembering to build on the criteria for the individual's successful learning.

BARRIERS TO TAKING UP APPROPRIATE EDUCATION OR TRAINING

Teachers should be sufficiently flexible to cater for learners with constraints that limit their access to education, such as time, dependents, limited funds and geographical distance. Increasingly, and particularly through systems responses to the COVID-19 pandemic, educational opportunities are moving online, with asynchronous elements. In addition to barriers to inter-professional learning (addressed previously), Box 3.4 outlines blocks and barriers to establishing a coherent education and training programme across a practice or healthcare organisation.

BOX 3.4 BLOCKS AND BARRIERS TO ESTABLISHING A COHERENT EDUCATION AND TRAINING PROGRAMME ACROSS A PRACTICE, UNIT OR HOSPITAL TRUST

- Isolation of healthcare professionals, even many who appear to work in a team.
- 'Tribalism' as different disciplines protect their traditional roles and responsibilities.
- Lack of incentives to take up learner-centred, interactive education as opposed to more passive modes of educational delivery.
- Various employed/attached/self-employed terms and conditions between staff employed in the same workplace, including differing rights to time and funds for continuing education.
- Lack of communication between healthcare organisations and individuals.
- Domination of the medical model over those of other disciplines.
- Rigid educational budgets of different professionals obstructing true multidisciplinary education.
- Lack of personal educational needs assessments, which means that education may not be targeted appropriately for individual or organisational needs.
- Practitioners being overwhelmed with service work, and therefore having little time for continuing education.
- Dissonance between individuals' perceived educational needs and service relevant needs.
- Lack of shared ownership of both education and development.
- The perception that all education should be paid for by someone else.
- Conservatism – reluctance to develop or accept new models of working and extended roles.
- Selection of educational activities according to preference rather than need.
- Mental ill health – depression, stress, burnout of learner or teacher, fear of and resistance to change.

APPROACHES TO THE DEVELOPMENT OF NEW EDUCATION AND TRAINING PROGRAMMES

The starting point for education and training programmes of many organisations is sometimes a poorly coordinated base of education and training – by individual practitioners themselves, across disciplines, between clinical and administrative staff, and between primary/community/secondary care settings. At practice or directorate level there may have been little strategic planning of the education and training needs of *all* staff, and if there has been some such planning at district or regional levels, those on the ground may not be aware of it.

Locality coordination of education and training should be arranged to ensure that programmes are networked into a district and sub-regional overview of the whole healthcare workforce. This should help to reduce duplication of resources and tailor educational provision to that needed to equip the workforce to be the most effective that the locality can afford.

When reorganising workforce training (see Box 3.5), learning environments should be:

- Suitable and offer opportunities to facilitate multidisciplinary learning
- Available in sufficient numbers to meet the training needs of the service
- Managed, supervised and assessed by appropriately experienced and qualified professional staff
- Quality assured and responsive to learner evaluation and feedback.

BOX 3.5 REORGANISATION OF WORKFORCE TRAINING

1. The healthcare organisation must be clear about service needs, and about the skills and staff required to deliver those services efficiently and effectively.
2. Workforce and resources should be considered together to ensure that plans and developments are consistent and coordinated.
3. There should be an appropriate mix between central (top-down) and local (bottom-up) planning.
4. Planning should cover the whole healthcare workforce, looking across sectors (primary, secondary and tertiary), employers (public, private and voluntary) and staff groups (nurses, doctors, dentists, other professions and other staff), and should take account of evolving roles.
5. Workforce planning arrangements should reflect clear and agreed responsibilities and accountabilities, with effective performance management systems.

All healthcare organisations should appoint an education and training, professional development and workforce planning lead, to ensure that the aforementioned recommendations are met.

Learning across the healthcare system should encompass the concept of lifelong learning and foster links between education, organisational development and human resources. Six themes emerging for education and training within a healthcare system are about developing a better understanding of the following:

- The nature and implementation of healthcare system changes among all staff
- The organisation and funding of health-related education and workforce planning systems
- Practical links between educational providers and healthcare providers to support staff
- The educational and development needs of healthcare providers

- The development of a population focus in healthcare providers by clinicians and managers
- Access and use of information to support learning.

Planning an appropriate education and training programme

Figure 3.1 illustrates the framework of a plan to shape an appropriate education and training programme for clinical and non-clinical healthcare staff, to meet the requirements of the healthcare system, the workforce and the local context. Start at the bottom of the page and work upwards, thinking about what the stages involve from the point of view of a healthcare provider director, manager and/or teacher:

1. Your starting point in terms of the budget, the numbers of staff, their skill base, and the extent and quality of education, training courses and activities available.
2. Preliminary identification of the education and training needs of the workforce that you are planning for. Take account of the gaps in the baseline resources that you identified, the short- and longer-term visions of development for your organisation, and how the national, district and local workforce planning strategies will affect you. Anticipate workforce trends, as there will be a lag phase of several years to recruit and train new staff.
3. Budget constraints will influence your education and training programme, as your preferred vision becomes your affordable vision. Other limitations that will influence the design of the education and training programme include the workforce's willingness to cooperate with the programme, and the need to make the programme relevant to service needs, other priorities and local issues. The design will be influenced by the historical education and training provision that the workforce are used to, the workforce's willingness to take it up, their preferences for particular modes of delivery, the opinions of others (e.g. the public and patients), current fashions (topics and type of delivery) and pressure from local champions or special interest groups.
4. Provision can be mapped out once plans have been agreed. Consider how to meet the needs of the entire workforce for generic knowledge and skills – for example, skills needed for interacting effectively with patients and the public, uni-professional education and training in specialty areas, inter-professional provision whenever appropriate and practicable, and managerial or organisational education and training for those whose roles and responsibilities indicate this.
5. Appraisal and evaluation of the skills, knowledge, attitudes and competence of the workforce with regard to the relevance to service needs should be a regular feature of any education and training programme, with feedback on achievements and gaps in provision at all stages in the cycle. The healthcare system will continue to develop and extend its focus of interest and capability, and any education and training programme should be proactive in this dynamic process, and capable of responding reactively to new directives and developments or public opinion.

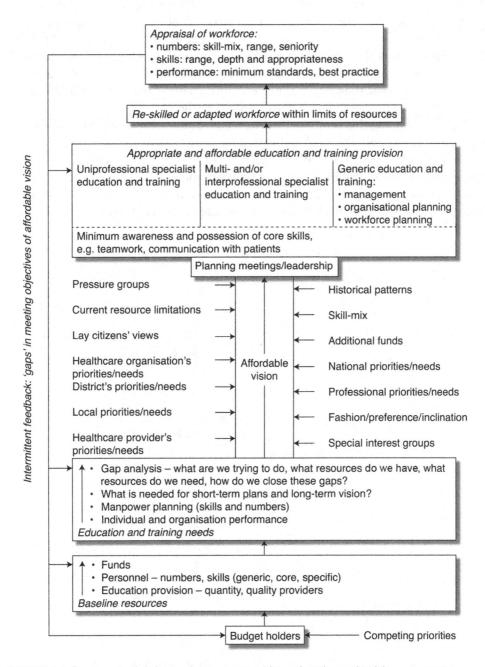

FIGURE 3.1 Framework of a plan to shape an appropriate education and training programme.

EDUCATIONAL PLAN FOR INDIVIDUAL PRACTITIONER

Assessment of your own or others' educational and training needs must include consideration of the differing priority areas of national bodies (e.g. the government), district bodies, your local organisation, your practice or unit and the general public. You need to decide how to weigh one priority against another, as education and training time is limited by competing service demands. This will involve actively looking at every educational or training event for an opportunity to make the activity as relevant as possible to healthcare needs as a whole.

One way of doing this is to visualise the planned educational activity as shown in Figure 3.2. If you 'join the dots' midway along those sides of the octagon that apply to any particular topic, the resulting surface area will give you a visual representation of the number of priority areas that the topic addresses.

In the octagon in Figure 3.2, all of the dots are joined when the educational topic is 'coronary heart disease (CHD)', because this subject is part of any national strategy

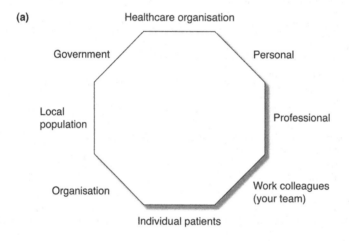

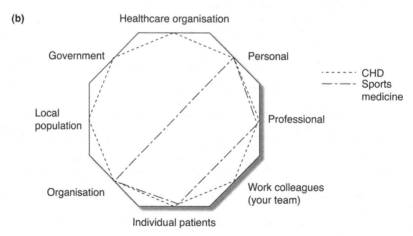

FIGURE 3.2 Visual representation of priority areas.

for prevention and management of CHD, and may also be a priority area of the district population (if standard mortality rates are relatively high), the practice, work colleagues and individual patients (if there has been a sudden death, or if there is particular interest in the quality of cardiac care as a work-based team), professional (if the focus is on the capability to resuscitate any person who arrests) and personal (if there is a wish to maintain competence in managing CHD and adopt best practice).

The surface area that you obtain as a result of joining the dots gives you some idea of the number of priority areas that a potential educational topic addresses, but no idea of the need or baseline depth of knowledge. If the surface area that you draw out is relatively small, as in the second example ('sports medicine'), think how you might teach or learn about the topic so that it is more relevant to priority areas for development of others as well as yourself.

EDUCATION IN A GLOBAL CONTEXT

Socio-economic and geo-political factors frequently cause healthcare professionals to shift from one setting to another and even from one continent to another. At the time of writing, war in Ukraine is causing disruption in medical schools and resulting in the movement of students as 'educational-migrants' to universities around the world. Refugee populations have specific needs, and large numbers of people on the move, fleeing natural disasters, conflict or persecution bring specific challenges for resident healthcare providers. Many of the principles for identifying educational needs and designing an educational environment for healthcare providers remain true in such situations, but rapid change, limited ability to plan and resource-poor conditions bring additional complexity.

Case study: establishing a postgraduate fellowship in humanitarian medicine – building capacity and ensuring sustainability for the health sector in the Rohingya Crisis

The refugee crisis in Cox's Bazar, Bangladesh, was responded to in 2017 by a UK-based humanitarian aid agency, Doctors Worldwide. Doctors in the region and from around the world had moved to the refugee camps, working with international agencies and local charities to set up healthcare facilities. The doctors that staffed these facilities ranged from experienced aid workers and healthcare professionals to junior medical officers, barely out of medical school. The infrastructure needs for clinic and hospital facilities were enormous, but so were the educational needs of these junior doctors who, motivated by altruism, but often un-sustained by any training or educational support, found themselves isolated. They felt out of their depth and found that medical school or internship had not prepared them for the roles they had entered.

Doctors Worldwide carried out an educational needs assessment and developed a rolling 13-week training programme, involving local faculty with context-specific knowledge, which incorporated mentoring, knowledge transfer, clinical skills updating and workplace-based communities of practice. When the COVID-19 pandemic struck, the programme evolved into a hybrid model with online support by international faculty. A key feature of the programme was a focus on quality improvement projects (QIPs) led by the junior doctors and based on changes they knew to be needed in their clinics.

The programme has further, organically, progressed to a cascade model of teaching where alumni from the initial cohorts have stepped up into leadership roles and now plan and deliver training on an interdisciplinary basis for colleagues.

Lessons learnt from developing the programme include the following:

1. Be sure to take advice from, and involve the ideas of, local experts both in healthcare and education.
2. Not all educational models travel well, and the prior experience of teaching and learning (and assessment) will influence how learners learn in new and uncertain settings.
3. The importance of communities of practice. Positive role models, testing of ideas, imagination, creativity and reflection are all important to push the boundaries of legitimate peripheral participation (LPP) through which novices become experienced members, and eventually leaders of, a community of practice or collaborative project (Wenger 1998; see also Chapter 9).

Source: Ahmad and Mohanna (2021).

SUPPORTING CLINICIAN COLLEAGUES TO BE ABLE TO WORK IN A NEW CONTEXT

Understanding the health and care system is key for clinical colleagues moving settings and hoping, or already started, to work in a new country. Their intelligent knowledge of the context will be as important as their medical knowledge and skills. They may, for example, come from a setting where general practice (or family medicine) is under-developed or not valued, so they may not have first-hand experience of a referral system such as the UK system with a GP 'gatekeeper' to healthcare services.

Many doctors moving from one country to another may have passed a formal language test but still not be confident applying that language in clinician-to-clinician interaction or direct clinician-to-patient engagement. The latter in the UK sometimes requires a less formal register than expected by some whose home societal structures might not, for example, incorporate small talk between doctor and patient (Mohanna 2019). Sometimes, clinicians trained in one country and working in another have difficulties with a rigid application of the 'rules' of patient conversations. For example, in the UK context, colleagues may have followed well-meaning guidance from private Professional and Linguistic Assessments Board (PLAB) courses which results in formulaic application of phrases. Perhaps they have been taught to interject if a patient were to say '. . . then my father died' with a reflex 'I'm sorry to hear that your father died' when the patient is in the midst of a personal description of their symptoms and situation.

The following suggestions to support colleagues who have been trained in a different context and moved to the UK. The principles may translate to other contexts:

- Encourage colleagues to develop less formal modes of communication by listening to and echoing the words and phrases that patients use.
- Work on developing patient-friendly vocabulary for day-to-day practice; this will likely be different from the technical terms learnt when they studied medicine.
- Consider using a translation app such as 'Google translate' for difficult phrases and concepts.
- Use trusted local medical websites to read up on clinical care and best practice clinical management for a wide range of medical conditions.
- Read books and discuss them with a friend in English.
- Listen to the radio, such as BBC radio 4 which has in-depth discussion of current issues.
- Utilise apps linked to good English conversation and discussions, such as TED and Times Radio, or those that help to improve pronunciation, such as the 'English Pronunciation' app recognisable with its Union Jack logo.

It's great if clinicians who are on a path to taking and passing an English language test can attract friends or a mentor (you??) who speaks good English and meet up regularly for informal catch ups where English is spoken as the main language. This embeds working language knowledge faster than speaking English whilst doing a course but then reverting to a different language for the rest of the day.

Gaining UK health professional registration

For a large number of overseas trained doctors, pharmacists, dentists and nurses, information on the structure of the health service and the alternative options open to them to practise as clinicians will provide a vital first step to working in the UK. The organisation of the NHS may differ significantly from the health service that they are used to in their country of origin, or where they trained as a clinician. They need information about the principles underlying UK clinical guidelines and protocols, referral pathways, patient expectations, the career structure for health professionals in different parts of the UK – as many will find these elements confusing.

International medical graduates (IMG doctors) and other internationally trained practitioners need information that is specific to their situation. Such information should cover their professional registration as a health professional in the UK, work permits and the limitations that moving to the UK from abroad will have on the career options open to them. Qualifications from different parts of the world should be discussed and the role of further training if needed. There are some reciprocal agreements in place with some countries.

This group of health professionals will require information on how to do the PLAB tests which is a necessary precursor to working in the UK for many. In addition, for those whose first language is not English and whose health professional degree was not taught in English, the IELTS examination (International English Language Testing System), or alternatively the Occupational English Test (OET) which many find easier to pass than IELTS, will be important. The OET is individualised to the specific health profession and recognised by the UK professional regulatory bodies such as the GMC, NMC.

If you are advising colleagues aiming to make the transition to UK practice, be sure they know how to access reliable and up to date information of the requirements, including visas, language and professional aspects. This varies from one profession to another and also within professions such as medical specialties.

At the time of writing, to obtain GMC full registration, a doctor who has trained overseas needs proof of the following:

- English language proficiency (IELTS/OET).
- Pass in PLAB 1 and 2 or an accepted postgraduate qualification.
- Details of internship in their Electronic Portfolio of International Credentials (EPIC) and Certificate of Good Standing.
- Successful application for GMC full registration.

SUPPORTING PATIENTS FROM OVERSEAS: TRANSFERABLE EDUCATIONAL SKILLS

Another important aspect of the impact of context on learning is when aiding non-English language speaking patients and their carers. According to Language Line Solutions, there are around 4.2 million UK citizens in this category whose primary language is not English as well as around 11 million who are deaf or hard of hearing (see www.languageline.com/uk/s). Some health and care organizations commission a translation service to be easily available by phone or video call that can be triggered by the responsible clinician for the consultation with a short connection time to a translator who speaks the language of the patient.

If the patient brings a carer or friend to translate, then the clinician will need to be very aware of information governance aspects relating to the consultation and that the patient is willingly giving informed consent to having an extra person in the consulting room hearing the clinical conversation, without duress. It is rarely appropriate to use family members as translators, however convenient it might be.

Be aware that if the patient has experienced trauma, torture and other violence in the past before they came to the UK, this may have diminished their trust in health professionals, if healthcare staff were involved somehow in their own country. So work hard to recreate that trust in the healthcare services you are providing, and ensure that they understand that they are entitled to NHS care. Many asylum seekers suffer from poor mental health as they await a decision about their asylum claim, which can be a very protracted process (Ahmad 2022; Arnold 2022). Patients who are migrants are moved around the country with little warning, and their medical care, treatment and investigations may be disrupted, with consequences for the individual's health and wellbeing.

In summary, this chapter has included principles and suggestions for adapting teaching to context. Whether facilitating the educational journey of formal or informal learners (students, trainees or colleagues) or adapting teaching for patients, some of these principles will be transferable across settings.

REFERENCES

Ahmad A. (2022) Recognise suffering and improve responses. *BMJ*, 376: 221.

Ahmad M.S. and Mohanna K. (2021) Establishing a postgraduate fellowship in humanitarian medicine – building capacity and ensuring sustainability for the health sector in the Rohingya crisis. *Education for Primary Care*. DOI: 10.1080/14739879.2020.1864782.

Arnold F. (2022) How can we help asylum seekers? *BMJ*, 376: 302.

Belbin R.M. (1981) *Management teams: Why they succeed or fail*. Oxford: Heinemann.

CAIPE (2016) Statement of purpose. Available at www.caipe.org/resource/CAIPE-Statement-of-Purpose-2016.pdf (Accessed 28.3.22).

Commission on Education and Training for Patient Safety (2016) *Improving safety through education and training*. London: HEE.

Frances Report (2010) Available at www.gov.uk/government/publications/independent-inquiry-into-care-provided-by-mid-staffordshire-nhs-foundation-trust-january-2001-to-march-2009 (Accessed 28.3.22).

Hammick M., Freeth D., Koppel I., et al. (2007) A best evidence systematic review of interprofessional education. *Medical Teacher*, 29: 735–751.

Mohanna K. (2019) *Liaquat National Journal of Primary Care*, 1(1): 6–12. https://doi.org/10.37184/lnjpc.2707-3521.1.9.

Wenger E. (1998) *Communities of practice: Learning, meaning and identity*. Cambridge: Cambridge University Press.

CHAPTER 4

Supporting learners in a changing multidisciplinary team

....

The UK Government prioritised growing and diversifying the workforce in England in the NHS Five Year Forward View (NHS 2014). New roles have been introduced, including nursing associates, advanced nurse practitioners and physician associates, and changes have been made to existing roles, for example, increasing the prominence of clinical pharmacists and the introduction of first contact physiotherapists (FCPs).

However, the optimal implementation and operationalisation of these roles has not always been made clear at the point of introduction. Some role descriptions outline proposed activities but do not completely bridge the gap in understanding how to train individuals to undertake them. In addition, at times, there has been confusion about the nature of some of the new roles, for example, in England, those funded by the Additional Roles Reimbursement Scheme (NHSE 2019). For all new roles this also applies to the balance between service delivery and requirements for training.

Due to the diversification of roles within the healthcare team, senior clinicians may now find themselves leading teams of, or delivering on-the-job training to, professionals that may have had initial training that is very different from their own and who follow a very different model of practice. The ability to identify and support the educational needs of a colleague in a different profession from your own is a key leadership skill.

FAMILIARISE YOURSELF WITH THE ROLE

While the need to familiarise yourself with your learner's role may sound obvious, it is not always easy to do. Role descriptors from national resources can

DOI: 10.1201/9781003352532-5

be high level and difficult to operationalise. For example, the NHS Health Careers website describes a physician associate role as providing 'support to doctors in the diagnosis and management of patients', which includes 'taking histories, performing examinations, diagnosing illnesses and developing management plans' (NHS 2022). Without a more granular description it is not clear how this differentiates such a role from many other clinical roles, and we do not always have a reference point to understand what that looks like in the real world. Indeed, it is not always clear how independent new practitioners are allowed to be and whether their role requires statutory registration and mandatory continuing professional development and re-licensing. Where does the clinical indemnity responsibility lie as more senior roles and responsibilities are taken up? New employers and/or supervisors will need to ensure that they are fully aware of and compliant with the legal requirements of their healthcare system in which they practice, and this may bring some extra emphasis on learning needs.

Role descriptions for newer roles may be developed from the literature from other health economies which might not directly translate to the NHS. For example, for physician associates much of the early information was derived from the United States of America, where physician associate roles are more embedded, more familiar and more senior. There they may be able to prescribe and order radiographs, and their role in decision making might require a different level of supervision than a UK-trained physician associate.

Among the newer roles, senior or established role models are few and far between. We therefore lose the ability to base our understanding of the role on experience and observation. If you are supervising a new or extended role practitioner, it is important to try and develop an understanding of their role, which may involve comparison with other professional groups. However, it is important to also try and gain an understanding of the role in its own right. For example, it is not uncommon for physician associates to be described, or describe themselves, as 'a bit like a doctor but cannot prescribe' or 'between a doctor and a nurse'. It is not clear that such comparisons really help to identify the needs and direction of development for the learner. When familiarising yourself with these new roles and how you will support them as an educator, it may be better to frame your understanding of your learner's role in terms of what they are experts in rather than which of the existing, familiar roles they can be compared to.

An additional aspect to bear in mind is that whilst the capabilities of different individuals within the same role may differ, there will also be some differences in the scope of practice between individuals within newer roles. For example, some First Contact Physiotherapists (FCPs) can prescribe and inject joints while others cannot, and this will need to be clarified. When conducting an initial learning needs assessment, optional capabilities that colleagues may hold within the role should be identified and explicitly explored.

Case study

The size of the task for understanding and optimising newer roles within the healthcare service should not be underestimated. The North Staffordshire GP Federation addressed the need to foster an understanding of new roles in primary care at a system level, through the development of a physician associate internship programme (NSGPF 2022). However, over its inception and development, it became clear that to really success-fully integrate this new role at scale within primary care, targeted documents, dedicated practice and physician associate support, a post-graduate physician associate teaching curriculum and ongoing feedback to practices and the physician associates was required and needed to be developed based on best practice.

Schemes such as this are not common-place nor provided for all new roles. Where such schemes do not exist, the onus is on educators and organisations to actively seek out the experiences of, and advice from, those who have previously hosted these newer roles. You might be able to identify professional champions from the same role as your learner, to establish how they have worked in settings such as yours, what tasks they have been doing (plus any governance requirements to support these) and the educational support they have required.

THE IMPORTANCE OF UNDERSTANDING GOVERNANCE REQUIREMENTS

If you are the supervisor of one of the newer healthcare roles, it is important to focus at all times on patient safety and governance. For example, as a non-prescriber, how can an advanced care practitioner be enabled to administer a joint injection? Clarity about the legal requirements for certain activities is not always clear. If we err on the side of caution unnecessarily, this may result in barriers or inefficient processes being introduced that undermine the value of these new roles. Being unaware of the legal and governance restrictions can leave supervisors and their organisations exposed to significant negative consequences.

There are differences in the supervisory requirements of the various new roles, with some professional groups being autonomous and others being reliant on senior clinical presence at all times. Some roles must be supervised by a doctor, others may be supervised by anyone who holds the necessary expertise. While it is important to know and meet the expectations and requirements of the roles you are supervising, you also need to be mindful of the negative impact of unnecessary over-supervision. If a professional does not need to discuss every case with you as the senior clinician, yet this is enforced, the learner's growth and development can be stunted through never needing to take full responsibility for their decision-making. Do not under-estimate the responsibility learners feel when they are the ones deciding on their own whether it is okay for the patient to leave the department. This responsibility is magnified in primary care, when healthcare professionals consult with patients alone and patients only come into contact with the healthcare professional they have been booked with. Your supervision style needs to facilitate a growth mindset through progressively tailoring your involvement to the individual learner and your own 'risk-thermostat' (Mohanna and Chambers 2001). You should actively review the level of supervision required as you and the learner become comfortable with an increasingly devolved responsibility for independent decision making.

The drive for increasing the workforce through diversifying professional roles has resulted in part from the problems of recruitment and retention. This at times has led to those very healthcare professionals who are facing additional workforce challenges becoming the ones to assume new teaching and supervisory roles. The training needs of learners must however be met, and it is important that there is clarity between the organisation and the learner about the balance between service delivery and learning. Early investment in the learner can reap rewards through service delivery later on; inadequate early support can result in stress, anxiety, lack of personal fulfilment, suboptimal attainment of the service delivery potential and early departure of the individual from the role.

WHAT DOES THE INDIVIDUAL NEED TO LEARN?

As with any workplace learning, you need to know both where the learner needs to get to and where they are now. This can present a challenge for some of the newer roles, for example, you may be faced with a lengthy curriculum as the only formal source of information about their training to date and a very high-level description of what is expected from your new colleague. Operationalising a training plan within the workplace can be challenging. Further, the direction of development for the learner is not determined simply by the documented roles they might undertake, but rather a combination of this, the requirements for revalidation (if needed), the requirements of the Trust or your organisation's service needs. This latter issue is important as the tasks required from a professional will depend on a balance with others in the team. For example, an advanced nurse practitioner in primary care may be required to do independent acute home visits, whereas in a Trust outpatients department this is unlikely.

When the supervisor is less familiar with the learner's role, there is a temptation for the learning plan to be very heavily led by the learner. While, in adult learning, it is appropriate for learners to identify their learning needs, the complicating factors for the newer roles are two-fold: (1) the learner may not be aware of the potential tasks and roles that may be available within the clinical setting, and (2) the learner may have insecurities about unfamiliar aspects of the role and avoid this being included in the learning plan, particularly if it is not known to you as the supervisor that this role or task would be appropriate. Such problems are compounded when the learner has had only very limited time in the clinical setting in their undergraduate or previous training. Where both the supervisor and the learner are unaware of the potential for the learner's role within their organisation, this can limit their growth and development and prevent them from exploring or reaching their full potential. This really underlines the need to familiarise yourself with your learner's role right from the beginning and to challenge and support the learner to push the limits of their potential within your organisation.

HOW TO ADDRESS AND DEVELOP THE INDIVIDUAL'S SCOPE OF PRACTICE

As with any learner, it is important to set up regular review meetings to ensure that development is an ongoing process. For some roles, the minimum number and interval of review meetings may be prescribed within their training curriculum or contract, however, where it is not, you should discuss with your learner an appropriate frequency with which to undertake such reviews. This allows goals to be set and a shared understanding to be developed about what the learning needs and potential roles of the individual are. It can be helpful to formally map the learner's current scope of practice and an aspirational scope of practice at each of your review meetings.

The use of Red Amber Green (RAG) ratings of tasks/activities/competencies have been used by some organisations to support both the administrative staff to allocate patients to the most appropriate professional and to ensure that the individual healthcare professional does not have appointments with patients for presentations outside of their scope of practice. This can be incredibly useful when your learner works within an unfamiliar professional role, has a very defined scope of practice (e.g. first contact physiotherapists), has current defined areas of inadequate expertise (e.g. a trainee nurse associate who has not been trained in phlebotomy) and where there are clear legal or governance restrictions. However, for the more generalist roles, RAG ratings, if they remain static and embedded, can risk limiting development and ongoing maintenance of competencies required for revalidation. The optimal way to use RAG ratings is therefore to view these as a support for administrative staff and service planning, but, from the educator's perspective, they should be viewed as a dynamic document that develops with the learner. RAG ratings should be regularly reviewed to identify areas for potential role expansion. Reviews should be undertaken individually with the learner but also cross-organisation to ensure the most appropriate individuals are always undertaking the most appropriate tasks and activities (as this may change as other professional roles develop and individuals come or go).

CONTEXT OF TEACHING

A recent first contact physiotherapist (FCP) programme evaluation identified that the variation in the way in which the roles were physically located impacted the outcomes of the integration, training and supervision (Stynes et al. 2020). Those FCPs working in a hub setting away from an associated base were less well integrated, understood, utilised and supported than those who were co-located within their base, where support for learning happened much more organically. If your learners are not co-located in your usual place of work, you may need to establish proactive strategies to mitigate against the difficulties and facilitate and optimise learning opportunities.

Traditionally healthcare professionals have been trained to undertake a specific professional role, for example, mental health nurse training, operating department practitioner training and so on. In this model, roles are more clearly defined. However, as we have seen, as the workforce has diversified, some tasks or procedures can be undertaken by a variety of professional roles. This means that a role-based approach to education may not always be the most appropriate, and usually, a mixture of role and task-based training will best meet the needs of the learner.

Task or topic-based training is learning and development to undertake certain activities or learn about particular themes. Examples might be prescribing, sonography, phlebotomy, end of life care or endoscopy. Learning for such tasks might be best organised jointly, drawing together insights from all different professional groups who carry out such activities to enhance the experience and also ensure that care provided is standardised through consistent training. Through task-based training, the coming together of different professional roles can enhance understanding of the skillsets and expertise of professional groups other than their own. This can foster better working relationships and better use of the roles through more accurate mapping of tasks to the most appropriately equipped professional. Multidisciplinary teaching sessions can be scheduled within organisations to support the delivery of service need priorities, for example, to learn from errors, complaints or identified problems. Protecting time within an organisation to deliver multidisciplinary training can result in valuable opportunities for professionals with a variety of experience and expertise to share experiences and support each other to find solutions that may not otherwise have been identified.

Role-based training, that is training or learning delivered to one professional group, has its value in that issues specific to that professional group can be identified and discussed with others with a shared understanding and expertise of that particular role. For example, providing information about preparing for professional revalidation is much better suited to role-based teaching. Role-based training may need to be cross-organisational, particularly for newer roles where there may be fewer individuals from that professional background. This has the added benefit of sharing of learning, information and processes which can be fed back into the individual learner's organisation. Supervisors who are not from the same professional background as the learner value the presence of centrally delivered role-based training delivered by experts of that professional group in their setting as an assurance that their learners were receiving training that is suitable to their needs and at their level. However, the value to the learner (and the learner's organisation) is determined by the applicability of the role-based teaching to the learner's current professional setting. Educators delivering role-based teaching must be selected carefully to meet, and be mindful of, the needs of the learners in their own contexts. For example, an advanced nurse practitioner with significant expertise who is working in a hospital delivering teaching about the management of heart failure may not be equipped to provide the insights required for those working in the community making decisions about when to admit a patient. For this reason, role-based training may not always need to be delivered by an expert from the same professional background as the learners; a clinical pharmacist might be best placed to deliver training on depo injections to new community mental health nurses, and an FCP may be an ideal person to deliver musculoskeletal assessment training to advanced nurse practitioners.

Within settings such as the emergency department and in primary care in which undifferentiated illness is commonly encountered and in which it is not possible to generate protocols to support learners across the entire breadth of their work, just-in-time learning and/or teaching should be factored into the timetables of learners and their supervisors. Ways to support just-in-time learning need to be tailored to the needs of the learner and service delivery requirements. Early introduction to reliable, high quality and easily accessible sources of clinical information and longer appointment times may be all that is required for some learners to enable them to seek information as they encounter new presentations or scenarios.

However, other roles may require dedicated supervision time throughout the day. As the workforce has become more diverse in primary care, for example, some practices have adopted the approach of a senior doctor who has no or few booked appointments to allow easy access to supervision and just-in-time teaching and support. In this way, one single general practitioner (GP) can supervise multiple staff and learners at any one time while completing what has been called their 'silent workload' – administrative or business leadership tasks – when not required for supervision (see Figure 4.1).

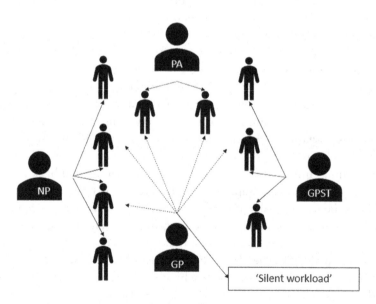

FIGURE 4.1 The 'silent workload' of non–patient-facing GP tasks.

In summary, the new and rapidly expanding range of clinical professions brings a need for a new and flexible approach to identifying and supporting learning needs. The effective supervisor will need an interest and curiosity about roles their learners can undertake and access to innovative and creative approaches to teaching and learning. If taken up, the opportunity for enhanced opportunities for multidisciplinary team joint training could also lead to increased job satisfaction and team working.

REFERENCES

Mohanna K. and Chambers R. (2001) *Risk matters in healthcare.* Oxford: Radcliffe Medical Press.

NHS Careers (2022) Medical associate professions roles. Available at www.healthcareers. nhs.uk/explore-roles/medical-associate-professions/roles-medical-associate-professions/ physician-associate (Accessed 28.3.22).

NHSE (2014, revised 2019) *NHS forward view.* London: NHSE.

NHSE and NHSI (2019) Network contract directed enhanced service: Additional roles reimbursement scheme (ARRS) guidance. Available at www.england.nhs.uk/wp-content/ uploads/2019/12/network-contract-des-additional-roles-reimbursement-scheme- guidance-december2019.pdf (Accessed 28.3.22).

North Staffordshire GP Federation (2022) Staffordshire physician associate internship. Available at www.nsgpfed.org.uk/2021/12/08/staffordshire-physician-associate-pa-internship- programme-update-december-2021 (Accessed 28.3.22).

Stynes S., Goodwin R. and Bishop A. (2020) *National evaluation of first contact practitioner (FCP) model of primary care.* Chartered Society of Physiotherapy CSP Charitable Trust. Available at www.csp.org.uk/system/files/documents/2020-11/final_fcp_phase_3_national_ evaluation_report.pdf (Accessed 28.3.22).

CHAPTER 5

Curriculum development

....

WHAT IS A CURRICULUM?

Recently, the term 'curriculum' has come to mean a document produced by a national body and handed down. For example, following the creation of the Postgraduate Medical Education and Training Board (PMETB) in 2005, medical education in the UK saw a flurry of activity within the Medical Royal Colleges, producing national postgraduate training curricula. After the PMETB merged with the General Medical Council (GMC) in 2010, the GMC started to work towards a unified curriculum for medical schools which has become Outcomes for Graduates (GMC 2018). At the time of writing, we are soon to see the introduction of a national handed down assessment as part of that curriculum, the Medical Licensing Assessment that all UK medical graduates will sit from 2024 (GMC 2022).

The term 'curriculum' is also used to refer to what teachers do – that is, plan, implement and evaluate their educational programmes. Some authors use the term *curriculum design* to refer to official processes, and the term *curriculum development* to describe what teachers do. Both meanings are practically important for course planners, because the presence of a national curriculum usually means that a large amount of control over planning, content and assessment has passed from a local level to a higher authority. Whether this is a good thing depends upon the quality of the official document and the values of the teacher. In healthcare, curriculum development at a local level must align with national requirements, which is not always a straightforward process when universities are used to designing and implementing their own assessment strategies and curricula.

Curriculum planning is not just a simple matter of fitting content into a timetable. A curriculum should support practitioners in order to make the transition from novice to expert (see Box 5.1).

DOI: 10.1201/9781003352532-6

BOX 5.1 PROGRESSION FROM NOVICE TO EXPERT

Level 1: Novice

- Rigid adherence to taught rules or plans.
- Little situational perception.
- No discretionary judgement.

Level 2: Advanced beginner

- Guidelines for action based on attributes or aspects (aspects are global characteristics of situations recognisable only after some prior experience).
- Situational perception still limited.
- All attributes and aspects are treated separately and given equal importance.

Level 3: Competent

- Coping with crowdedness (the number of patients, activities, pieces of information, etc. competing for the individual's attention).
- Now sees actions at least partially in terms of longer-term goals.
- Conscious deliberate planning.
- Standardised and routinised procedures.

Level 4: Proficient

- Sees situations holistically rather than in terms of aspects.
- Sees what is most important in a situation.
- Perceives deviations from the normal pattern.
- Decision making is less laboured.
- Uses maxims for guidance, whose meaning varies according to the situation.

Level 5: Expert

- No longer relies on rules, guidelines or maxims.
- Intuitive grasp of situations based on deep tacit understanding.
- Analytical approaches used only in novel situations, when problems occur or when justifying conclusions.
- Has a vision of what is possible.

Source: Adapted from Eraut (1994).

HOW SHOULD I START TO PLAN MY EDUCATIONAL PROGRAMME OR COURSE?

First, identify the broad *aims* of the course. Clarity will help subsequent course design and also explanation of the course to stakeholders. The more clearly learners understand your intentions, the greater will be their ability to take control of their own learning.

After deciding on the big picture, chunk down these aims into a medium-level *course outline*. This will depend on the decisions that you make on content, so concept mapping (Harden 2001; Novak and Canas 2008) may be helpful here.

As well as designing blocks of content, identify one or two themes that run through the whole course or through several elements. This gives unity to the course, allows learners to appreciate the interconnectedness of items, breaks down barriers and undermines fixed perspectives. An alternative approach to linear curriculum planning is the concept of a spiral curriculum (Harden and Stamper 1999). This addresses the lack of integration within healthcare education, and involves revisiting topics and subject areas over time.

Once you have a broad outline, think about *course objectives* (see Box 5.2). These are more specific than aims.

BOX 5.2 CLARIFYING CURRICULUM OBJECTIVES

Step 1. Decide what kind of knowledge is to be involved.

Step 2. Select the topics to teach.

Step 3. Decide the purpose of teaching the topic and hence the level of knowledge that it is desirable for learners to acquire.

Step 4. Put the package of objectives together and relate them to assessment tasks.

Source: Biggs (2003).

After the curriculum objectives have been finalised, you can write *schemes of work*. Following these, the final units of design are individual *lesson plans*. These will depend on local circumstances and your own preferences.

The questions in Box 5.3 highlight the choices to be made in setting course aims and objectives.

BOX 5.3 QUESTION 1: WHAT IS THE CONTEXT WITHIN WHICH YOU ARE PLANNING?

- Is there a 'handed down' curriculum that you need to take into account?
- Are you planning part of a larger curriculum and need to take account of other educators?
- Are you free to make your own decisions?
- Are there resource issues?

Context

Early decisions in curriculum planning

Curriculum planning rarely starts with a blank sheet of paper. You should be prepared for other educational activity, such as a written curriculum, a previous curriculum or examination syllabus, or the views of other departments with which you may have to compete for the learner's attention.

If there is a national curriculum, you must first decide what purpose it serves for you. If you have a 'handed down' curriculum (see Box 5.4), power resides in a higher authority. The other two options see power being exercised locally or even shared by the learner.

BOX 5.4 WHAT IS YOUR ATTITUDE TO A 'HANDED DOWN' CURRICULUM?

- It is a blueprint (from which we intend to make replicas).
- It is like a play (as directors, we follow the text but interpret it in our own way).
- It is like a springboard (a point of departure from which teachers and learners launch themselves).

Teachers may find themselves in one of two basic positions. One position cedes all authority to the national document for content, planning and the curriculum is used as a blueprint. In the other, the national curriculum is used as an authoritative resource, but teachers maintain their own judgement about suitable content and methods. Teachers may also want to retain a say in evaluation.

This decision will depend on many factors, such as the quality of the national curriculum, the wishes of the learners, the wishes of teachers and the resources available. In the health professions, as with all regulated professions, there may be little flexibility.

Designing a curriculum from scratch

If you get the opportunity to design a curriculum from scratch, don't waste it. This can be an opportunity for creativity and ownership. Three areas of activity have been identified in the production of a curriculum, each of which plays a part in creating the success of the end product (Bowe et al. 1992; see Figure 5.1).

The burden of history

Another context problem that curriculum writers face is the burden of history. Both teachers and learners will often be attached to familiar content, teaching methods and assessments. The management of change, and negotiations involved, in introducing a curriculum is complex. This is not a new problem as identified by Abrahamson who listed nine 'diseases of the curriculum' (Abrahamson 1978):

1. Curriculosclerosis or 'hardening of the categories' – departments vie to ensure the contribution of their specialty persists unchanged.

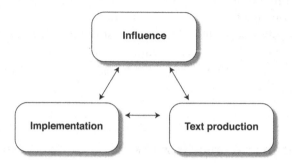

FIGURE 5.1 If you are a curriculum writer, responsible for producing the text, be aware of the requirements of regulators (e.g. government, regulatory organisations) and other outside bodies (e.g. professional organisations, student bodies, pressure groups).

2. Carcinoma of the curriculum – rapid and seemingly uncontrolled growth in certain areas due to drivers such as research interests, grant funding or political imperatives.
3. Curriculoarthritis – problems affecting the articulation of adjacent areas of the curriculum. This can be horizontally such as at the end of one year and the start of the next or vertically e.g. between subject leads in different years. Often resulting from poor communication.
4. Curriculum 'diesthesia' or malaise. Something is 'just not right'. This might precede another more specific disease after a few more investigations, through curriculum evaluation.
5. Iatrogenic curriculitis – The constant shifting, changing, modifying and adjusting allow no opportunity for thoughtful review let alone evaluative research.
6. Curriculum hypertrophy – the expansion of scientific progress increases demand for curriculum time but nothing gets dropped.
7. Idiopathic curriculitis – something is 'not quite right', but this time it is 'pedagogic insufficiency', the teaching that is to blame, not the curriculum itself.
8. Intercurrent curriculitis – occurring alongside any of the conditions above but not related to it and arising from incompatibility of the curriculum with the needs of society.
9. Curriculum ossification – the curriculum becomes fixed in stone because 'we studied like this and we turned out ok'.

Content

There are many methods of determining content (see Box 5.5), including the Delphi technique (expert panel), critical incident survey (educational lessons of good and bad practice), task analysis (observation of practitioners), epidemiology (mortality and morbidity rates) and gap analysis (identifying what is missing from current practice).

**BOX 5.5 QUESTION 2: HOW WILL YOU DECIDE ON THE CONTENT
OF YOUR CURRICULUM?**

- What do you want learners to know?
- What skills do they need to acquire?
- What functions do you want learners to be able to perform by the end of the course?

Topics to include are those that:

- Directly contribute to course objectives
- Are essential building blocks to understanding later learning
- Develop intellectual abilities such as critical thinking
- Make connections between elements of the curriculum

(Harden 1986)

Content specification can be difficult. Although most learners and teachers are satisfied with broad brushstrokes, some want everything to be specified in detail. Such hyperspecification can result in a vast curriculum document that no one will read. Another disadvantage of a detailed syllabus is that it often produces the command that there shall be no teaching or assessment of anything that is not written into the curriculum. Given the rapid rate of change in the world of healthcare, you need to be able to incorporate new developments in healthcare professionals' training.

Structuring your content description

Traditionally, medical curricula were based on catalogues of diseases mapped on to body systems. Today, this biomedical, pathology-based approach is being abandoned in favour of a classification that addresses the relationship between the patient and the healthcare professional and takes into account a more holistic understanding of the patient's world.

We can distinguish between 'discipline' or 'organ systems' curricula and those that used a problem-based approach to learning. Today, the organisational structures of curricula take into account the relationship between healthcare professionals and society. Issues such as ethics, trust, accountability, healthcare professionals' self-awareness, their relationships with colleagues, the nature of healthcare services, health economics and leadership are often grouped under the term 'professionalism'. For example, see CanMEDS (RCPSC 2015).

Healthcare workers often overvalue factual knowledge, and this can have a distorting effect on curriculum planning. Biggs (2003) defines various forms of knowledge:

- Declarative knowledge:
  - Knowing about things
  - Knowledge that we can declare to someone in writing or verbally

TABLE 5.1 Distinction between Professional and Academic Knowledge

Professional knowledge	Academic knowledge
Functioning, specific and pragmatic	*Declarative, abstract and conceptual*
Deals with executing, applying and making priorities	*Deals with labelling, differentiating, elaborating and justifying*

Source: Adapted from Biggs (2003).

- Functioning knowledge:
  - Knowledge that we put to work in problem solving, analysing or designing something, or in making an argument

Functioning knowledge depends not only on knowing *facts* (declarative knowledge), but also on knowledge of *how* (procedural knowledge) and *when* and *why* (conditional knowledge).

Another useful distinction is between academic and professional knowledge (see Table 5.1).

Tension arises between the knowledge of the 'ivory towers' of academia and the practice-bound practical 'know-how' of the professional, not only in the content but also in the way that knowledge is used. Learners can have problems transferring knowledge from abstract, academic discourse to real-world problems.

Established, expert practitioners cannot always explain their decision-making processes. Their knowledge is unconscious, intuitive or tacit. A large proportion of the knowledge that healthcare professionals use is implicit or tacit. This 'action knowledge' (Eraut 2000) is quicker to access and more intuitive, making it more useful than explicit knowledge, which would be slow and cumbersome in many clinical situations. A curriculum that puts the emphasis on the teaching and assessment of factual knowledge can have an adverse effect on the learning of less tangible professional qualities, such as creativity, imagination, enquiry, values and attitudes.

Learner-perceived needs and stakeholder needs

Carrying out a thorough learning needs assessment has clear advantages, not least the avoidance of teaching people what they already know. However, a major disadvantage is that it can allow learners to limit their learning to what they are interested in, rather than what they need to know.

At the curriculum level, you should define what needs to be known and highlight the relative importance of each topic area, rather than solely focusing on learning gaps. With the shift towards self-directed learning, learners often decide which events to attend in order to achieve their learning aims. Clear statements of intended outcomes help the learner with this.

Curriculum mapping can clarify thinking in planning and help explain a curriculum both to learners and faculty. Decide whether to cover all possible content superficially or selected topics in depth. Remember that 'the greatest enemy of understanding is coverage' (Biggs 2003). Course planners must be prepared to omit enough topics to create the space needed to do justice to key areas. An effective map can help learners locate learning resources and content when looking back on teaching (see Harden 2001 and Figure 5.2).

Assessment (see also Chapters 16 and 17)

Traditionally, assessment and course evaluation occur at the end of the course. The argument for this has been that learning continues throughout the course and is expected to be maximal at the end.

Deeper analysis of the nature of professional learning however indicates that although knowledge is important, it is not sufficient for the kind of complex decisions that professionals need to make.

Beyond knowledge testing

Knowledge testing is beloved by psychometricians, as candidates' scores remain fairly constant over time, and it is thus the best predictor of success.

This makes it a strongly desirable feature of selection processes. However, it is overvalued for end-point assessment. Knowledge of something does not directly translate into capability. For example, it is one thing to be able to demonstrate a high degree of knowledge about patient-centred consulting in an essay; actual application of this knowledge into patient-centred behaviour that can be observed is a different type of capability and requires a different type of assessment Miller's pyramid (1990; see Figure 5.3).

Miller argues that although knowledge is an important foundation for learning, professional assessments require methods that assess the application of knowledge to real-life situations and those in which the healthcare professional can demonstrate competence at complex tasks. Although testing competence is a useful assessment of learning, learners can demonstrate competence in examination situations by exhibiting behaviours that they do not use in real life.

The strongest educational argument for assessment over time is that, unlike competence, performance can only be measured over time.

Aligning curriculum and assessment

Aligning the curriculum with assessments is very important, not least because learners will be dissatisfied if they are not taught what they are assessed on. If you have control over assessment, this is much easier. However, assessment methods may be chosen without reference to the curriculum, pre-date the curriculum or be chosen by

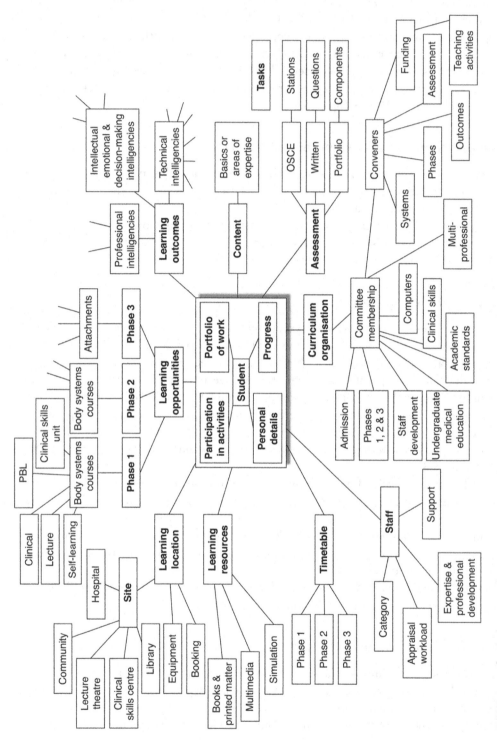

FIGURE 5.2 Curriculum mapping.

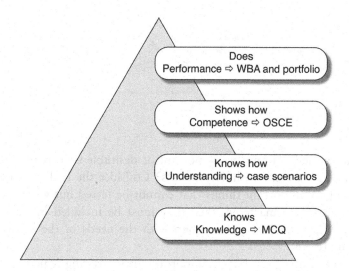

FIGURE 5.3 Miller's pyramid.

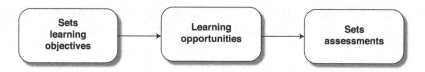

FIGURE 5.4 Setting assessments aligned with outcomes.

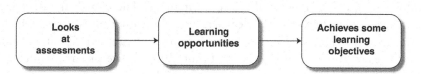

FIGURE 5.5 Assessments drive learning.

a different body of people. Fitting a curriculum to assessments is a common problem for teachers.

If curriculum items are not tested in a formal assessment, they are likely to be unpopular with (or ignored by) learners. In Figure 5.4 the teacher identifies learning objectives and creates learning opportunities for these objectives to be achieved, which are then assessed. The learner, on the other hand, as in Figure 5.5, is more likely to first look at the assessments and then, from the same learning opportunities, achieve some of the objectives that the teacher set.

Unless the curriculum and the assessments are perfectly aligned, the learning that is achieved will be a subset of the original intended learning outcomes.

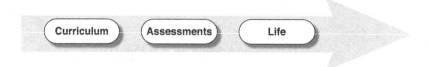

FIGURE 5.6 Alignment for the future.

Should the curriculum sacrifice important or desirable aspects of education just to achieve good alignment with assessments? Consider the reality of life after the course. If there are important things that cannot be tested but which are essential for the learner to have mastered, then they must be included in the curriculum. Curriculum and assessments should align with the needs of the learner after the course (see Figure 5.6).

Modes of assessment are hugely important in improving learning (assessment *for* rather than *of* learning), but this is often ignored in the education of healthcare professionals. Often the emphasis is on high stakes assessment, which has little positive effect and many adverse effects on learning. Biggs has highlighted assessments that provide useful guidance to course planners about what is being learnt and also guide learners to learn, not just check whether they have (see Table 5.2) (Biggs 2003).

The classroom and the workplace

The clinical setting is not primarily designed for teaching, it is designed for patients. Clinical teaching can thus be challenging to manage. The conflicting demands on clinical teachers may be why some learners prefer learning on courses rather than in the workplace. Learners also prefer things to be black and white, rather than the various shades of grey of real-life events. Eraut (2000) however has highlighted the richness of the workplace for learning (see Table 5.3).

Activities

Activities have more uses than just delivering content. They can be important in motivating learners, conveying attitudes or getting learners to respond to curricular content. Be careful to place the focus of activities on those that the learners need, rather than those that you need to use to teach. Examples might include interdisciplinary/interprofessional scenario-based teaching where learners from different healthcare professions take their own future role in a large group exercise. This can range from the every-day such as discharge planning to large exercises such as a mass casualty simulation.

Aligning activities with your curriculum aims is essential (see Chapter 10 for further information on *matching methods with message*).

TABLE 5.2 Alignment of Assessment Modalities with Types of Learning

	Assessment mode	Most likely kind of learning assessed
Extended prose, essay type	*Essay exam*	*Rote, question spotting, speed structuring*
	Open book	*As above but less memory, coverage*
	Assignment, take-home	*Read widely, interrelate, organise, apply, copy*
Objective test	*Multiple choice*	*Recognition, strategy, comprehension*
	Ordered outcome	*Hierarchies of understanding*
Performance assessment	*Practicum*	*Skills needed in real life*
	Seminar, presentation	*Communication skills*
	Posters	*Concentrating on relevance, application*
	Interviewing	*Responding interactively*
	Critical incidents	*Reflection, application, sense of relevance*
	Project	*Research skills*
	Reflective journal	*Reflection, application, sense of relevance*
	Case study, problems	*Application, professional skills*
	Portfolio	*Reflection, creativity, unintended outcomes*
Rapid assessments (large class)	*Concept maps*	*Coverage, relationships*
	Venn diagrams	*Relationships*
	Three-minute essay	*Level of understanding, sense of relevance*
	Gobbets	*Realising the importance of significant detail*
	Short answers	*Recall units of information, coverage*
	Letter-to-a-friend	*Holistic understanding, application, reflection*
	Cloze test (passages of text with missing words to be completed)	*Comprehension of main ideas*

TABLE 5.3 Learning in the Workplace

Work processes with learning as a by-product	Learning activities located within work or learning processes	Learning processes at or near the workplace
Multidisciplinary team processes	Asking questions	Being supervised
	Listening	Being coached
Working alongside others	Observing	Being mentored
Consultation	Obtaining information	Shadowing
Tackling challenging tasks and roles	Learning from mistakes	Visiting other sites
	Reflecting	Independent study
Problem solving	Locating resource people	Conferences
Trying things out	Giving and receiving feedback	Short courses
Working with patients		Working for a qualification

INSIGHTS FROM CURRICULUM THEORY: MUCH OF WHAT IS LEARNED IS NOT IN THE CURRICULUM

Hafferty delineates two useful categories beyond 'the stated, intended, formally offered and endorsed curriculum' (Hafferty 1998):

1. The informal curriculum – the unscripted, highly interpersonal ad hoc teaching
2. The hidden curriculum – the 'set of influences that function at the level of organisational structure and culture'

Both of these categories of unstated aims have both beneficial and adverse effects.

Teachers often assume a causal relationship between teaching and learning. However, much of what is learned is not taught. Even when what is learned is what you intended, it may not be learned from you. Learners may use sources other than your teaching for their knowledge. Sadly, even though learners don't always learn what is intended, they often learn lessons that teachers would not intend or might reject. Your behaviour is the model upon which your learners base theirs.

The 'hidden curriculum' describes the implicit way in which social norms are conveyed by academic institutions – the unofficial expectations relating to social attitudes and behaviours. For example, the hidden curriculum has been used to explain how, contrary to the expressed intention of the curriculum, medical students can be socialised by the prevailing culture into treating patients as objects:

Today's medical care, while being technologically advanced, is experienced by many patients as impersonal and dehumanizing. Medical schools have

TABLE 5.4 Essential and Ideal Features of Activities

Essential features	Ideal features
Built around key curriculum ideas	Motivational
Feasible and cost-effective	Address multiple goals
Time and resource efficient	Topic currency related to what is current or recently taught or experienced
Pitched at the right level	
Challenging – encourage higher-order thinking (e.g. analysis, interpretation, synthesis)	Related to real world
	Connect declarative knowledge (know that) with procedural knowledge (know how)
Not frustrating	Encourage self-directedness

Source: Brophy and Alleman (1991).

responded by trying to teach the human dimensions of care. These efforts, however, are often thwarted by the culture of medicine, which places a premium on technology at the expense of interpersonal relationships.

(Haidet and Stein 2006)

In a similar way, aspiring to cultivate collaboration and team working in junior doctors whilst simultaneously encouraging competition by ranking medical students at the end of their studies to compete for their first jobs seems doomed to fail ('The educational performance measure', UKFO 2022).

Learners are aware of the hidden curriculum, and they know that it has a profound effect on their learning, but its lessons can be unclear to them (Ozolins et al. 2008). They often associate facts with the formal curriculum, and 'learning how to be a doctor' with the hidden curriculum. Hidden lessons on behaviour are often worked out through oral and written narratives, such as the story in Box 5.6.

BOX 5.6 AN ERROR OF OMISSION

The patient, an elderly lady, was blind and deaf without speech. She had been brought in as an emergency case, clutching her abdomen and moaning. She had been like that for a couple of hours, and had also vomited several times. On examination she had some epigastric tenderness, her heart and lungs were normal, and her blood pressure was slightly low. Routine investigations were ordered; a drip was set up, and the team moved on.

On the next round the patient was still in severe pain. Nothing new had turned up. Her serum haemoglobin concentration, blood biochemistry, and chest and abdominal radiographs were normal. We hesitated over whether to provide pain relief. Antispasmodic drugs had been ineffective.

An ultrasound scan ruled out problems with the patient's gallbladder. Endoscopy took another day to organise and produced negative results. The patient's pain and sickness continued. On the fifth day she died, with the causes undiagnosed, and her suffering unrelieved.

As house officer on the ward I had to prepare a case summary. Fishing in the pack of X-ray films for the reports, I caught the long strip of an electrocardiogram. It bore the date of admission. I had asked a nurse to do it as part of the routine work-up, but had not remembered to check the results. The textbook signs of an extensive acute myocardial infarction were plain even to my untrained eye.

I took the tracing to the senior consultant's office. He cast a glance over it and then stared at me for two uncomfortably long seconds.

'Making a fuss about this won't bring her back', he said. He tore off the old date and then in a firm hand wrote the current date under the patient's name.

'She has died of an acute myocardial infarction. *But let this be a lesson to all of us.*'

Source: Singer et al. (2001).

How should a curriculum or course writer manage an informal and hidden curriculum?

Can these two concepts be of any use to the planner given that, by definition, they are outside what is intended and stated? There are two ways in which the planner should anticipate informal and hidden elements in the curriculum, even though neither will be entirely predictable or under their control. Firstly the informal curriculum offers opportunities to develop learning in unplanned but beneficial ways if generic guidance is given. Second, the hidden curriculum is difficult to predict or influence, but transmission of social values is likely, so should be anticipated and influenced in a positive way.

Importance of case studies and narratives

Stories can be powerful learning tools. Build them into your courses to help learners to become aware of hidden aspects of their work. Learning occurs when stories and experiences are interweaved with knowledge and theory.

Others emphasise the importance of emotional involvement in this process:

Unless the trainee stays emotionally involved and accepts the joy of a job well done, as well as the remorse of mistakes, [they] will not develop further, and will eventually burn out trying to keep track of all the features and aspects, rules and maxims that modern medicine requires. In general, resistance to involvement and risk leads to stagnation and ultimately to boredom and regression.

(Dreyfus and Dreyfus 2005)

Importance of values

Some curricula are written without reference to values, yet in the end, it is the values that the curriculum expresses and how they relate to the values of teachers and learners that will determine the success of the curriculum. If the values expressed in the curriculum are not in line with those of the faculty who deliver the teaching, the curriculum will fail (see also Chapter 24).

Choosing from the many options: what type of curriculum am I aiming for?

Education can be seen as a product, a process, or research and discovery (see Table 5.5).

When planning a course, you can choose between these three perspectives while being mindful of what kind of healthcare professional is needed. Remember the distinction between training and education:

> Training . . . prepares the learner to perform tasks already identified and described, by methods which have gained general approval. . . . Education teaches us to solve problems, the nature of which may not be known at the time when the education is taking place, and the solutions to which cannot be seen or even imagined by the teachers.
>
> *(Marinker 1992)*

> Education . . . deals with unknown outcomes, and circumstances which require a complex synthesis of knowledge, skills and experience to solve problems. Education refers its questions and actions to principles and values rather than merely standards and criteria. . . . Training . . . has application when: a) there is some identifiable performance and/or skill that has to be mastered; and b) practice is required for the mastery of it. . . . Effective learning in medical education . . . includes elements of training set in the context of lifelong learning.
>
> *(Brigden and Grieveson 2003)*

The success of your curriculum should be evaluated, but that evaluation depends on the model of curriculum you proposed. If you are using the product version, evaluation could be by means of a questionnaire designed by you, and will be answered anonymously. If you see education as a process, there may be a discussion among learners and teachers about what worked and what did not work, in order to develop an outline for next time. Those who see curriculum as research will not use evaluation, because they assess their experience throughout the course and change the content and methods to suit their needs. They will point out to you that evaluation at the end of a course is only a snapshot reaction to recent events, and they will only find out how good it has been in the months and years ahead.

TABLE 5.5 Three Approaches to Education and Their Effect on Curriculum Design

	Education as a product	Education as a process	Education as research
Intention	Teacher transmits knowledge	Teacher promotes knowledge	Learners explore understanding
Locus of knowledge	Teacher	Teachers and learners	Learner group
Student activities	Passive learners	Active learners	Aware of selves as active learners and negotiators
Motivation via	Teacher	Own active learning	Group learning and active learning
Sees learner as	Receiver of knowledge	Active seeker of knowledge	Discoverer or reconstructor of own knowledge
Sees teacher as	Teller Instructor	Seeker Catalyst	Facilitator Neutral chair
Teaching activities	Lecturing	Facilitates learning Sets up problems Probably knows answers	Teacher is leader within group but learns alongside them
Sees assessment as	End-of-course tests Summative teacher assessment	Part of teaching Part of learning Formative – and summative	Self-assessment Group assessment Aiding understanding
Plans by means of	Aims, objectives, detailed method for whole session, summative assessment	Aims, intentions, principles of procedure, list of content, assessment as part of this process	Aims, intentions, a negotiated agenda, counselling-type methods, assessment within this process
View of professional	Teacher is a performer whose performance is significant in the quality of the learner's education	Teacher is a facilitator who sets up learning for learners, and whose input features less in the sessions	Teacher is a facilitator who learns alongside learners, but this can only be on a highly disciplined basis

Source: Adapted from Fish and Coles (2005).

Tips from experienced teachers

- Planning a course (curriculum) involves blending content with timetable.
- When dealing with a 'handed down' curriculum, you should make decisions on structuring and what to emphasise or omit.
- Curriculum decisions can be problematic, and choices may depend on your values.
- When planning education, consider what view of learning you wish to promote.
- Professional knowledge is complex and cannot be transmitted as a product. Education is distinct from training.
- Healthcare professionals need to make creative decisions. To be effective, their learning must be based on their practice.
- You must understand the relationship between theory and practice.
- Look beyond the course to the world that learners will be entering, and create learning outcomes that are relevant to life outside the classroom.

REFERENCES

Abrahamson S. (1978) Diseases of the curriculum. *Journal of Medical Education*, 53: 951–957.

Biggs J.B. (2003) *Teaching for quality learning at university: What the student does.* Maidenhead: Society for Research into Higher Education and Open University Press.

Bowe R., Ball S.J. and Gold A. (1992) *Reforming education and changing schools: Case studies in policy sociology.* London: Routledge.

Brigden D.N. and Grieveson B. (2003) Lifelong learning. *Prime Dental Care*, 10: 31–32.

Brophy J. and Alleman J. (1991) Activities as instructional tools: A framework for analysis and evaluation. *Educational Researcher*, 20: 9–23.

Dreyfus H.L. and Dreyfus S.E. (2005) Peripheral vision: Expertise in real world contexts. *Organization Studies*, 26: 779–792.

Eraut M. (1994) *Developing professional knowledge and competence.* London: Routledge Falmer.

Eraut M. (2000) Non-formal learning and tacit knowledge in professional work. *British Journal of Educational Psychology*, 70: 113–136.

Fish D. and Coles C. (2005) *Medical education: Developing a curriculum for practice.* Maidenhead: Open University Press.

GMC (2018) *Outcomes for graduates.* Manchester: GMC. Available at www.gmc-uk.org/education/standards-guidance-and-curricula/standards-and-outcomes/outcomes-for-graduates (Accessed 2.4.22).

GMC (2022) Medical licensing assessment. Available at www.gmc-uk.org/education/medical-licensing-assessment (Accessed 2.4.22).

Hafferty F. (1998) Beyond curriculum reform: Confronting medicine's hidden curriculum. *Academic Medicine*, 73: 403–407.

Haidet P. and Stein H.F. (2006) The role of the student-teacher relationship in the formation of physicians. The hidden curriculum as process. *Journal of General Internal Medicine*, 21(Suppl. 1): S16–S20.

Harden R.M. (1986) Ten questions to ask when planning a course or curriculum. *Medical Educational*, 20: 356–365.

Harden R.M. (2001) AMEE Guide No. 21: Curriculum mapping: A tool for transparent and authentic teaching and learning. *Medical Teacher*, 23: 123–137.

Harden R.M. and Stamper N. (1999) What is a spiral curriculum? *Medical Teacher*, 21: 141–143.

Marinker M. (1992) Assessment of postgraduate medical education – future directions. In Lawrence M. and Prichard P. (eds) *General practitioner education: UK and Nordic perspectives*. London: Springer Verlag, pp. 75–80.

Miller G.E. (1990) The assessment of clinical skills/competence/performance. *Academic Medicine*, 65: S63–S67.

Novak J.D. and Canas A.J. (2008) *The theory underlying concept maps and how to construct and use them*. Pensacola, FL: Florida Institute for Human and Machine Cognition.

Ozolins I., Hall H. and Peterson R. (2008) The student voice: Recognising the hidden and informal curriculum in medicine. *Medical Teacher*, 30: 606–611.

Royal College of Physicians and Surgeons of Canada (2015) CanMEDS physicians competency framework. Available from https://canmeds.royalcollege.ca/en/framework (Accessed 2.4.22).

Singer P.A., Wu A.W., Fazel S., et al. (2001) An ethical dilemma: Medical errors and medical culture; An error of omission; Commentary: Learning to love mistakes; Commentary: Doctors are obliged to be honest with their patients; Commentary: A climate of secrecy undermines public trust. *BMJ*, 322: 1236–1240.

UKFO (2022) Available at https://foundationprogramme.nhs.uk/faqs/educational-perfor mance-measure-epm-faqs/.

CHAPTER 6

Evaluation

....

There is much confusion about the three terms *evaluation, assessment* and *appraisal*. All three have specific meanings within health professions education.

- **Evaluation** is the topic of this chapter and is about measuring the teaching process.
- **Assessment** is about testing the learners (and this might form part of an evaluation of our teaching) (see Chapters 16 and 17).
- **Appraisal,** or formative assessment, is a process to help develop personal, professional and educational needs (see Chapter 18).

Part of the confusion may be because in everyday life these words can be used interchangeably. In addition, in North America the word *evaluation* is sometimes used instead of *assessment* to mean assessing the learners. An example of this is in the mini-CEX (mini clinical evaluation exercise) for testing junior doctors' history taking and examination skills (Norcini et al. 2003). However, this paper is titled '*The mini CEX: a method of assessing clinical skills*'.

PROGRAMME EVALUATION

Programme evaluation focuses on questions relating to whether a programme is working as planned or if there are any unintended consequences (Lovato and Wall 2014). The term *programme* can refer to a curriculum, a course, session, student service, event, guideline or a policy in healthcare education.

Evaluation questions which may be asked could be as follows:

- What did nursing students think of their placements in care homes?
- What elements of the cross-cultural communication skills course were most useful in practice?

DOI: 10.1201/9781003352532-7

- What is the educational climate like for medical students in the operating theatre?
- Was the six-day faculty development course effective, and did people go on to put the lessons into practice?
- What was the impact of operating room experiences in oral surgery on the confidence of dental students?
- How reliable was our shortlisting and interviewing for paediatrics trainees?
- What new skills were achieved by nursing students during the online learning for practical skills during the COVID-19 pandemic?

Evaluation is not merely about handing out feedback questionnaires to students and trainees at the end of our teaching sessions; although this is an important element, it is much more than this. Evaluation should be wide ranging and all-encompassing in education. Much of this uses maps, models and theoretical frameworks and concepts applied to the asking and answering of questions about curriculum design.

Purposes of evaluation

There are many purposes of evaluation. One way to conceptualise this is to think in terms of the curriculum, teaching and learning, and assessment.

In terms of curriculum, evaluation may be incorporated into curriculum development in measuring if the curriculum is fit for purpose, looking at the alignment between curricula goals and outcomes and the wider implications of curriculum choices.

In terms of teaching and learning, evaluation may be used to measure and ensure that teaching is meeting the learners' needs and the needs of the professions. Did the learners learn from the teaching programme? It is often used to identify areas where the educational experience (in its widest sense) needs to improve. It is used to see if an educational programme is of an acceptable standard, so it may be approved for training and accreditation purposes. It may be used to give feedback to teachers, to managers and to faculty on the programmes being run in the organisation. It may be used as part of the information presented at the annual appraisal process for medical teachers, and for promotion and career development.

In terms of assessments, evaluation may be used to gather outcome measures on pass rates for qualifying and professional examinations. Also, increasingly it is used in the field of psychometrics, evaluating the development, uses, reliability and validity of assessment tools (see Chapter 16 on assessment). Often this has reached very sophisticated levels, using complex statistical theory, including generalizability theory, to see if assessment tools are fit for purpose. Finally, evaluation may be a way to see if the correct assessments are being used for the right purposes.

In summary, these purposes of evaluation appear in this chapter.

Curriculum

- Curriculum development
- Fitness for purpose
- Curriculum outcomes

Teaching and learning

- Meeting learners' needs
- Identifying poor teaching
- Approval of teaching programmes
- Feedback to teachers and the organisation
- Annual appraisal for teachers
- Promotion and career development

Assessment

- Outcome of assessments
- Assessment tools development and use
- Appropriateness of assessment strategies

Characteristics of a good evaluation question

A good evaluation question is:

- Appropriate – relevant to the educational programme
- Intelligible – can be understood clearly
- Unambiguous – means the same thing to everybody
- Unbiased – does not trigger one response selectively
- Simple – contains only one idea per question
- Ethical
- Pitched at the higher levels in the Kirkpatrick Hierarchy (see Section 6.1.10)

Such questions should be valid, reliable, simple, practical and probably anonymous. They may be either qualitative (descriptive) or quantitative (numerical), or a mixture of both.

Some conceptual models in evaluation

It is helpful to have simple models to use in understanding evaluation. The evaluation cycle is one such model. The Task model, CIPP (Content, Input, Process, Product) model, the Logic Model and the Kirkpatrick Hierarchy are others for looking at different levels of evaluation and evaluating change. The use of the long-established Harden's Ten Questions when evaluating a course or curriculum may also be helpful.

The evaluation cycle

A simple four step model of the evaluation cycle is presented here (Wilkes and Bligh 1999). It begins with *planning and preparation*, then the *teaching and learning activity*, then the *collection of data about the activity*, and then *reflection and analysis*. Diagrammatically the cycle is presented in Figure 6.1.

A model of the evaluation cycle

Musick (2006) suggested a model with five steps, which was called a task orientated model of programme evaluation in graduate medical education.

1. Examine the evaluation need – why are you doing it and for whom?
2. Determine the evaluation focus – what is going to be evaluated?
3. Determine the evaluation methodology – when, where and how, what sorts of analyses?
4. Present the evaluation results – who are key stakeholders, and how should results be presented?
5. Document the evaluation results – how are results documented and fed into programme improvement?

The CIPP (context – input – process – product)

This model can be applied to any stage of an educational programme development. This could include planning a new course, evaluating an existing programme, or measuring the results after completion of the course (see Figure 6.2). It is non-linear,

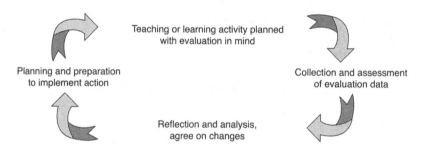

FIGURE 6.1 The task orientated model of programme evaluation.

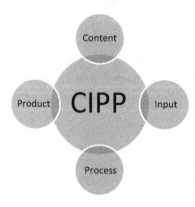

FIGURE 6.2 The CIPP model.

in contrast to other models. However, it needs a lot of work as multiple data collection methods are often needed (Ferris and Collins 2015).

The logic model

The Logic Model (Ferris and Collins 2015) is a linear evaluation tool for planning and evaluation educational programmes. It is a simple design, of Inputs, Activities, Outputs, Outcomes and Impact.

Kirkpatrick Hierarchy

The Kirkpatrick Hierarchy was first described in 1967 as a hierarchy of levels of evaluation on which to focus questions (Kirkpatrick 1967; Dent and Harden 2013, p. 19):

- Level 1 – Reaction – What did the participants think? Did they complete the course?
- Level 2 – Knowledge – What did the participants learn?
- Level 3 – Behaviour – Did the participants change their behaviour as a result?
- Level 4 – Results – Did clinical care or practice improve as a result?

The Kirkpatrick Hierarchy has been modified for use in medical education (Belfield et al. 2001). Here, the new lowest level was now a description of participation or completion of the learning, next reaction or satisfaction of participants, the learning or knowledge, then health professionals' behaviours, performance or practice, and finally, at the top of the hierarchy, healthcare outcomes.

This is a widely used evaluation tool in healthcare education, even if questions are not often used to explore the important, but harder to access, higher order outcomes of transfer into and impact on patient care. Belfield et al. (2001) found that in a study of 305 papers evaluating teaching interventions, only 1.6% had looked at healthcare outcomes.

Following are some examples of evaluation questions mapped to the levels in Kirkpatrick's Hierarchy:

Satisfaction

- Did the day meet your expectations?
- What went well for you today?
- What could have gone better?

Knowledge and skills

- What do you know now that you did not know before?
- What helped the learning to happen?
- What got in the way of learning?

Transfer of skills

What will you do differently now in your teaching or clinical practice?

Impact

How will your learners/patients be affected by what you have learned?

This could form the basic design for a feedback form. If you include a section for free text comments you may gather useful ideas to assist your evaluation.

The Best Evidence Medical Education (BEME) Collaboration has used this model in its various projects which have evaluated particular educational strategies. These may be accessed on the BEME website on www.bemecollaboration.org/ together with the projects undertaken, coding sheets for evaluation, published papers and so on.

Evaluation methods

Methods include questionnaires, interviews, focus groups, site visits, administrative records and group methods (such as the snowball review and the nominal group technique – described in Chapter 21 on research). Often more than one method may be used. For example, interviews and focus groups may be used to generate key themes for the construction and administration of a questionnaire to a larger group of learners.

Survey Monkey® (2023) is a useful way to use an online questionnaire, send it out and receive evaluation data by email. Within the survey monkey healthcare section, there are many purpose-made questionnaires, or one may be designed. It has the advantages of not needing postage, reply envelopes and so on, but you will of course need email addresses for all participants, and your respondents need to be able to access and use the internet.

Naturalistic evaluation considers participants' views of key concerns and issues. Data collection is qualitative, from interviews, focus groups and documents. The language used and the method of presentation of the findings are intended to be accessible to participants.

Sources of evaluation evidence

There are many potential sources of evidence for the evaluation of educational programmes in the health professions. These include information from students, clinical supervisors, staff members, faculty and patients. In terms of teaching, a central part of the evaluation of educational programmes, Berk (2006) bemoaned the fact that student ratings have dominated the evaluation of teaching effectiveness for many years. He urged that a variety of sources could be studied to widen the evaluation and to make decisions on teaching effectiveness.

He suggested 13 sources of evidence, using a wide variety of evaluation strategies. These were as follows:

Student/Learner ratings	Evaluation questionnaires
Peer ratings	Sitting in, observing, reading and reviewing teaching materials
External expert ratings	Looking at the teaching programme
Self-ratings	Self-evaluation and reflection on one's own efforts
Video recordings	Widely used in general medical practice teaching
Student interviews	Interviews with groups of students
Exit and alumni ratings	Feedback but from a different viewpoint – such as fit for purpose
Employer ratings	Are new graduates fit for the job?
Administrator ratings	Senior academics evaluation of faculty for teaching excellence
Teaching scholarship	Academic contribution made to medical education
Teaching awards	Rewards for teaching excellence
Learning outcome measures	Results in professional examinations
Teaching portfolios	Containing one's best work as an educator

In addition, remember that patients' views are another important source of evaluation evidence. After all, they often have valuable insights into the clinician's performance.

Some examples of evaluations

Evaluation of the educational climate experienced by undergraduate and postgraduate learners

Educational climate is about what it is like to be a learner within that organisation. It may be considered in three parts, the physical environment (safety, food shelter, comfort, accommodation), the emotional climate (security, supportive feedback, absence of bullying and harassment) and the intellectual climate (learning and teaching, relevance to patients, active participation by learners).

The Centre for Medical Education in the University of Dundee has made a major contribution in researching and developing questionnaire tools for the evaluation of educational climate. The DREEM (Dundee Ready Educational Environment Measure) was designed to evaluate the medical student climate (Roff et al. 1997). The PHEEM (Postgraduate Hospital Educational Environment Measure) followed on, to look at the climate for postgraduate doctors and dentists in the training grades (Roff et al. 2005). A detailed evaluation of PHEEM confirmed the original three domains of the tool, namely teaching, role autonomy and social support. In addition, the reliability was 0.928 – an extremely reliable result (Wall et al. 2009). The STEEM (Surgical Training Educational Environment Measure) was designed to look at the climate in the operating room for surgical trainees (Field et al. 2012). From this was developed the Mini-STEEM, a shortened version to evaluate the medical students' views in the operating room (Nagraj et al. 2006, 2007). All of these have been validated, are reliable and have been evaluated by psychometric testing. DREEM and PHEEM have been translated into many languages and are used in many countries now. DREEM has been translated and validated in Persian, Swedish, Greek, Spanish, Chinese, Arabic, Malay, Portuguese, Norwegian and Thai languages (Bakhshialiabad et al. 2019).

The UK General Medical Council national training survey

Each year, trainees give their views on their training and the environments where they work (General Medical Council 2021). Also, trainers give their views as clinical and educational supervisors. For the 2021 survey, 63,000 doctors in training and trainers responded. The questions in their survey are organised around five main themes, namely:

- Learning environment and culture
- Educational governance and leadership
- Supporting learners
- Supporting educators
- Developing and implementing curricula and assessments

The results of the 2021 study showed positive responses on teaching, supervision and overall training experience. However, intense workplace pressures with the COVID-19 pandemic showed burnout rates to increase to their highest levels ever in the survey, with one third of trainees feeling burnt out to a high or very high degree.

Evaluating a course or curriculum in medical education with Harden's Ten Questions

These questions are useful in planning a course or curriculum, and for evaluating an existing course in a systematic manner, to ensure that a wide coverage is employed.

1. What are the needs in relation to the product of the training programme?
2. What are the aims and objectives?
3. What content should be included?
4. How should the content be organised?
5. What educational strategies should be adopted?
6. What teaching methods should be adopted?
7. How should assessment be carried out?
8. How should details of the curriculum be communicated?
9. What educational environment or climate should be fostered?
10. How should the process be managed?

(Harden 1986)

Evaluating online learning in medical education

During the COVID-19 pandemic, there was a rapid increase in the amount of remote learning happening worldwide. This brought online learning from being one option among many modalities to the only existing solution if education in clinical subjects was to continue (see also Chapter 11).

This has raised the issue of how evaluation of online courses can take place and quality assurance be maintained. Wasfy et al. (2021) developed a set of descriptors for best practice in online medical education. Using qualitative methods, including a question guided focus group, thematic analysis, Delphi technique and an expert consensus session with triangulation, sets of standards were developed with input from 32 institutions in 19 countries. Detailed checklists were developed for organisational capacity, educational effectiveness, and assessment and human resources (Wasfy et al. 2021). These will enable educators, institutions and evaluators of educational practices to tackle this new and rapidly expanding area of clinical educational practice.

In particular, see Table 4 in the cited paper which is proposed as a comprehensive self-assessment checklist for quality practices in educational effectiveness (https://bmcmededuc.biomedcentral.com/articles/10.1186/s12909-021-02752-2/tables/4).

The challenges in educational evaluation

There are several pitfalls to try to avoid in educational evaluation. They fall under the headings of doing what the client wants, following one methodology only, not giving equal weight to all opinion without bias, and elitism – allowing more powerful voices to be given greater weight. In addition, following are some other of the pitfalls experienced over many years work in evaluating medical educational programmes both in hospital and in general practice.

Only measuring what is easy to measure

It is easy to send out a questionnaire, and more difficult to do case studies where problems of bullying or negative feedback, for example, might be uncovered. Only gathering one source of evidence rather than trying to triangulate the evidence from three different areas can be problematic, and Berk's 13 methods of evaluating teaching effectiveness, discussed previously, can help with this (Berk 2006).

Low response rates

The lower the response rate, the greater the potential bias from not knowing what the non-responders think. This may have a serious effect. So, aim for a good response rate of perhaps over 70%, and state what the response rate is in any analysis of evaluations carried out.

Poor reliability

Some evaluation instruments have not been properly tested for reliability, or if they have, have been found wanting. Methods include reliability statistical testing using Cronbach's alpha and generalisability theory (see Chapter 16 on Assessment). In shortlisting and appointment procedures, evaluating the strength of such high stakes processes is essential.

Generally it is important to use the literature to help you find evaluation tools which have already been developed, as with many you will find validity and reliability have already been researched. This is far easier than trying to develop and validate your own efforts.

Taking your eye off the ball

A significant challenge in evaluation strategies is in assuming if it was good last year, it will remain so. For example, changes of programme director, changes in the hospital Trust organisation, government targets for healthcare delivery or changes in staffing levels can all affect teaching.

Taking too much notice of the individual with a misplaced grievance

Beware placing undue emphasis on disaffected and sometimes dysfunctional individuals. Eliciting the views of learners is fundamental to a thorough evaluation of a learning environment, but outliers should be treated with caution. Is this learner a lone voice because others are afraid to speak up, or are they out of step with the overall experience? Aim to ensure you cross check your conclusions with other respondents.

CONCLUSION

Evaluation is an essential process in medical education, and it needs to be carried out rigorously and correctly. It is not all 'small scale and intended for local use' as some may claim (Morrison 2003). Some evaluations have required international collaboration and participation (Wall et al. 2009). Effective scrutiny of educational activities is vital to ensure probity in allocation of resources, cost effectiveness and ongoing educational impact.

REFERENCES

Bakhshialiabad H., Bakhshi G., Hashemi Z., Bakhshi A. and Abazzari F. (2019) Improving students' learning environment by DREEM. – An educational experiment in an Iranian medical sciences university (2011–2016) BMC medical education, Bakhshialiabad et al. *BMC Medical Education*, 19: 397. https://doi.org/10.1186/s12909-019-1839-9.

Belfield C.R., Thomas H.R., Bullock A.D., Eynon R.E. and Wall D.W. (2001) Measuring effectiveness for best evidence medical education – a discussion. *Medical Teacher*, 23: 164–170.

Berk R.A. (2006) *Thirteen strategies to measure college teaching.* Sterling, VA: Stylus Publishing LLC.

Dent J.A. and Harden R.M. (2013a) *A practical guide for medical teachers.* 4th edn. London: Churchill Livingstone Elsevier.

Ferris M.E. and Collins H.A. (2015) Research and evaluation in medical education. *International Journal of Higher Education*, 4(3): 104–111.

Field M., Mitchell S., van Dellen D., Wall D. and Roff S. (2012) Training in theatres are bigger hospitals better? *Annals of the Royal College of Surgeons of England* 94(6): 1–4.

General Medical Council (2021) National training survey. Available at www.gmc-uk.org/education/how-we-quality-assure/national-training-surveys (Accessed 30.4.22).

Harden R.M. (1986) Ten questions to ask when planning a course or curriculum. *Medical Education*, 356: 365.

Kirkpatrick D.I. (1967) Evaluation of training. In Craig R. and Mittel I. (eds) *Training and development handbook*. New York: McGraw Hill.

Lovato C. and Wall D. (2014) Programme evaluation: Improving practice, influencing policy and decision making. In Swanwick T. (ed) *Understanding medical education: Evidence, theory and practice*. 2nd edn. Oxford: Wiley Blackwell, pp. 385–399.

Morrison J. (2003) Evaluation. *British Medical Journal*, 326: 385–387.

Musick D. (2006) A conceptual model for program evaluation in graduate medical education. *Academic Medicine*, 81: 759–765.

Nagraj S., Wall D. and Jones E. (2006) Can STEEM be used to measure the educational environment within the operating theatre for undergraduate medical students? *Medical Teacher*, 28: 642–647.

Nagraj S., Wall D. and Jones E. (2007) The development and validation of the mini-surgical theatre educational environment measure. *Medical Teacher*, 29: e192–e197.

Norcini J.J., Blank L.L., Duffy F.D. and Fortna G.S. (2003) The miniCEX: A method of assessing clinical skills. *Annals of Internal Medicine*, 138: 476–483.

Roff S., McAleer S. and Harden R.M. (1997) Development and validation of the dundee ready education environment measure (DREEM). *Medical Teacher*, 19(4): 295–299.

Roff S., McAleer S. and Skinner A. (2005) Development and validation of an instrument to measure the postgraduate clinical learning and teaching environment for hospital-based doctors in the UK. *Medical Teacher*, 27: 326–331.

Survey Monkey (2023) Healthcare survey center. Available at www.surveymonkey.co.uk/mp/healthcare-surveys/ (Accessed 6.5.22).

Wall D., Clapham M., Riquelme A., Viera J., Cartmill R., Aspegren K. and Roff S (2009) Is PHEEM a multi-dimensional instrument? An international perspective. *Medical Teacher*, 31: e521–e527.

Wasfy N.F., Abouzeid E., Nasser A.A., Ahmed S.A., Youssry I., Hegazy N.N., Shehata M.H.K., Kamal D. and Atwa H. (2021) A guide for evaluation of online learning in medical education: A qualitative reflective analysis. *BMC Medical Education*, 21: Article 339. https://bmcmededuc.biomedcentral.com/articles/10.1186/s12909-021-02752-2 (Accessed 21.5.22).

Wilkes M. and Bligh J. (1999) Evaluating educational interventions. *British Medical Journal*, 318: 1269–1272.

SECTION 2

For healthcare educators in relation to teaching and facilitating learning

CHAPTER 7

The theory behind the practical aspects of teaching and learning

···

SELF-DETERMINATION THEORY (SDT)

First formulated in 1985, self-determination theory (SDT) is offered by the authors as a framework for the study of human motivation (Deci and Ryan 1985). It enables reflection on the interaction between internal and external motivators to drive actions or learning. SDT focusses on how social and cultural factors facilitate or undermine people's sense of their own self-drive and ability to make choices, and thence how those factors might be modified in the teaching environment. The model identifies three key elements: autonomy (doing things my way), competence (doing things well), and relatedness (doing things with and for others) and proposes that it is the balance between these three key psychological needs that supports learning. Thus achievement will be impacted by the balance between, and the extent to which, these three psychological needs are met within a social context. 'Human beings can be proactive and engaged or, alternatively, passive and alienated, largely as a function of the social conditions in which they develop and function' (Ryan and Deci 2000). The Six 'Mini-Theories' of SDT propose the following:

1. Intrinsic motivation is based on the satisfactions of learning or acting 'for its own sake'. It is supported or reinforced by conditions that facilitate competence and autonomy. This is a helpful theory for thinking about individual pursuits such as learning a surgical skill, including how hard it can be to learn something unless you yourself are interested to do so.
2. Extrinsic motivation drives behaviours that are instrumental – that aim toward outcomes beyond learning itself and might include external regulation. It is reinforced by factors that support autonomy and relatedness, and the more internalised the goals or values of extrinsic motivators (such as mandatory training or patient safety initiatives), the more autonomous the person will feel.

DOI: 10.1201/9781003352532-9

3. People can orient toward environments and regulate behaviour in three ways:
   - The autonomy orientation in which persons act out of interest in and valuing what is occurring
   - The control orientation in which the focus is on rewards, gains and approval
   - The impersonal or amotivated orientation characterised by anxiety concerning competence and being 'good enough'.
4. The fourth theory of basic psychological need suggests that optimal learning is predicated on autonomy, competence and relatedness all being equally in balance.
5. Motivation, action and learning are equally able to find support by a focus on goals, which may be extrinsic goals such as examination success or intrinsic goals such as good relationships or patient satisfaction.
6. Relatedness has to do with the development and maintenance of close personal relationships, but not only is the 'relatedness need' satisfied in high-quality relationships, but the 'autonomy need' and to a lesser degree the 'competence need' are also satisfied.

USING SDT TO ENHANCE TEACHING AND LEARNING

As educators we can create, or engineer, learning environments that are more or less likely to provoke effective motivators. Factors such as heavy workload, long hours and few team building activities (little time to build effective relationships), emphasis on examination success (external goals) and few opportunities for choice or selection in learning activities (thus minimising the benefit of autonomy in learning) sustain environments that might not support the three key psychological needs.

Pause for a moment . . .

Think back to a time when you experienced an educational event where you felt unmotivated to learn, or the outcome was not good. On reflection, were there any elements of the learning environments that seem now not to support the three psychological needs identified in SDT? What might you or the teachers have done differently to create a different outcome?

Focussing on these three key psychological needs is one way to ensure we build safe and effective educational environments for learners (see Section 7.3).

THE PSYCHOLOGY OF LEARNING

In the first half of the twentieth century there were two main schools of thought about learning theory, namely behaviourist and cognitive. A third group, the motivational theorists, had less pre-eminence.

The behaviourist school reflected a mechanistic view of teaching and learning – a given stimulus produces a certain reaction in the learner. A simple example is the rat in a box with a lever that, when pressed, releases food. The rat quickly learns the result of pressing the lever, and the action is thus reinforced. At a higher level, on a resuscitation course there may be a particular procedure to be learned, which if performed according to the manual is correct and if performed another way is incorrect. Learners are taught to react in a certain way to specific situations, and not necessarily to think out their actions first. In emergency situations, where split-second reactions are important, this may be reasonable. In another context this is akin to when cabin crew teach about safety actions in the event of a crash landing, this is done by instruction not experimentation.

Cognitive theorists rejected this mechanistic view and argued that individual learners were not passive organisms who responded to stimuli in a certain way, but rather that they thought about things, selected out and processed information, and then acted in different ways to altered circumstances. They believed that prior knowledge and skills were important and new ideas were built on old ones. Thus learners could reorganise their existing knowledge to solve new problems, and 'latent learning' – learning that takes place along the way and does not show itself until much later, when it is needed – could also occur.

The importance of the motivation of learners has been in the forefront of teaching practice for over 60 years, and it is interesting to look back at McGregor's 'Theory X and Theory Y' model, originally applied to workers, characterising the assumptions made about individuals and consider how that has influenced teaching strategies (McGregor 1960).

Box 7.1 shows how, by assuming one or other to be the case, it might influence how we respond as teachers.

BOX 7.1 THEORY X AND THEORY Y OF LEARNING

- Theory X: Learners are irresponsible and immature.
- Theory Y: Learners are motivated and responsible.

Characteristics of learners according to Theory X

- Learners hate work and avoid it if they can.
- They need to be coerced to work by control, direction and punishment, or they need to be coerced by reward, praise and privileges.
- Learners wish to be directed, avoid any responsibility, have no ambition but want security.
- Few learners have any imagination, ingenuity or creativity.
- The intellect of the average learner is already all used up.

Characteristics of learners according to Theory Y

- Learning is a natural activity, and learners will try to succeed in achieving objectives to which they are committed.
- Commitment to learning is a function of rewards associated with that achievement.
- Learners learn to accept and seek out responsibility for their own learning.
- Most learners have imagination, ingenuity and creativity.
- The intellectual potential of the average learner is only partly utilised. There is a lot more in there!

These three early theories of learning – behavioural, cognitive and motivational – have been summarised and matched against 13 educational strategies (Beard and Hartley 1984; see Box 7.2).

BOX 7.2 EARLY THEORIES OF LEARNING

Behaviourist mode

- Activity: learning by doing, where active is better than passive learning (students will learn more when they are actively involved).
- Repetition, generalisation and discrimination: frequent practice in a variety of situations helps (especially when learning new skills).
- Reinforcement: positive is better than negative. Rewards, praise and successes are more effective reinforcers than failures.

Cognitive mode

- Learning with understanding: meaningful and fits in with what learners already know.
- Organisation and structure: logical and well-organised material is easier to follow and learn from.
- Perceptual features: the way in which a problem is displayed to learners is important (e.g. a handout accompanying a lecture).
- Cognitive feedback: it is important to know how well you are doing.
- Individual differences: differences in ability, personality and motivation all affect learning.

Motivational mode

- Natural learning: learners are naturally curious and learn from all kinds of situations.
- Purposes and goals: learners have needs, goals and purposes, which are relevant to motivation in learning.

- Social situation: the group atmosphere and whether there is cooperation or competition with others affects success and satisfaction in learning.
- Choice, relevance and responsibility: learning is more effective when the material is relevant, chosen by the learners and delivered when they want to learn it.
- Anxiety and emotions: when learning involves emotions, learning is more significant; it is most effective in a non-threatening environment.

EDUCATIONAL CLIMATE

Educationalists refer to the 'atmosphere' or 'ambience' of an organisation as the 'climate' or sometimes the 'press'. Knowles states that the first requirement for adult learning is to establish the physical and psychological climate or ethos with regard to learning (Knowles 1984).

Teachers must consider all aspects of the 'educational environment':

> The crucial knowledge concerns the overall atmosphere or characteristics of the classroom; the kind of things that are rewarded, encouraged, emphasised; the style of life that is valued in the classroom or school community and is most visibly expressed and felt.
>
> *(Pace 1963)*

The educational climate may be subdivided into three parts:

1. Physical environment (facilities, comfort, safety, food, shelter, etc.)
2. Emotional climate (security, positive methods, reinforcement, etc.)
3. Intellectual climate (learning with patients, reflective practice, evidence-based, up-to-date knowledge and skills).

Looking back to earlier chapters, remember learners' likes and dislikes with regard to educational climate.

Likes include:
- Encouragement and praise
- Learning on the job
- Discussing cases, including best management practice, a chance to present the case and describe their management
- Challenge
- A relaxed atmosphere
- Group discussions
- Positive feedback
- Approachable seniors who are up to date, enthusiastic about their subject and able to say 'I don't know, let's look it up'

Dislikes include:

- Just looking at mistakes
- Humiliation, especially in front of patients and staff
- Being shouted at
- Being frightened
- Teachers not appreciating that they have knowledge gaps
- Irrelevant teaching about rare conditions
- Senior colleagues who are out of date and unable to admit that they do not know everything

The educational environment must be considered in healthcare, as it encourages important abstract behaviours such as 'professionalism' or 'bedside manner'. By giving attention to aspects of the learning environment and offering yourself as a role model, you can contribute to the likelihood that such behaviours will be fostered.

Consider the questions posed in Box 7.3 in relation to the environment that you cultivate for your learners (Pace 1963).

BOX 7.3 CUES (COLLEGE AND UNIVERSITY ENVIRONMENT SCALES) TO THE EDUCATIONAL ENVIRONMENT

- *Scholarship:* what am I doing to encourage scholarly, intellectual and academic pursuits?
- *Practicality:* how much attention do I give to the pragmatic and the practical, and to business-like efficiency?
- *Community:* is there concern for fostering friendliness and a sense of community both between teacher and students and among students?
- *Awareness:* what do I do that might encourage the development of a sense of personal identity, self-expression and social responsibility?
- *Propriety:* to what extent do I place emphasis on the environment being a polite and considerate sort of place, where 'proper' behaviours are called for, and where there is some emphasis on rules and regulations?

CONSTRUCTIVISM

Constructivism is a long-standing theory from the early 20th century, which describes learning as the process of integrating new information or experiences into an existing model built of prior knowledge. The teacher acts not as a transmitter of knowledge but rather as a guide who facilitates this integration. Learners 'construct' their own knowledge on the basis of what they already know. Teachers should provide learning opportunities that challenge previously held opinions and current understanding. Following the constructivist model involves engaging students actively in learning activities, probably in small group settings, performing tasks that are taken from life experiences. Adequate time (and encouragement) must be given for reflection on new experiences. The acquisition of new knowledge follows in-depth critique of the new information, and involves active judgements by learners about when and how to modify their existing knowledge.

This process of reflection is prompted by new information, surprises or unexpected events, and can be of two kinds (Schon 1987):

Reflection in action: this occurs immediately, as the 'ability to learn and develop continually by creatively applying current and past experience and reasoning to unfamiliar events whilst they are occurring'.

Reflection on action: this occurs later, as the 'process of thinking back on what happened in a past situation, what may have contributed to it, whether the actions taken were appropriate. and how this situation may affect future practice' (Kauffman 2003).

Reflection does not come naturally to all learners. Effective teachers encourage learners to look critically at both the learning process and outcomes to increase their level of self-directedness (see also Chapter 8).

THE EXPERIENTIAL LEARNING CYCLE

Constructing new models and learning from experience can be powerful. The experiential learning cycle is a model for thinking about the process by which the experiences we have are integrated to construct the foundations of new knowledge, and is conceptualised as a cycle of four stages (Kolb 1984).

The model predicts that if the learner completes all the stages of the cycle, learning will be more effective. The stages are described as:

- Action (having the experience)
- Reflection (thinking about how it went)
- Conclusion (integrating one's reflections with existing knowledge and information from other sources, and forming a conclusion about how it went)
- Planning (deciding whether to do it the same or differently next time)

Depending on personality, previous experience and motivational context, learners tend to be more comfortable in one or other of the stages of the experiential learning cycle. Some like to be busy and have lots of new experiences, and will need teachers to encourage them to plan or reflect more. Others may tend to prevaricate and overplan new activities, and may require a gentle push to start new projects. Yet others quickly draw conclusions from events, and may need encouragement to reflect fully on outcomes and integrate this with other opinions before reaching a conclusion. Finally, some learners think long and hard about past experiences and are paralysed by indecision about what to do next time. They need to be encouraged to reach and test a conclusion.

LEARNING STYLES

A strongly contested theoretical model is one of learning 'styles'. Proponents suggest that individuals learn in different ways and have preferences for certain kinds of information and ways of processing that information to learn. The theory predicts that if teachers match the way they present information, for example, visually compared to aurally, or if different types of activity are proposed, for example, private reading compared to group work, then learning will be enhanced. Critics point out that although learners certainly do express preferences for which way they like to learn, there is little supporting evidence that if teachers adjust their teaching to these preferences, it makes any difference to the efficiency of learning. They point to the absence of an evidence base for an effect, or a neuro-psychological basis for these assumptions and particularly decry the validity of 'diagnostic tools' to determine an individual's learning style.

Several models have been described, and although there is far from a consensus on whether any of these theories make accurate predictions about future learning, all of the models are useful when thinking about variety in teaching design. In particular, what seems to be helpful is an understanding of the importance of matching methods with intended learning outcomes (see Chapter 10).

Another particular way in which the concept of 'learning styles' can be helpful however is by mapping activities to the experiential learning cycle to try to enhance learning from experience. Let us consider probably the most famous model, Honey and Mumford's four learning styles (Honey and Mumford 1986). We include it here because it might be considered ubiquitous in teaching and learning settings and does have a place in thinking about how you organise teaching if we set to one side some of the controversy about whether 'style' is a fixed characteristic of a learner, or can be 'diagnosed'. It is also important to remember that with learners from diverse backgrounds – geographically, culturally and educationally, or for differently-abled learners – these 'styles' become even more vulnerable to attacks on validity.

Honey and Mumford have done an enormous amount of work to suggest the type of activities through which different people learn best. They suggest it is possible to determine your learning style, and this can be done with a 10-minute, 80-item, self-assessment questionnaire. The outcome divides learners into four different styles, described below, which map directly on to the stages of the experiential learning cycle. Individuals may have a combination of two styles, possess features of all four styles in similar proportions, or may have the features of one style only.

- **Activists** like to be fully involved in new experiences, are open-minded, and are happy to try anything once, thriving on the challenge of new experiences, but soon get bored and want to move on to the next challenge. They are gregarious and like to be the centre of attention. Activists learn best with new experiences, short activities, situations where they can be centre stage (e.g. chairing meetings, leading discussions), when they are allowed to generate new ideas, have a go at things or brainstorm ideas.

- **Reflectors** like to stand back, think about things thoroughly and collect a lot of information before reaching a conclusion. They are cautious, take a back seat in meetings and discussions, adopt a low profile, and appear tolerant and unruffled. When they do act it is by using the wide picture of their own and others' views. Reflectors learn best from situations where they are allowed to watch and think about activities, think before acting, carry out research first, review evidence, produce carefully constructed reports and reach decisions in their own time.
- **Theorists** like to adapt and integrate observations into logical maps and models, using step-by-step processes. They tend to be perfectionists, detached, analytical and objective, and reject anything that is subjective and flippant in nature or that involves lateral thinking. Theorists learn best from activities where there are plans, maps and models to describe what is going on, time to explore the methodology, structured situations with a clear purpose, and when they are offered complex situations to understand and are intellectually stretched.
- **Pragmatists** like to try out ideas, theories and techniques to see whether they work in practice. They will act quickly and confidently on ideas that attract them, and are impatient with ruminating and open-ended discussions. They are down-to-earth people who like problem solving and making practical decisions. Pragmatists learn best when there is an obvious link between the subject and their job. They enjoy trying out techniques with coaching and feedback, practical issues and real problems to solve, and when given the immediate chance to implement what has been learned.

Proponents suggest that it is also useful to determine your own style so that if you have a trainee who has a very different style to yours, you can accommodate your differences. You may for example have a reflector-theorist learning pattern. If you have a new learner who is an activist, they may not respond to your ideas, principles, maps and models of things. They may get bored easily and will want to proceed with the task and try new experiences. Unless you realise what is going on, you may not realise why conflict may arise.

Box 7.4 describes some other well-known ways in which learners are said to differ, and claims made about their strengths. All of them have critics and supporters but none are evidence based. These are included here to illustrate a range of ways of thinking about learning and to stimulate thinking about learner-difference. We do not offer them in any way to be seen as incontrovertible truths about learning or learners but rather that you might debate and discuss these ideas with colleagues and learners!

BOX 7.4 THE CONTESTED CONCEPT OF 'LEARNING STYLES' AND CLAIMS MADE ABOUT THEM (FOR DISCUSSION)

VARK: visual, aural, reading, kinaestheic learners

- Visual learners learn best from graphic displays such as charts, diagrams, illustrations, handouts, and videos.
- Aural (or auditory) learners learn best by hearing information. They tend to get a great deal out of lectures and are good at remembering things they are told.
- Reading and writing learners prefer to take in information that is displayed as words and text.
- Kinaesthetic (or tactile) learners learn best by touching and doing or hands-on experience.

Convergent and divergent thinkers

- Convergent thinkers tend to find a single solution to a problem that is presented to them. Science students might be more convergent.
- Divergent thinkers tend to generate new ideas, expand ideas and explore widely.
- Arts students might be more divergent.

Serialists and holists

- Serialists learn best by taking one step at a time.
- Holists learn best by first obtaining the big picture and then filling in the steps.
- Individuals appear to learn best when teaching is matched to their learning style. Some people are able to use either approach. Therefore if you expect learners to make their own way through learning material, it needs to be arranged so that it can be followed by both serialists and holists.

Introverts and extroverts

- Introverts (who are internally referenced) do better with well-structured situations.
- Extroverts (whose locus of stimulation is external to themselves) do better with less structured situations.

Deep and surface processors

- Deep processors like to focus on the main points of an article in order to understand it.
- Surface processors like to read through the material, remembering as much as possible.
- Studies on the reading and summarising of text do seem to suggest that deep processors look for the main ideas and principles and can summarise text well. Surface processors read through the text from start to finish and often fail to grasp the main points but have a clearer grasp of the overall picture.

DEEP AND SURFACE APPROACHES TO LEARNING

Although it is our belief that it is unlikely that individual learners can be described as deep or surface learners, it is certainly a concept that can be applied to learning environments. Most learners know the difference and will adopt whichever approach seems appropriate, but what seems to be appropriate might be informed by an individual's understanding of learning. The development of this understanding can be described in five levels:

1. Learning is understood by the learner to be an increase in knowledge – something done to the learner by the teacher.
2. Learning is memorising – the learner actively memorises information but does not transform it in any way.
3. Learning is the acquisition of facts and procedures to be used.
4. Learning is making sense – the learner makes an active search for abstract meaning.
5. Learning is understanding reality – knowledge acquired by the learner enables them to see the world differently.

Learners who understand learning at a surface level (levels 1–3) are unlikely to take a deep approach to learning. Unsurprisingly, a relationship exists between understanding of learning and expectations of teaching. Learners in the reproducing group (levels 1–3) expect teaching to be 'closed' (i.e. teachers select the content, present it to the learners and then test them to see whether it has 'stuck'). Learners in the 'making sense' levels (levels 4–5) feel that teaching should be 'open' (i.e. the learner functions independently, with facilitation).

Often learners are at levels 1–3 simply because they have only been exposed to closed teaching, especially that involved in examination preparation. Assessment systems can dictate the way in which learners learn. Development of tasks that make different demands on learners can develop their understanding of what learning is.

The characteristics of learning activities that could foster a surface approach to learning include:

- Heavy workload
- Relatively high number of teacher-contact hours
- Excessive amounts of course material
- Lack of time to pursue subjects in depth
- Lack of choice with regard to subject matter and study methods
- Threatening and anxiety-provoking assessment systems.

How can we use this concept of learner difference to help learners to find approaches that suit them? There are four main approaches to tailoring learning to individual needs:

1. **Matching:** trying to offer learning activities you think this learner prefers.
2. **Allowing choice:** since learners come from a range of backgrounds and have different ways of learning, and varying aims, you should aim for flexibility in your provision.
3. **Providing several different methods of learning on the same course:** that way learners can mix and match, or will always find something that suits them.
4. **Independent study:** complete freedom to study, whilst threatening to those that need structure, can give good results, especially with more mature learners.

THE EDUCATIONAL CYCLE

Not to be confused with the experiential learning cycle, the principles of the educational cycle are applicable to most, if not all, teaching and learning situations within healthcare education. The cycle builds on the traditional approach to organising teaching, namely the 'training triangle' of *aims*, *methods* and *assessment*.

This educational cycle is a four-step model:

1. Assessment of the individual's needs.
2. Setting educational objectives or outcomes.
3. Choosing and using a variety of methods of teaching and learning.
4. Assessing whether learning has occurred and evaluating the teaching.

APPLYING THE EDUCATIONAL CYCLE

1. What does the learner need to know? Assess what the learner has done before and knows about already, while making reference to the appropriate training curriculum. Encourage the learner to use a tool to self-rate their levels of knowledge and skills in various areas. Using this, you may agree with your learner some key topics that they need to address during their time with you. You are now ready to progress to the next step of the cycle.
2. Educational outcomes describe what it is intended the learner will know or be able to do at the end of the course, or how that learner is expected to change through the learning in the areas of need identified. They are often written in behavioural terms. For many educational activities, the objectives model fits very well, particularly in terms of practical skills. Once the learner and teacher have consulted the curriculum and have assessed needs, they can devise and agree a plan, listing a set of learning outcomes to be achieved. Remember also that thinking about assessment begins with the stage of setting learning objectives.
3. There is no single teaching method that is best. Different methods suit different situations, learners and teachers. However, there are optimum methods for teaching different things (see Chapter 10).

Most people learn best by 'doing', using active methods of learning, rather than sitting passively in a lecture theatre. This is not news – it was recognised by an ancient Chinese proverb:

- I hear and I forget
- I see and I remember
- I do and I understand.

4. How do you know whether learning has occurred? One simple approach is to base assessments (see Chapter 16) on learning objectives set at the beginning. If you have established good, achievable learning objectives and chosen appropriate learning methods, the learner will progress through the course and learn what you expected. So after setting learning objectives at the start, check the learner's progress using regular appraisal meetings, and assess completion of learning at the end.

RETURNING AGAIN TO MOTIVATION OF LEARNERS

At the start of this chapter, we discussed self-determination theory and how that can help us think about the learning process. We might summarise some of these ideas in the following four principles of motivation:

1. We all have an inbuilt urge to attempt to achieve things.
2. Our needs are related to specific goals. Factors such as self-image, group bonding and security are all relevant.
3. The relationship between needs and goals is complex and unstable. The same needs produce different behaviours in different individuals.
4. We all have many needs, but only a few are subject to conscious action at any one time.

Intrinsic and extrinsic factors influence motivation. Intrinsic factors come from within the individual, and include wanting to succeed at something, achieving a career goal, satisfying curiosity and accepting a challenge. Such intrinsic motivational forces may be very strong. Extrinsic factors, from outside influences, include competition, respect for others, not wishing to let the side down, and admiration of one's peers. Extrinsic motivational forces may be positive or negative. Competition among students may be helpful to some but may demotivate others, especially with regard to many types of assessment. These may produce an underlying fear and anxiety, which force the student to learn a certain amount in order to pass the test, but the material is often learned superficially and soon forgotten.

Another foundational theory underpinning an effective approach to learning that draws together some of these ideas is Maslow's motivational theory (Maslow 1970). Maslow described a hierarchy of needs, with the most basic needs at the bottom and the need for self-realisation at the top (see Figure 7.1).

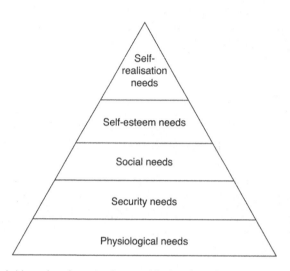

FIGURE 7.1 Maslow's hierarchy of needs. *Source*: Maslow (1970).

Physiological needs, such as food, clothing and shelter, are necessary for any living creature to survive. Safety and security issues come next, and are related to the survival needs lower down in the hierarchy. If these fundamental needs are not met, perhaps because of instability or a transition in a learner's life, the learner will not progress. Since for most of our learners these needs are usually well satisfied however, they rarely help to motivate them. In cultures where autonomy and independence are valued, generally the higher needs, the self-realisation needs (or 'doing your own thing') are much more powerful motivating factors.

In between the need for self-realisation at the top and safety and security at the bottom of the pyramid are two needs, the order of which might depend on cultural norms. In Figure 7.1 relational or social needs are positioned lower than esteem needs. In many cultures individual esteem – the need to be recognised, to be valued for one's own uniqueness, abilities and achievements, are considerably higher than social ones. However social needs – related to being part of a group, belonging and having a collective responsibility are key drivers in other cultures.

How can an understanding of what generally motivates learners be applied to our teaching? There is a recognition that motivation waxes and wanes, including in response to past achievements and current goals. As we achieve a goal, we might experience a reduction in the drive to learn or change. This can be represented cyclically as in Figure 7.2. This 'motivational cycle' may be of help in understanding where learners are in a particular situation. It might inform a conversation both at the needs assessment stage of planning learning or when there appears to be a block or barrier to engaging in learning.

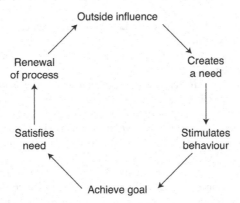

FIGURE 7.2 Motivational cycle.

In Chapter 8, we will continue with this theoretical look at some of the principles of effective teaching.

Finally, in conclusion to this chapter in which we have looked at some of the long-standing and respected theories of how learners learn, Box 7.5 includes some practical ideas. These are drawn from the theories described and are tips about how you can motivate your trainees to learn more, to be enthusiastic learners, and to take control of and responsibility for their own learning.

BOX 7.5 TIPS FROM EXPERIENCED TEACHERS

- Think of positive ways to motivate your learners. What matters to them?
- Make learning interesting.
- Encourage the active contribution of learners to the learning process.
- Make learning relevant to learners' needs.
- Give regular constructive feedback on progress.
- Allow time, and build the skills required, for reflection.
- Reinforce positive aspects, not negative ones.
- Learning feeds on success.
- Give students responsibility for learning.
- Ensure that the right learning environment is provided.
- Reward good performance and good discipline.
- Goals should be translated into specific objectives.

REFERENCES

Beard R.M. and Hartley J. (1984) *Teaching and learning in higher education.* 4th edn. Newcastle upon Tyne: Athaeneum Press.
Deci E.L. and Ryan R.M. (1985) *Intrinsic motivation and self-determination in human behavior.* New York, NY: Plenum.

Honey P. and Mumford A. (1986) *Using your learning styles.* Maidenhead: Peter Honey Publications.

Kauffman D.M. (2003) Applying educational theory in practice. ABC of learning and teaching. *BMJ*, 326: 213–216.

Knowles M.S. (1984) *Androgogy in action: Applying modern principles of adult learning.* San Francisco, CA: Jossey-Bass.

Kolb D.A. (1984) *Experiential learning: Experience as the source of learning and development.* Englewood Cliffs, NJ: Prentice Hal.

Maslow A.H. (1970) *Motivation and personality.* New York: Harper and Row.

McGregor D. (1960) *The human side of enterprise.* New York: McGraw-Hill.

Pace C.R. (1963) *College and university environmental scales. Technical manual.* Princeton, NJ: Education Testing Service.

Ryan R.M. and Deci E.L. (2000) Self-determination theory and the facilitation of intrinsic motivation, social development, and well-being. *American Psychologist*, 55: 68–78.

Schon D.A. (1987) *Educating the reflective practitioner: Toward a new design for teaching and learning in the professions.* San Francisco, CA: Jossey-Bass.

CHAPTER 8

Adult learning and supporting self-directed learners

··

Knowles coined the term 'androgogy' to refer to the art and science of teaching adults (Knowles 1984). This should not be considered a theory, but more a set of assumptions based on experience and observation about supporting adult learners.

The five assumptions of adult learning are as follows:

1. Adults are independent and self-directing.
2. They have accumulated a great deal of experience, which is a rich resource for learning.
3. They value learning that integrates with the demands of their everyday life.
4. They are more interested in immediate, problem-centred approaches than in subject-centred ones.
5. They are more motivated to learn by internal drivers than by external ones.

Healthcare is too broad for all the content to be delivered by teachers and, if such an attempt were made, an opportunity would be missed to develop learners for the time when formal education has ended. Our role as teachers is to equip learners with the skills to solve problems and continue learning throughout their careers:

Education teaches us to solve problems, the nature of which may not be known to us at the time the education is taking place, and the solutions to which cannot be seen or even imagined by our teachers (Marinker 1992).

It can sometimes be frustrating when learners appear not to take responsibility for their own learning and appear to expect to be 'spoon-fed'. Underlying this frustration is often a failure to recognise that the capacity to be self-directed is not an all-or-nothing function that develops overnight. Learners act at different levels or stages of self-direction depending on for example, previous teaching, learning and assessment experiences, the subject matter and context of learning. Not all learners are ready to take responsibility for their own learning.

DOI: 10.1201/9781003352532-10

Effective teachers recognise this and realise that adult learning is *facilitated* by the teacher. Consider learning to be like a voyage in a boat. As the teacher you do not stop being the rudder, but you avoid being the oars or the engine. Brookfield (see also Section 8.8) has debated the subject of adult learning at length, providing many examples (Brookfield 1986).

GROW'S STAGES OF SELF-DIRECTED LEARNING (SSDL) MODEL

Grow's SSDL model builds on the work by Hersey, co-author of the Situational Leadership Model® and is a helpful way to look at tensions that can arise if the learner's and teacher's levels are not matched (Hersey and Blanchard 1982; Grow 1996). By kind permission of the author, who has also given us permission to use his illustrations, we reproduce here the essential features of this model.

The SSDL model describes four developmental stages for students (S1–4):

1. Dependent learner
2. Interested learner
3. Involved learner
4. Self-directed learner

and four styles of teaching (T1–4):

1. Authority, coach
2. Motivator, guide
3. Facilitator
4. Consultant, delegator

Grow has depicted these four styles of teaching with the following four cartoons (Figure 8.1).

For each learning stage, some ways of delivering teaching and activities are better suited than others (see Table 8.1).

Tensions can arise if the learner's stage and delivery of teaching are mismatched – for example, when dependent learners are placed with non-directive teachers and when self-directed learners work with highly directive teachers (see Table 8.2).

T1/S4 MISMATCH

When self-directed students (S4) are paired with an authoritarian teacher (T1), problems may arise, although some S4 learners develop the ability to function well and retain overall control of their learning, even under directive teachers. However, other S4 learners will resent the authoritarian teacher and rebel against the barrage of low-level demands. This mismatch may cause the learner to rebel or to retreat into boredom.

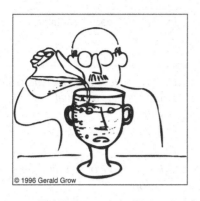

T1 TEACHER

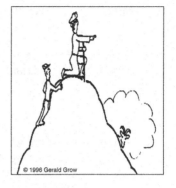

T3 TEACHER

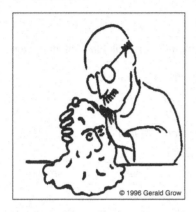

T2 TEACHER

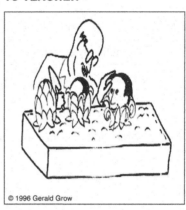

T4 TEACHER

FIGURE 8.1 The four teaching styles of SSDL.

TABLE 8.1 Stages of Development of Learning and Teaching, Leading to Self-directed Learning

Stage or level of development of learner	Learner	Teacher	Examples of teaching activities
Stage 1	*Dependent*	*Authority, coach*	*Coaching with immediate feedback* *Drill* *Informational lecture* *Overcoming deficiencies and resistance*
Stage 2	*Interested*	*Motivator, guide*	*Inspiring lecture plus guided discussion* *Goal-setting and learning strategies*

(continued)

TABLE 8.1 (Continued)

Stage or level of development of learner	Learner	Teacher	Examples of teaching activities
Stage 3	Involved	Facilitator	Discussion facilitated by teacher who participates as equal Seminar Group projects
Stage 4	Self-directed	Consultant, delegator	Dissertation Individual work or self-directed study group

TABLE 8.2 Mismatch of Levels of Self-direction of Learning with Type of Delivery of Teaching

	T1: authority expert	T2: motivator	T3: facilitator	T4: delegator
S4: Self-directed learner	Severe mismatch Students resent authoritarian teacher	Mismatch	Near match	Match
S3: Involved learner	Mismatch	Near match	Match	Near match
S2: Interested learner	Near match	Match	Near match	Mismatch
S1: Dependent learner	Match	Near match	Mismatch	Severe mismatch Learners resent freedom they are not ready for

Furthermore, the T1 teacher will probably not interpret such rebellion as the result of a mismatch. Instead that teacher is likely to see the learner as surly, uncooperative and unprepared to concentrate on learning basic facts. Extreme over-control by any leader results in stress and conflict, and in the follower engaging in behaviour designed to get the leader out – or to escape from under the leader.

T1/S3-S4 MISMATCH

Learners who are capable of more individual involvement in learning are relegated to passive roles in authoritarian classrooms.

Adults who return to education may find themselves in this position. Their life experiences and learning skills generally enable them to learn at the S3 or S4 level, but they may be placed with teachers accustomed to using Stage 1 and 2 methods on adolescents.

Furthermore, after many years of responsibility, adults may experience difficulty learning from T1 teachers. Adults may be accustomed to having authority, and unused to blindly doing what they are told without understanding why and consenting to the task.

Adults returning for postgraduate study, in particular, may run aground on courses like statistics, which are often taught by briskly directive teachers using the Stage 1 mode. The more appropriate Stage 3 mode is not always used with experienced learners when teachers lack experience in this type of teaching.

T4/S1 MISMATCH

When dependent learners (S1) are paired with a T3 or T4 teacher, they may be delegated responsibility for learning that they are not equipped to handle.

Such learners may be unable to make use of the 'freedom to learn' because they lack the following necessary skills for self-directed learning:

- Goal setting
- Self-evaluation
- Project management
- Critical thinking
- Group participation
- Learning strategies
- Information resources
- Self-esteem

Learners may resent the teacher for forcing upon them a freedom for which they are not ready. These dependent learners expect close supervision, immediate feedback, frequent interaction, constant motivation, and the reassuring presence of an authority-figure telling them what to do. Such learners are unlikely to respond well to the delegating style of teaching, a hands-off delegator, or a critical theorist who demands that they confront their own learning roles.

Grow describes the results of this mismatch as a kind of 'havoc' that occurs when the followers do not receive the guidance that they need, and:

> Lacking the ability to perform the task, [they] tend to feel that the leader has little interest in their work and does not care about them personally. This form [of teacher leadership] makes it difficult for these followers to increase their ability, and reinforces their lack of confidence. If the leader waits too long but then provides high amounts of structure, the followers tend to see this action as a punitive rather than a helping relationship.
>
> *(Grow 1996)*

The learner's stage of self-direction is often a result of the teaching that they have previously experienced. Consider Grow's quote from a hypothetical learner:

> I am the product of a system built around assignments, deadlines, and conventional examinations. Therefore, with this course graded by the flexible method and four other courses graded by the more conventional methods, I tend to give less attention to this course than it merits, due to a lack of well-defined requirements.

This learner has made a strategic decision about study. Other learners in this position may experience shock and resentment when faced with the necessity of making unguided, responsible choices.

THE FALSE STAGE 4 LEARNER

Some students appear to be Stage 4 self-directed learners, but turn out to be highly dependent students in a state of defiance. The one who strongly insists on doing it 'their way' might be a 'false independent' learner who may have not mastered the necessary details of the subject and instead be 'winging it' at an abstract level. They may also have erected a high façade, to prevent their lack of experience showing.

False independent learners need help to raise their knowledge and skills to the level of their self-belief. They may need to master how to learn productively from others, and may benefit from a strong-willed teacher who challenges them to become autonomous and effective.

DEPENDENT, RESISTANT LEARNERS AS A PRODUCT OF THE EDUCATIONAL SYSTEM

The way in which much teaching has been organised in the past can produce learners who resist direction. A group of highly resistant learners can coerce teachers into an authoritarian mode, and then frustrate them, at the same time being both dependent on teachers and resentful of being taught. So the resistant form of Stage 1 is probably not a natural condition. It results from years of dependency training. Most children are naturally Stage 3 or 4 learners when undirected. Even when taught in a directive manner, they are generally available, interested and excitable, and have a spontaneous creative energy that they are willing to direct into satisfying projects under the guidance of a capable teacher.

Resistant dependent learning may be a product of culture and upbringing, as well as of the education system. Sources of resistance in adult learners may include threats to cultural identity that might have been generated by the (hopefully now changing) pressures of hierarchical medicine. As teachers we need to understand dependency in context – certain forms of help may make the problem worse.

We will return to these styles of teaching again in Chapter 9.

KNOWLES' GUIDELINES ON TEACHING SELF-DIRECTED ADULTS

We started this chapter on adult learning with the work of Malcolm Knowles. He has defined seven fundamentals that have stood the test of time as guidelines to encourage adult learners (Knowles 1984):

1. Establish an effective learning climate in which learners feel safe and comfortable expressing themselves.
2. Involve learners in mutual planning of relevant methods and curricular content.
3. Trigger internal motivation by involving learners in diagnosing their own needs.
4. Give learners more control by encouraging them to formulate their own learning objectives.
5. Encourage learners to identify resources and devise strategies for using resources to achieve their objectives.
6. Support learners in carrying out their learning plans.
7. Develop learners' skills of critical reflection by involving them in evaluating their own learning.

Following these guidelines might encourage learners to move up through the stages of self-direction that Grow has defined.

BROOKFIELD'S PRINCIPLES OF ADULT LEARNING

Some of the most respected work on adult learners has been done by Steven Brookfield, and he proposed six principles of adult learning that if incorporated into teaching can support the growth of self-directedness (Brookfield 1986).

1. Participation is voluntary – the decision to learn is that of the learner.
2. There should be mutual respect – shown by teachers and learners for each other, and by learners for other learners.
3. Collaboration is important – between learners and teachers, and among learners.
4. Action and reflection – learning is a continuous process of investigation, exploration, action, reflection and further action.
5. Critical reflection – this brings awareness that alternatives can be presented as challenges to the learner to gather evidence, ask questions and develop a critically aware frame of mind.
6. Self-directed adult individuals need to be nurtured.

HOW TO PUT THE PRINCIPLES OF ADULT LEARNING INTO PRACTICE

What can busy healthcare professionals do to help themselves and their learners to develop into self-directed, independent adult learners? Brookfield gives ten tips on doing this (see Box 8.1).

BOX 8.1 HOW TO CREATE AN ADULT LEARNER

1. Progressively reduce the learner's dependence on the teachers.
2. Help the learner to understand the use of learning resources, including the experiences of fellow learners.
3. Help the learner to use reflective practice to analyse their practice and define their learning needs.
4. Help the learner to define their learning objectives, plan their programmes and assess their own progress.
5. Organise what is to be learned in terms of personal understanding, goals and concerns at the learner's level of understanding.
6. Encourage the learner to take decisions, and to expand their learning experiences and range of opportunities for learning.
7. Encourage the use of criteria for judging all aspects of learning, not just those that are easy to measure.
8. Facilitate problem posing and problem solving in relation to personal and group needs issues.
9. Reinforce progressive mastery of skills through constructive feedback and mutual support.
10. Emphasise experiential learning (learning by doing, learning on the job) and use of learning contracts.

WORK-BASED LEARNING

Work-based learning aligns with the principles of adult learning and represents the most accessible opportunities for self-directed learning during clinical work. Clinical experiences offer a vast range of learning opportunities. Health professions educators can encourage self-directed work-based learning by promoting and enhancing the quality of the following:

- Reflection
- Management of complaints
- Significant events and critical incidents
- Audit
- Handover

REFLECTION

All healthcare practitioners and teachers should regularly reflect on their practice to ensure a mindful consideration of features of their practice and to ensure they are staying up to date. Processes of reflection, including *reflection in action* and *reflection on action* (Schon 1987) were introduced in Chapter 7. Formal evidence of reflection is required for clinical and academic professional portfolios and revalidation, and these skills are often sought in job recruitment processes. Learners sometimes struggle to see the worth of reflection and, anecdotally, this can be a problem among undergraduates. You must undertake regular reflection on your own work, be able to assist learners with reflection, and highlight the benefits of doing so.

The important benefits of reflection are as follows:

- Keeping abreast of changes to the healthcare system, patient expectations and/or medical knowledge
- Helping to understand why things went well or why they didn't – this can help both clinical practice and self-esteem, particularly if things have gone wrong
- Helping you to make sense of a difficult situation, to prevent a knee-jerk reaction and unfair attribution of causation
- Improving practice for the next time by taking a more informed and thought-out approach
- Identifying learning needs to direct progress with personal development plans

Although documented evidence of formal reflective practice is usually required, not all reflection needs to be written down. For example, it is possible to take learners through the process of reflection through discussion (e.g. of a specific case or after role play).

MODELS OF REFLECTION

Reflection is about dissecting a situation and understanding the whys and the hows, rather than just stating what happened. A number of models outline stages of reflection:

- Gibbs' (1988) model of reflection
- Johns' (1995) model of reflection
- Atkins and Murphy's (1994) model of reflection

Perhaps the most familiar model of reflection is Gibbs' (see Figure 8.2 and Box 8.2).

Figure 8.2 summarises the key points from each one to provide a cycle of prompts and processes that should be considered for effective reflection. However, not all of them will be applicable in every case.

Identify situation, event or experience upon which you can reflect

Awareness of uncomfortable feelings
   and thoughts
New experience
Previously difficult experience

Describe situation, event or experience

What happened?
What were the key points?
Why did you act in this way?
What were the consequences for you,
   colleagues, patient, learner and/or family?

Make a plan

What would you do next time if you
   find yourself in the same situation?
What further learning is required?
How are you going to address this?

Analyse situation, event or experience

Thoughts and feelings
- At the time and since
- Of you, colleagues,
  patient/learner/family
- How do you know what others were
  feeling?
Knowledge
- What did you need to know?
- What did you know?
- What did you not know that you needed
  to?
Actions
- What did you do? Why?
- What did others do? Why?
Influencing factors
- Internal factors
- External factors
Options
- What were your other options?
- What would have been the result of
  taking any other option?

Draw conclusions about the situation, event or experience

What went well?
What did not go well?
What else could be done by you
   and others to improve the current
   and/or similar future situation, event
   or experience?
What have you learnt?
How do you make sense of the event?

FIGURE 8.2 Gibbs' cycle of reflection.

BOX 8.2 GIBBS' STAGES OF REFLECTION, OR 'DE-BRIEFING'

Description: What happened? Don't make judgements yet or try to draw conclusions; simply describe.

Feelings: What were your reactions and feelings? Again, don't move on to analysing these yet.

Evaluation: What was good or bad about the experience? Make value judgements.

Analysis: What sense can you make of the situation? Bring in ideas from outside the experience to help you. What was really going on? Were different people's experiences similar or different in important ways?

Conclusions: (general) What can be concluded, in a general sense, from these experiences and the analyses you have undertaken?

Conclusions: (specific) What can be concluded about your own specific, unique, personal situation or way of working?

Personal action plans: What are you going to do differently in this type of situation next time? What steps are you going to take on the basis of what you have learnt?

(Gibbs 1988, p. 50)

REFLECTING AND LEARNING AS QUESTIONS ARISE

Reflection in action can be encouraged by teachers until it becomes self-directed. For example, in the clinical environment a learner may detect a condition that they have little experience of managing. Rather than stepping in and taking over, you can establish what the learner already knows and encourage them to address any knowledge gaps. Learners could trial a management approach or research missing knowledge in the clinical setting (e.g. by consulting evidence-based guidelines). This helps the learner to reach a conclusion through careful reasoning. The learner can direct their subsequent personal study to read up about their case and any remaining knowledge deficits. Maintaining a notebook to record questions, uncertainties or knowledge gaps may ensure that personal study can be directed appropriately.

FOLLOWING UP CASES THAT HAVE BEEN SEEN

To promote *reflection on action* and to prevent worthwhile reflective cases or situations being missed, learners should be encouraged to follow up cases that they have seen. Often the cases in which unforeseen circumstances arose are those from which the most can be learned. This may not necessarily mean that a mistake occurred, but rather that a patient's condition was not what it first appeared to be, or problems within healthcare system delivery prevented the originally planned management. Such cases may not be routinely brought to the attention of the learner if no mistakes were made or the patient has not been harmed. However, for the learner there may be a wealth of learning opportunities to address. The self-directed learner will take note of the patients they see and find out what subsequently happens during the care episode. Any cases in which unforeseen circumstances arose could be used for a learning event analysis (see Section 8.16).

COMPLAINTS

You may feel defensive, disheartened and/or defeated upon receiving a complaint. However, complaints can be a useful stimulus for reflection and professional development. All professionals have to answer complaints that arise against them. As a junior, this may consist of providing a statement to senior staff, who may handle the situation from then on, or a formal response may be required. The skills learned through developing your reflective practice will assist with the production of such documents and also with the explanations that are provided to patients.

It is often a quality assurance requirement of a clinical setting that a complaints record should be held. This helps aid detection of any patterns of problems. As an educational supervisor or mentor you can help learners to consolidate what they have learned from a complaint by considering the following:

- Description of the event
- Concerns expressed by the complainant
- Assessment of the complaint
- Actions resulting from the assessment
- Outcome, including the response to the complainant
- Reflection on the experience and description of the learner's own involvement

LEARNING EVENT ANALYSIS

Learning event analyses, often referred to in the past as either significant event analyses or critical incident reporting, are increasingly becoming ingrained in the normal working practice of every healthcare professional and are recognised conduits for identifying problems in services, initiating change to improve the quality of practice and patient safety, and influencing professional development through reflective learning.

Learning events are cases in which an adverse, unforeseen or undesired (clinical, administrative or teaching) event has occurred or where a good outcome has occurred worthy of celebration and congratulations. Often they involve situations in which harm or potential harm has resulted, but learners and junior colleagues in particular need to be encouraged and reminded to reflect on positive achievements to ensure the learning is captured and best practice shared. Learning events are now commonly required for appraisal, revalidation and professional accreditation.

Although the term 'critical incident' may be synonymous with 'significant event', it can also describe situations that the professional has identified as being important in their professional development. Thus the event may not have posed a threat to patient safety, but may have been challenging or particularly rich in learning points. The latter situation should be addressed in the same manner as reflection (see Figure 8.2).

The following steps are involved in learning event analysis:

1. Identify the case or situation for consideration.
2. Collect and collate data. This includes both factual information and gathering the thoughts, opinions and impressions of those involved.
3. Organise a meeting of relevant team members to discuss and analyse the learning event.

4. Agree and implement changes and organise follow-up.
5. Keep a written record.
6. Obtain peer review of the process and outcomes.

Formal reporting and analysis of learning events, like the management of complaints, are tasks that require good reflective skills and are useful catalysts for learning. However, all members of the team should feel free to participate in discussions and analysis of the event. Evidence that changes have occurred and the results of these changes are also usually required when reporting learning events, particularly for appraisal or revalidation purposes.

AUDIT AND QUALITY IMPROVEMENT PROJECTS (QIPS)

Audit is the process whereby actual practice (organisational, clinical or educational) is compared with pre-defined standards and/or expectations of practice. In contrast to the individual case nature of learning event analysis, audits examine data of multiple cases, procedures or actions in order to obtain an overview of service provision. Data regarding your personal or service's practice are gathered and compared with the expected, pre-defined standards, and any deficits are identified. Formal reflection can help to explain areas that require attention and/or improvement to better meet the standards, and a plan should be made to initiate change. Once the change has been initiated, the whole process should be repeated to establish signs of improvement in adherence to expected practice. Thus a cycle is created that should be worked round repeatedly.

Increasingly our learners are attached to our clinical settings for shorter periods of time, and it may not be possible to complete the whole audit cycle, since time has to be allowed to pass in order to check whether changes have worked and whether standards are being adhered to. Quality improvement projects (QIPs) enable demonstration of the same skills of reflection and analysis of practice and also those of leadership, change management and team work. A QIP might be a short time limited action to implement a change in policy or practice with evaluation of impact. Examples of the process and ideas for implementation of QIPs can be found by registering here: www.rcgp.org.uk/clinical-and-research/our-programmes/quality-improvement.aspx

HANDOVERS

Handovers are an excellent opportunity for work-based learning. They affect clinical care, and due to shortened working hours, they have become increasingly frequent. Handovers if done poorly can be the weak link of the patient care chain. Failure to hand over adequately can result in medical errors, wasted time and/or money, poor patient care, patient dissatisfaction and potentially patient death. Help learners to identify areas for development through robust and informative handover processes. Formal handovers involving seniors at each shift change provide an ideal platform for ensuring appropriate and adequate handover by junior staff, and for questioning and exploring patient management.

Tips from experienced teachers

Consistent reflection is the single most important skill to impart to a learner. It will lead to a change in attitudes as well as updated knowledge and new technical skills, and will enable them to maintain a consistently good performance throughout their health professional career.

REFERENCES

Atkins S. and Murphy K. (1994) Reflective practice. *Nursing Standard*, 8: 49–56.

Brookfield S.D. (1986) *Understanding and facilitating adult learning.* Milton Keynes: Open University Press.

Gibbs G. (1988) *Learning by doing: A guide to teaching and learning methods.* Oxford: Further Education Unit, Oxford Polytechnic.

Grow G.O. (1996) Teaching learners to be self-directed. *Adult Education Quarterly*, 41(3): 125–149.

Hersey P. and Blanchard K. (1982) *Management of organizational behavior: Utilising human resources.* Englewood Cliffs, NJ: Prentice-Hall.

Johns C. (1995) Framing learning through reflection within Carper's fundamental ways of knowing in nursing. *Journal of Advanced Nursing*, 22: 226–234.

Knowles M.S. (1984) *Androgogy in action: Applying modern principles of adult learning.* San Francisco, CA: Jossey-Bass.

Marinker M. (1992) Assessment of postgraduate medical education – future directions. In Lawrence M. (ed) *Significant event analysis.* NHS Education for Scotland. Available at www.nes.scot.nhs.uk/pharmacy/CPD/sea.

Schon D.A. (1987) *Educating the reflective practitioner: Toward a new design for teaching and learning in the professions.* San Francisco, CA: Jossey-Bass.

CHAPTER 9

Developing teaching style and enabling communities of practice

······································

An effective teacher does not just support an increase in knowledge and skills, but does so in a way that engages learners and creates a sense of 'belongingness'. The effective teacher empowers a student to want to learn more and to put their learning into practice. Most of our health professions learners will be high achievers, used to doing well in education and training. It might not be too much of an over-generalisation to say that for the most part they achieve despite us, rather than because of us! Perhaps one of the worst things that can happen however is that our style of teaching actively undermines a learner's confidence or demotivates them and leaves them feeling that they do not belong. This can certainly affect their mental health and wellbeing but will also risk leaving them without the skills for life-long learning that they will need in an ever-changing healthcare world.

In nursing much work has been done, notably by Levett-Jones and her colleagues, to look at strategies that learners use to 'fit in', 'get the work done', and 'learn the rules'. Belongingness is characterised as a pre-requisite for, and an active component of, becoming an effective learner in nursing (Levett-Jones and Lathlean 2008).

How does such belongingness develop? Consider Box 9.1 that shares, with the permission of the student, a comment on social media that followed a belittling experience:

BOX 9.1 SOCIAL MEDIA TWEET

'Such a shame when some healthcare staff and teachers choose to take their frustration out on med students rather than strive to break the cycle. Picking on the people lower down on the ladder is only going to create bitter future doctors.'

DOI: 10.1201/9781003352532-11

West and Coia were commissioned by the General Medical Council to carry out a UK-wide review into the factors which impact on the mental health and wellbeing of medical students and doctors (West 2019). A recurring theme, along with workload and pastoral issues, throughout their document was the impact of poor teaching and supervision: 'In our engagement across the UK we heard of examples of a minority of doctors treating trainees and medical students aggressively or rudely' (p. 56). They stated that 'Some interactions with other professionals made medical students feel at the "bottom of the ladder" undermining their confidence and wellbeing' (p. 72). As a teacher you are in a leadership position, not always by virtue of position or title but through your opportunity to role-model professionalism and facilitate communities of practice (Lave and Wenger 1991). Lave and Wenger noted that after entry to a new field, such as the transition of healthcare students into the healthcare setting, a socialization process starts as learners observe existing practice, gain new knowledge, skills and behaviours and adjust themselves to join as full members of that community of practice. They start to 'belong'. Through a process they named legitimate peripheral participation, learners start to develop the competences required for the role and assume a professional identity. This is a crucial point where the teachers with whom they come into contact, and the style of teaching they experience, can shape their development and expectations of the sort of healthcare professional they should become.

The medical student in Box 9.1 went on to say 'at least I know I will never be that sort of teacher'. We would add that none of us should be that sort of teacher.

West and Coia call for 'compassionate leadership across all healthcare sectors' (West and Coia, 2019, p. 17):

> Central to doctors' sense of belonging is the quality of team working and the culture and leadership within their teams and organisations. It is of critical importance that such cultures are inclusive and take account of the needs of all.
>
> *(p. 49)*

Case study

Contrast the experience in Box 9.1 with this example from Lancashire Teaching Hospitals NHS Foundation Trust, cited in West and Coia (2019), pp. 73–74.

The Trust introduced clinical placement facilitators (CPFs), band six or seven nurses, who work closely with medical students and clinical placement supervisors (CPS) in identifying struggling students and supporting, guiding and teaching them within each placement. Students say they are excellent mentors who help organise their placements based on their needs.

'CPFs make a huge difference and are invaluable for learning and support. They go out of their way to make your placement run smoothly. I feel lucky I got a placement at Preston' (Medical student 1).

'Excellent CPFs in organising medical students' learning, so we can make the most out of our placement' (Medical student 2).

Wenger suggests that three 'modes of belonging' are important aspects of learning in communities of practice, and these can be supported and facilitated by an effective teaching style (Wenger 1998, p. 217; see Figure 9.1).

The three modes, which Wenger named engagement, alignment and imagination, come together in different combinations depending on teacher guidance (see Figure 9.2).

Reflective practice results from the effective combination of engagement plus imagination. Wenger points out that the presence of an outside view, such as provided by peers, educational and clinical supervisors enables a learner both to engage fully with the reality of their experience, for example, by having attention brought to unconscious aspects of practice, but also to trigger new interpretations enabling the imagination of other futures – where clinical practice might be enhanced.

Imagination and creativity however must be combined with alignment to context to ground it. Teachers can ensure this alignment by supporting access to observation of practice and facilitating discussions of the realities of patient care. This combination situates learning into practice. Additionally, the learning that can result from combining alignment with imagination ensures that practitioners remain adaptable when situations change, for example, when protocols do not apply, or resources do not allow a preferred course of action.

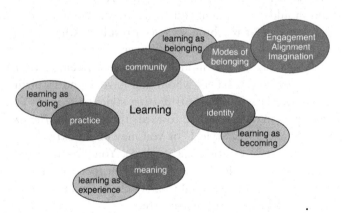

FIGURE 9.1 Adapted from Wenger's model of a community of practice. *Source:* Wenger (1998, p. xvi).

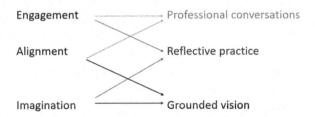

FIGURE 9.2 Learning through modes of belonging. *Source:* Developed from Mohanna (2018), after Wenger (1998).

Combining the modes of belonging of engagement plus alignment within a community of practice leads to professional conversations that can fully exploit variation in practice. In negotiating and defending our practice with colleagues, we can come to see ambiguities, inconsistencies and perhaps mutually develop new ways of doing things.

West and Coai make this recommendation:

> Organisations responsible for education and training of doctors and medical students should ensure they have an appropriate level of high-quality educational and clinical supervision provided by well-trained and compassionate supervisors. Approach and practical solutions should include: quality and accessibility of education and clinical supervision; ensuring training and working environments are safe for patients and supportive for learners and educators; they should adhere to the GMC's 'Promoting excellence – standards for medical education and training'.
>
> *(Recommendation 7, p. 95)*

BE AWARE OF YOUR OWN TEACHING STYLE(S)

During formal teaching, your appearance, voice and what you say are vitally important components of your teaching style. Your gestures and body language should not be distracting, and should complement your voice and the messages of your teaching. You will have developed your teaching style as a result of what comes naturally to you, the training and feedback that you have received, and your experience. There may have been some particular role models who have influenced your style, as you have unconsciously emulated teachers whom you have found inspiring, or deliberately avoided being like those with an off-putting style (or worse). You might have a quiet, introverted personality and tend towards the *all-round flexible and adaptable* teaching style (Section 9.2, Style 1) or you may be an extrovert and enjoy the *big conference* teaching style (Section 9.2, Style 5). Your healthcare discipline may also influence your teaching style. In the past at least, perhaps doctors might have adopted a dominating style and expected to be in charge, whereas nurses and allied health professionals may be more learner-centred.

You will become more aware of the nature of the style that you are using and how effective it is from continuing reflection, feedback and evaluation of your teaching over the years. However, good performance in teaching, just as much as in learning, requires a supportive teaching environment, sufficient time to deliver the required scope and level of learning, a reasonable teacher/learner ratio and a good match between learners' needs and your expertise/knowledge. Non–work-related worries, such as health or financial concerns, working in unfamiliar settings or being generally harassed, may affect your performance and awareness of your teaching style. These factors may affect your concentration, restrict your intuitive powers and limit your reflective insights.

You may not feel comfortable using all teaching styles. However, your ability to vary your teaching style according to learners' needs and stage of development and the purpose of the learning activity will depend on your insight. Exploit those styles that you are good at, and practise the other styles for delivering learning when there is minimal pressure and you can obtain constructive feedback.

INVESTIGATE YOUR TEACHING STYLE

One way of considering the varied range of teaching styles is the Staffordshire Evaluation of Teaching Styles (SETS) approach (Mohanna et al. 2008).

The underpinning original research for this model determined six main styles.

1. The all-round flexible and adaptable teacher can use many different skills, can teach both peers and juniors, and is very aware of the whole environment both of teaching and of the learners.
2. The student-centred, sensitive teacher is very learner-centred, teaches in small groups, with emotions to the fore, using role play and drama, and is not comfortable doing straight presentations.
3. The official formal curriculum teacher is very well prepared, accredited, is very aware of and teaches to the formal curriculum, and follows external targets.
4. The straight-facts, no-nonsense teacher likes to teach the clear facts, with straight talking, concentrating on specific skills, and much prefers not to be involved with multi-professional teaching and learning.
5. The big conference teacher most enjoys standing up in front of a large audience and does not like sitting in groups or one-to-one teaching.
6. The one-off teacher likes to deliver small self-contained topics, on a one-to-one basis, with no props to help and no follow-up.

Try working out your preferred teaching style(s) by completing the four steps of the next exercise:

- Step 1. Fill in the questionnaire in Section 9.4.
- Step 2. Score your answers.
- Step 3. Rate each of the six teaching styles.
- Step 4. Plot your ratings to compare and contrast your preferences for each of the six teaching styles.

STEP 1: WORK OUT YOUR PREFERRED TEACHING STYLE(S) BY ANSWERING THE QUESTIONS

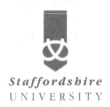

Staffordshire
UNIVERSITY

WEST MIDLANDS

DEANERY

THE STAFFORDSHIRE EVALUATION OF TEACHING STYLES (SETS)

This short questionnaire is designed to find out about your preferred teaching styles. Please rate how much you agree with each of the following statements on the five-point scale. Remember that 1 is not agreeing at all through to 5 which is very strongly agree. So the more you agree, the higher the score.

	not agree at all			strongly agree
Q1. I vary my approach depending on my audience	1	2	3	4	5
Q2. I am less comfortable giving straight presentations than teaching through games and exercises	1	2	3	4	5
Q3. I prefer to teach through games to relay learning	1	2	3	4	5
Q4. I like having external targets to determine the course of learning	1	2	3	4	5
Q5. I prefer teaching sessions that are self-contained with no follow-up.	1	2	3	4	5
Q6. Props often detract from a talk	1	2	3	4	5
Q7. I am comfortable addressing large audiences	1	2	3	4	5
Q8. Preparation for my teaching focuses on me and my role	1	2	3	4	5
Q9. I am usually standing up when I teach	1	2	3	4	5
Q10. The best teaching sessions convey straight facts in a clear way	1	2	3	4	5
Q11. I avoid being distracted from running sessions the way I plan to run them	1	2	3	4	5

Q12. I am happy teaching general skills	1	2	3	4	5
Q13. I put no value on being formally employed as a teacher	1	2	3	4	5
Q14. I dislike one to one teaching (e.g. as a tutor or mentor)	1	2	3	4	5
Q15. I am consistent in delivery of a topic, whatever the audience	1	2	3	4	5
Q16. I like to give learners opportunity to explore how to learn	1	2	3	4	5
Q17. I have developed my own style as a teacher	1	2	3	4	5
Q18. I prefer one-to-one teaching (e.g. as a tutor or mentor)	1	2	3	4	5
Q19. Eliciting emotions through role play or drama is a valuable aspect of teaching	1	2	3	4	5
Q20. I am comfortable using humour in my teaching	1	2	3	4	5
Q21. I am rarely sitting down when with the learners	1	2	3	4	5
Q22. It is important to me that my teaching is accredited by an official body	1	2	3	4	5
Q23. I am uncomfortable when I have multi-professional groups of learners to teach	1	2	3	4	5
Q24. I am at my best when organising my teaching to fit an external curriculum or organisational structure	1	2	3	4	5

THE STAFFORDSHIRE EVALUATION OF TEACHING STYLES

Scoring grid

Once you have filled in your own scores for all of the 24 questions on the SETS questionnaire, you will now need to score each question into the six teaching styles. The questions on the SETS have been randomly allocated on the SETS questionnaire, so it is important that you allocate the marks correctly to each teaching style.

Please fill in your score for each of the questions in the correct boxes, then add the columns up, and you will then obtain your score for each of the six teaching styles (out of a maximum of 20 marks).

Question	Style one	Style two	Style three	Style four	Style five	Style six
Q1	Q1 =					
Q2		Q2 =				
Q3		Q3 =				

(continued)

(Continued)

Question	Style one	Style two	Style three	Style four	Style five	Style six
Q4			Q4 =			
Q5						Q5 =
Q6						Q6 =
Q7					Q7 =	
Q8			Q8 =			
Q9					Q9 =	
Q10				Q10 =		
Q11				Q11 =		
Q12	Q12 =					
Q13						Q13 =
Q14					Q14 =	
Q15				Q15 =		
Q16		Q16 =				
Q17	Q17 =					
Q18						Q18 =
Q19		Q19 =				
Q20	Q20 =					
Q21					Q21 =	
Q22			Q22 =			
Q23				Q23 =		
Q24			Q24 =			
TOTALS						

Next, please fill in your scores obtained from the chart totals above into the six boxes against each of the teaching styles below.

Your scores

Style one.   The all-round flexible and adaptable teacher

This teacher can use lots of different skills, can teach both peers and juniors, and is very aware of the whole environment both in teaching and of the learners.

Style two.   The sensitive student-centred teacher

This teacher is very student-centred, teaches in small groups, with emotions to the fore, using role play and drama, and is not comfortable doing straight presentations.

Style three.   The official formal curriculum teacher

This teacher is very well prepared as a teacher, accredited, is very aware of and teaches to the formal curriculum and follows external targets for teaching.

Style four.   The straight facts no nonsense teacher

This teacher likes to teach the clear facts, with straight talking, concentrating on specific skills, and much prefers not to be involved with multidisciplinary teaching and learning.

Style five.   The big conference teacher

This teacher likes nothing better than to stand up in front of a big audience. This teacher does not like sitting in groups or one-to-one teaching.

Style six.   The one-off teacher

This teacher likes to deliver small self-contained bits of teaching, on a one-to-one basis, with no props to help and no follow up.

So now you have the scores out of 20 for your own self-evaluation of your preferred teaching styles. Now please go onto the diagram to plot your own scores on the SETS hexagon, along the six axes, using a cross where your own scores lie. Next, join up the crosses, and you will see where your own teaching styles lie diagrammatically.

Step 2: complete your scoring grid

Write your score for each of the questions in the correct boxes, then add up the columns to obtain your score for each of the six teaching styles (out of a maximum of 20 marks).

Step 3: rate each teaching style

Fill in your scores, obtained from the chart totals in Step 2, in the six boxes against each of the teaching styles listed below. Now you have the six scores out of 20 for your self-evaluation of your preferred teaching styles.

Step 4: plot your preferred teaching style(s) on the sets hexagon

Plot the marks, from the rating sheet in Step 3, with a cross along each of the six axes to represent your score for each of the six teaching styles. Join up the crosses to produce a shape that represents your own combination of styles.

- The Staffordshire Hexagon
- A diagrammatic representation of your preferred Teaching Styles
- Please take the marks (out of 20) from the scoring sheet and put a cross along each of the six axes to represent your score in each of the six teaching styles.
- You may wish to join up the crosses to produce a shape of your own combination of styles.

Remember that the six teaching styles are:

1. The all-round flexible and adaptable teacher 2. The sensitive student-centred teacher
3. The official formal curriculum teacher   4. The straight facts no nonsense teacher
5. The big conference teacher   6. The one-off teacher

TAILORING YOUR TEACHING STYLE(S) TO STUDENTS' LEARNING STYLE(S)

Consider whether your preferred teaching style suits the learning needs of your learners for a particular teaching episode. If it does not, you should switch or adapt your teaching style to engage with your learners better and, hopefully, to improve their understanding, knowledge and skills. The main approaches to tailoring your teaching style to learners' needs might be as summarised in Sections 9.7–9.11, but these do include wide generalisations to assist in illustrating our points.

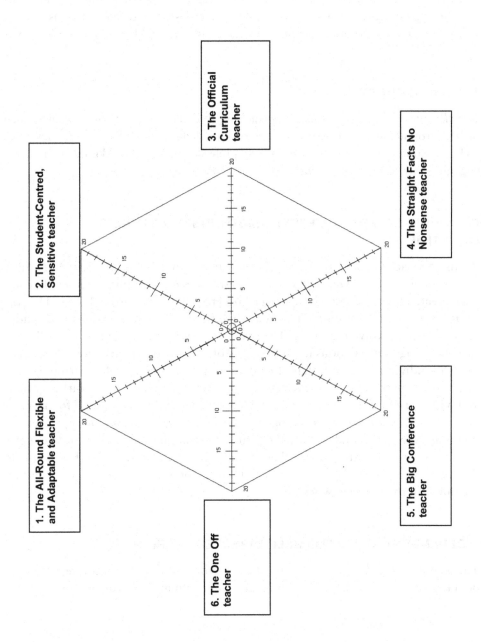

2. The Student-Centred, Sensitive teacher

3. The Official Curriculum teacher

4. The Straight Facts No Nonsense teacher

1. The All-Round Flexible and Adaptable teacher

5. The Big Conference teacher

6. The One Off teacher

MATCHING

This will encourage learners to be interested and involved. Perhaps your learner prefers well-structured situations, so a *straight-facts, no-nonsense* teaching style might suit this type of learner. An extrovert might prefer less structured situations maybe, so the *all-round flexible and adaptable* teaching style could be suitable for these learners.

ALLOWING CHOICE

The *all-round flexible and adaptable* teaching style should suit learners from a range of backgrounds and with various levels of knowledge and skills, as you vary your style and content to match their needs and preferences. You should guide them in an engaging way using your *sensitive, student-centred* style.

PROVIDING SEVERAL DIFFERENT METHODS OF LEARNING OVER TIME

If this approach is used, all of the learners should find something that suits them during their attachments, or during a programme of teaching, whether they are dependent, interested, involved or self-directed learners (Grow 1996). The *all-round flexible and adaptable* teaching style fits well, as it motivates and guides interested and involved learners. The *sensitive, student-centred* teacher will craft their teaching to the various learning styles of a group of learners and the specific needs of individual learners, handling dependent learners as well as firing up self-directed learners. The *official curriculum* teaching style is more authoritarian, and will be useful for covering the formal content of a course required for accreditation. The *big conference* teaching style could be useful for providing variety to all kinds of learners, and a *one-off* teaching style might make the most of experts brought in as external speakers. The *straight-facts, no-nonsense* style could help during revision sessions for dependent learners or for students who are falling behind with their course work.

INDEPENDENT STUDY FOR SELF-DIRECTED LEARNERS

The *all-round flexible and adaptable* teacher will facilitate and encourage the freedom to study as independent learning, especially with more mature learners.

TABLE 9.1 Grow's Teaching Delivery Styles Matched against the Six SETS Teaching Styles

Teaching delivery	SETS teaching styles					
	All-round flexible	Student-centred	Official curriculum	Straight facts	Big conference	One-off
T1 Authority	✓		✓	✓	✓	
T2 Motivator	✓	✓	maybe		maybe	maybe
T3 Facilitator	✓	✓				✓
T4 Delegator	✓	✓				✓

MATCHING YOUR TEACHING STYLE TO LEARNERS' NEEDS AND PREFERENCES

Another way of thinking about different teaching styles relates to your teaching *personality*. We shall return to Grow's stages of self-directed learning (SSDL) model with his four types of delivery of teaching (see Chapter 8).

T1: authority; coach
T2: motivator; guide
T3: facilitator
T4: consultant; delegator

These four different ways of delivering teaching (authoritarian, motivational, facilitatory and delegator) can be applied to the six different SETS teaching styles and situations (see Table 9.1).

The SSDL model suggests why 'good teaching' is widely misunderstood. Often people think that there is only one way to teach well – and usually it is their way! Awards generally go to teachers who are outstanding in one of the first two stages, either the one who provides copious structured information and instruction (sometimes called 'bucket filling', where the learner is seen as a vessel ready to be filled with information from the teacher) or the one who leads and motivates learners. Awards less often go to teachers who encourage learners to develop independently, or those who engage the most advanced learners with deep, open-ended problems.

'Good teaching' for one learner may not be 'good teaching' for another, or even for the same learner at a different stage of development. Good teaching does two things: it matches the learner's stage of self-direction, and it empowers the learner to progress towards greater self-direction. Good teaching is situational, yet it promotes the long term development of the learner.

MISMATCH BETWEEN TEACHING STYLE AND STAGE OF LEARNING

Even if teachers recognise that adult learners are not all necessarily self-directed learners, it is widely assumed that adults will become self-directed after a few sessions of explaining the concept.

However, not all adults become self-directed just because they have been told to do so. Adult learners can be at any of the four learning stages, but the literature on adult education is dominated by advocates of what the SSDL model would call a T3 style – a facilitative approach, emphasising group activity. However, teachers may sometimes need to approach certain learners in a directive, authoritarian style, and then gradually equip those learners with the skills, self-concept and motivation necessary to pursue learning in a more self-directed manner.

Every stage involves balancing the teacher's power with the learner's emerging self-direction.

THE TEMPTATIONS OF EACH TEACHING STYLE

The temptation for the T1 style teacher is to be authoritarian in a controlling way that stifles initiative and creates resistance and dependency. (Is this what happened in Box 9.1?)

The temptation for the T2 style teacher is to remain on centre stage, inspiring all who will listen but leaving them with no more learning skills or self-motivation than when they started.

The T3 style teacher can disappear into the group and demoralise learners by 'accepting and valuing almost anything from anybody'.

The T4 style teacher can withdraw too much from the learning experience, lose touch, fail to monitor progress, and leave learners struggling with a freedom they are unaccustomed to handling.

In each instance, the teacher may falter in the immensely difficult juggling act of becoming 'vitally, vigorously, creatively, energetically, and inspiringly unnecessary' (Grow 1996).

RECURSIVE TEACHING

The SSDL model describes a progression of stages, but the progress of a learner will rarely be linear, and most groups of learners will contain learners at different stages of self-direction. A more realistic version of the model would be non-linear and iterative.

Consider a course designed according to the T3 teaching style with stage 3 learners. The teacher serves as group facilitator, with the job of empowering learners to take greater charge of their learning and making certain that they master advanced levels of the subject matter. Most of the work takes place in this style where the teacher attempts to phase out external leadership and empower more self-direction.

However, there will be times when other learning modes are necessary. When the group (or some of its members) are deficient in basic skills, they may require drill and practice, a T1 style. (Even advanced learners sometimes choose T1 teachers who push them to achieve goals that they cannot achieve under their own motivation.) Sometimes the T3 teacher may determine that coaching or confrontation is necessary to reach a learner. The learner may loop back to the Stage 1 mode for a while before returning to Stage 3.

Continued motivation and encouragement may sometimes be supplied by members of the class, but it may require the teacher to shift to the T2 style and provide it.

At times the teacher's knowledge matters more than anything else; lecturing may be the best possible response at that point. During the lecture, the class loops back to the Stage 1 or Stage 2 mode, and then returns to the group interaction and subtle facilitation of the T3 style.

When individuals or subgroups become ready to exert self-direction and leadership, these learners can go into the S4 mode, independently carry out a project and then come back to the group and teach the results. With the Stage 3 facilitated mode of teaching as a base, the class can loop out to the other three stages when appropriate. A class that is focused on any stage of learning from S1 to S4 can draw support from the experiences in earlier stages and lean towards the later stages. Many courses centre around a series of T1/T2 style lectures, but have a weekly discussion group that is more effective when learners are in the Stage 3 mode. 'Looping' may be a more effective way to use the SSDL concept than trying to follow a sequence of linear stages.

Tips from experienced teachers

- Remember how it felt when you were new to the clinical setting. When did you start to feel you belonged? How did that happen?
- Don't become lazy. Continue to adapt your teaching style for your learners, and put their needs first. Is recycling your favourite annual lecture the best approach for these learners, now?
- Specify the requirements for an assignment in a supportive way so that dependent learners can more easily progress to being self-directed as they plan and apply their newly acquired knowledge and skills.

- Stay humble. Welcome (and seek) all feedback from learners (especially that which you could not have predicted), and continue to reflect on how you might improve your future delivery of teaching to different groups of learners.
- Listen, listen, listen . . . to your learners.

And perhaps, in the end, the only effective teaching style you need to create a community of practice and inculcate a sense of belonging in your learners is flexibility. And compassion.

REFERENCES

Grow G.O. (1996) Teaching learners to be self-directed. *Adult Education Quarterly*, 41: 125–149. Further detail available at www.longleaf.net/ggrow (Accessed 2.4.22).

Lave J. and Wenger E. (1991) *Situated learning: Legitimate peripheral participation.* Cambridge: Cambridge University Press.

Levett-Jones T. and Lathlean J. (2008) Belongingness: A prerequisite for nursing students' clinical education. *Nurse Education in Practice*, 8: 103–111.

Mohanna K. (2018) Belongingness: A commentary. *Education Primary Care*, 29(5): 276–277. DOI: 10.1080/14739879.2018.1522238.

Mohanna K., Chambers R. and Wall D. (2008) *Your teaching style: A practical guide to understanding, developing and improving.* Oxford: Radcliffe Publishing.

Wenger E. (1998) *Communities of practice: Learning, meaning and identity.* Cambridge: Cambridge University Press.

West M. and Coia D. (2019) *Caring for doctors caring for patients: How to transform UK healthcare environments to support doctors and medical students to care for patients.* Manchester: General Medical Council. Available at www.gmc-uk.org/-/media/documents/caring-for-doctors-caring-for-patients_pdf-80706341.pdf (Accessed 2.4.22).

CHAPTER 10

Matching methods with message

....

SELECTING TEACHING METHODS

In this chapter we will cover:

- Ad hoc teaching
- Teaching a practical skill
- Giving a lecture
- Running a workshop
- Working in small groups
- Running a learning group
- Problem-based learning
- Using audiovisual aids
- Writing educational materials
- Organising educational activities

The first steps when planning an educational session are to carefully and explicitly define the learning objectives, preferably in negotiation with or taking into account the views of learners; consider the domain of learning (knowledge, skills or attitudes) and then align your teaching strategy. Pragmatically, the teaching method is usually dictated, or at least influenced, by the available resources. Often you are invited to give a lecture, so the method is set for you. However, effective teachers show flexibility and creativity. If there is just you, one room and 50 learners, you will probably use a lecture format. But even within a lecture theatre, small group discussions are still possible by simply asking people to discuss specific points with their neighbour. If you ask the organisers in advance to arrange the room in 'cabaret style', you can run small groups around individual tables.

DOI: 10.1201/9781003352532-12

AD HOC TEACHING

Much of your teaching will probably occur while you are working in busy clinical settings. Often learners ask for explanations relating to their experiences as they go along, and you must manage this situation without the luxury of prior research or preparation of visual aids. Prepare for this by having a framework in mind that can be applied as appropriate. The five 'microskills' of the one-minute preceptor model listed in Box 10.1 can help you to assess, instruct and give feedback more efficiently.

BOX 10.1 THE ONE-MINUTE TEACHER: FIVE MICROSKILLS
FOR CLINICAL TEACHING

1. Get a commitment. Ask 'What do you think is going on here?' Ask the learner how they interpreted the situation to establish their learning needs.

2. Probe for supporting evidence. Ask 'What led you to that conclusion?' Ask the learner for their evidence before offering your opinion. This will allow you to find out what they know and identify knowledge gaps.

3. Teach general rules and principles: 'When this happens, do this . . .' Instruction will be better remembered if it is given as a general rule or principle.

4. Reinforce what was right and be specific: 'You did an excellent job of . . .' Learners' skills that are not well established need to be reinforced. Praise motivates people.

5. Correct mistakes: 'Next time this happens, try this instead . . .' Mistakes that are not addressed have a good chance of being repeated.

Source: Gordon et al. (1996).

TEACHING PRACTICAL SKILLS AND TECHNICAL PROCEDURES

Teaching skills requires an encouraging and supportive environment so that learners feel confident to practise and can reach the high quality of skills performance that is required to ensure patient safety and optimal health outcomes.

Research into improving the performance of other learners such as athletes and musicians gives a clear idea of what works in skills training, and it is usually not 'See one, do one, teach one'. The cognitive processes of a novice engaging in a practical skill are quite different to those of an expert. A seasoned expert is able to easily adapt existing procedures, to new or special circumstances. The goal of the novice is to achieve competence in the skill and feel comfortably proficient. The expert may think little about each step, but consciously slows down and increases their attentiveness when unexpected challenges arise. A novice must be able to perceive the various aspects of the procedure before learning to actually do it.

You will initially guide learners, allowing them safe opportunities to try the basic steps and to engage in repeated supervised practice. Observation and feedback is essential – practice involving repetition of errors does not lead to expertise. Later, you should provide opportunities to practise the new skill in increasingly complex situations. See Simpson's Taxonomy of the psychomotor domain (Box 10.2; Simpson 1972).

BOX 10.2 THE STEPS OF PSYCHOMOTOR SKILL ACQUISITION

Perception:	being aware.
Set:	getting ready.
Guided response:	following instructions.
Mechanism:	following habitual steps in action.
Complex response:	demonstrating coordination and efficiency of activity.
Adaptation:	adjusting procedures to new and special circumstances.
Origination:	creating new procedures.

Source: Simpson's taxonomy (Simpson 1972).

Eventually the learner will develop correct habits from repeated accurate practice and will be able to reproduce the expected steps unassisted. With repeated practice the learner will work more quickly in a coordinated time and energy efficient manner. By this stage the learner can begin to teach others how to perform this procedure.

Several educational models should be considered when teaching a specific practical skill or procedure. One of the most popular models is the *five-step method* (George and Doto 2001; see Box 10.3). For short procedures it can be followed directly. Longer, more complicated operations can be broken down into several shorter components and the model then applied for teaching possibly over an entire training programme.

BOX 10.3 FIVE-STEP METHOD

Step 1: Overview discussion

The learner's interest is stimulated by discussing why and how the particular procedure fits into healthcare.

Step 2: Demonstration without narration

The teacher shows the procedure completely and accurately at the usual pace of completion without descriptions to watching learners (conversation with the patient and other team members is continued as usual).

Step 3: Demonstration with discussion

The teacher performs the procedure while explaining each action and answering any questions from learners.

Step 4: Demonstration with learner narration

The teacher undertakes the procedure with learners advising the teacher how to perform each action.

Step 5: Learner performs the procedure

The learner performs the procedure with the teacher watching carefully and coaching as necessary.

A similar model from Walker and Peyton has four steps (see Walker and Peyton 1998):

1. Demonstration by the teacher.
2. Deconstruction of the task by the teacher into smaller practice components.
3. Assessing learner comprehension.
4. Learner performance.

'Advance mental practice': Mental practice, or rehearsal in one's mind prior to a performance, can help during both early and later stages of learning. Its effects are primarily in the cognitive and psychological preparedness aspects, rather than in physical muscle reactions (Feltz and Landers 1983).

GIVING A LECTURE

The advantages of the lecture include the following:

- Expertise is shared with many learners within a short period of time.
- It is relatively cheap in terms of resources, as one room is used, with one lecturer to many learners.
- Quick syllabus coverage can be achieved with a series of lectures.
- Expert clarification of difficult concepts can be achieved.
- It is a good format for a new topic and/or one about which little has been written.
- It allows a more meaningful description of feelings, and the potential for infectious enthusiasm to be transmitted from lecturer to learner, motivating learners to find out more.

There are however many disadvantages to the lecture format (see also Box 10.4):

- Passivity of the audience may shorten their concentration span to ten minutes or so.
- There may be little or no opportunity to ask questions.

- Learners' natural reticence prevents them from asking questions, due to fear of appearing stupid.
- Information is delivered at the same pace for all learners, which may be too fast or too slow for some audience members.
- It is difficult to assess content balance and reliability when faced with a single view of an enthusiastic expert.

BOX 10.4 THINGS THAT CAN GO WRONG WITH LECTURES

- Misjudging learners' prior knowledge – assuming too much or too little.
- Delivery inappropriate – too fast, boring, monotonous, challenging, funny or difficult to hear the words clearly.
- Format of teaching is mismatched with learners and/or content, such as a lecture when interaction is required, too little discussion or small group work that is too threatening.
- Dependence on audiovisual aids, causing panic when they fail to function properly.
- Poor preparation for questions.
- Lack of familiarity with the venue delaying the presentation while the teacher arranges lighting, seating, ventilation or audiovisual equipment.
- Being late due to not allowing sufficient travelling time.
- Poor lighting – too dark, causing the audience to fall asleep, or too bright, making slides illegible.
- Presentation appears disjointed because it lacks a logical flow.
- Too many speakers are involved, causing confusion to the audience.
- The lecturer looks down, avoids eye contact or continually turns their back to the audience to look at the slides on the screen.
- The topic is so difficult that learners risk leaving the session either ill-informed or more confused than they were before.
- Poor time keeping, particularly when the session is part of a tight programme.
- Inadequate structuring around learning outcomes that are relevant, necessary or important to the learners and match their preferences or needs.

You may avoid problems with giving a lecture if you consider the following:

- Establish the exact nature of the audience and their likely levels of knowledge and experience.
- Practise your talk. Time it carefully, making sure that you leave enough time to focus on the main points. Consider recording your practice talk and asking colleagues for constructive comments.
- Link your lecture into previous presentations by arriving early enough to hear them or arranging a private briefing from the course organiser before you speak.

- Open your lecture by sparking the attention of the audience in some way – with a prop, a challenging remark or a rhetorical question. Do not open by apologising for your lack of knowledge or for being there or keeping them from food, drink or freedom.
- 'Say what you are going to say, say it and then repeat what you said.' It has become a cliché because it works.
- Do not anxiously rock backwards and forwards when speaking into a static microphone, or your voice level will ebb and flow.
- Arrive early enough to check that your audiovisual aids are functioning and to establish how to operate the controls.
- Take a pointer with you in case one is not available at the venue.
- Fix your notes together if they are on different cards or pages, to maintain the correct order.
- Use a highlighter pen over key points of your lecture notes to enable you to pick out important phrases at a glance.
- Regularly raise your eyes to scan around the audience. Fix on one or two people when you are talking. Look at the back rows to prevent them feeling disconnected from the lecture.
- Develop your own style. Don't try and be funny if telling jokes makes you quake. Don't be crude or swear in a professional setting.
- Wear comfortable and appropriate clothes.
- Have water available if you are a nervous speaker.
- Write yourself big notices in your lecture notes saying 'slow down' if you tend to speak too fast, or timings if you often run behind schedule.
- Place your watch in a prominent position to remind you of the time.
- Inform the audience at the start whether you will take questions during or at the end of your lecture.
- Think positive, and imagine yourself giving a lecture and everything going well. Exude an air of enthusiasm and confidence about the subject.
- Finish with a well-polished, relevant conclusion. Perhaps use the answer to the rhetorical question posed at the beginning, the end of a story that was half told earlier in the presentation, or a challenge or action plan for the future. Don't just tail off and stop abruptly.

HOLDING YOUR AUDIENCE

An unresponsive audience can unnerve even experienced teachers. People behave differently when speaking in a one-to-one situation from when they give a lecture to a large number of people or run a workshop with groups of more than four or six people. In normal conversation the listener actively supports and encourages the speaker by giving non-verbal signs, making a suggestion if the speaker is lost for a word, and synchronising facial expressions and body posture with what the speaker is saying. When a lecturer addresses a large audience, this supportive interaction is lost and audience behaviour may even be off-putting. Learners' stares can seem threatening rather than the expressions of concentration which they might be. You may mistakenly interpret uninhibited comfort movements (e.g. head-propping, shuffling and yawning) as signs of boredom and disrespect. Neill termed this 'diffusion of responsibility' if there is 'no one responsible for supporting and providing feedback to the speaker, who may feel, from the lack of apparent response, as if he or she is throwing stones into treacle' (Neill 1999).

After a few minutes audiences tend to relax and display inattentive behaviour. When audiences are primed to put lecturers off by appearing to be inattentive, lecturers tend to perform worse than when audiences are primed to appear supportive and interested. To some extent, audiences should take responsibility for the quality of the lecture that they receive. Expect this type of behaviour, and either resolve not to be put off by it or take it personally and press on regardless despite the lack of feedback or support, or actively engage the audience by asking them questions, triggering discussion, setting challenges and using other interactive exercises.

RUNNING A WORKSHOP

A workshop format is useful if you want to exchange ideas and experiences about a relatively new area. It encourages interaction and discussion in response to a short, targeted expert input. A workshop relies on learners being willing to contribute and to think about how what they have heard applies to their situation and justify why they may or may not make changes. Workshops sometimes follow a lecture, providing the audience with an opportunity to think the topic through and challenge the speaker. If a workshop stands alone, the workshop leader will usually give a short presentation to introduce the subject and discussion points. Sometimes a workshop format is used for classroom teaching, such as learning critical appraisal skills or learning how to use new computer software. In these cases the leader often remains as an instructor and responds to questions throughout the session.

You may avoid problems with running a workshop by considering the following:

- Choose a title that is explicit and unambiguous, so that learners are unlikely to be misled about its content.
- Ensure that learners receive an abstract of the workshop prior to the session and are well primed about the topic and content of the workshop and the background of the facilitator.
- Hold a practice session first, especially if there is more than one workshop facilitator, to make sure that the facilitators share the same approach to the workshop, understand the learning objectives, agree roles and responsibilities, have small group facilitation skills and keep to time.
- Plan and keep to a timetable. Place it in a prominent position so that you and the other speakers or facilitators can keep an eye on the time. Be in a position to alert speakers who run over time.
- Establish the nature and likely prior knowledge of the audience.

- Inform the course or conference organiser of the upper limit of numbers of learners for your workshop prior to the event.
- Produce a sufficient number of copies of the small group discussion topics, so that delegates can remind themselves easily about the nature of the task in hand.
- Don't assume a flipchart with plenty of paper will be available for each small group, or flipchart pens. Take Blu-Tack® to help you to display flipchart reports to all learners.
- If the workshop involves representatives of small groups feeding back what they have discussed, make sure that these reporters keep to time and stay focused on presenting the discussion of their tasks.
- Round up the final plenary discussion with a conclusion based on the small group discussions that relates back to the objective of the workshop.

SMALL GROUP TEACHING: WHY USE SMALL GROUP TEACHING?

Small groups encourage learners to interact, explore and develop ideas. You might run a small group after a lecture, to allow the learners to debate the points that they have just heard, the extent to which these apply to their own circumstances and how they could change their professional practice or personal behaviour in response. A small group might be a forum for the exchange of different ideas to help learners to share tips and experiences that stimulate reflection and forward thinking. Small group work encourages learners to think independently, develop their own ideas and challenge preconceived beliefs. This is active learning, and it is often more effective than more passive methods (e.g. lectures).

Small group work is usually based on a task that is wide enough to encourage the learners to own and develop the topic themselves, but focused enough to restrict the ensuing discussions to the matter in hand. In small group work it is the learners who are key to the subsequent discussion, rather than the facilitator (see also Edmunds and Brown 2010).

BOX 10.5 THINGS THAT CAN GO WRONG WITH SMALL GROUP FUNCTIONING

- Groups are not well balanced (e.g. everyone sticks with friends or close colleagues instead of mixing with others). This can stifle discussion and limit the exchange of ideas.
- Members of the group do not introduce themselves, so no one knows who anyone is or what their backgrounds are.
- Conduct rules about confidentiality or the boundaries of discussion are not discussed or agreed, so that people feel they cannot speak about sensitive information. Even worse, group members confide sensitive information which is subsequently relayed outside the group.

- Too many small groups are packed into one room, so group members have difficulty hearing what others are saying and are distracted by what other groups are doing.
- Too little time is allowed for the small group discussion, preventing all of the tasks from being addressed.
- One or two members dominate the group while others sit quietly and unengaged.
- At the report-back session the group member presents their own views instead of the essence of the group's discussions.

If there is sufficient time, a small group evolves through five stages of development in group dynamics (Tuckman 1965). Especially if the small group is meeting frequently over time, it is worth monitoring which stage the group is at to help monitor and respond to difficulties.

1. **Forming:** getting to know one another.
2. **Norming:** the norms, roles and goals of the group are worked out through informal discussion, possibly checking out the task with the facilitator. There may be expressions of uncertainty about the task and some frustrations about lack of progress.
3. **Storming:** leaders emerge and some learners are perceived by the other group members as having special talents. There may be emotion, anger and impatience, requiring facilitation skills to hold the group together.
4. **Performing:** decisions are reached, and tasks are sorted out with a lot of mutual support and individual satisfaction. The group ends by reviewing and summarising its achievements.
5. **Mourning:** the group begins to disband as time runs out and members reluctantly leave the group. The facilitator may need to lighten the gloom and bereavement responses at this stage.

You may avoid problems with small group teaching by doing the following.

- Limit the numbers in a small group to 12, but preferably six or eight.
- Arrange the chairs facing each other in a circle, so that all members feel equally part of the group and can easily see everyone else.
- Remove any empty chairs so that the group feels complete.
- Appoint a facilitator who is skilled at handling group dynamics.
- Start the small group work by welcoming everybody, to create a positive atmosphere. Introduce yourself and ask the others to do the same.
- Agree ground rules about confidentiality at the beginning, and listen respectfully to each others' views and comments.
- Ensure that everyone knows what the task(s) involves. Have plenty of copies of the task(s) written out, or display them on a flipchart or project them from a computer.

- Brief the facilitator so that they know what main points should emerge and can guide the group members back to the central task if they become side-tracked.
- Encourage a group member to report the group's discussion back at a subsequent plenary session. Choose this person at the beginning so that they have ample warning and can take notes of everyone's contribution. This discourages reliance on the facilitator and maximises the engagement of the learners in addressing the task.
- If asked for information or an opinion, the facilitator should reflect questions back to the group rather than being seen to act as an expert.
- Ensure that everyone has a chance to have a say and contribute.
- Keep to time. The facilitator should have a general sense of the time allocated for each stage of the expected discussion, and should move the group on accordingly so that there is sufficient time to talk about alternative solutions and reach conclusions. Leave five minutes at the end so that the reporter can write down the main points for presenting at the plenary session.

RUNNING A LEARNING GROUP

There can be confusion about the terms 'learner set', 'learning group', 'learner group' and 'action learner set', and no general consensus about the different meanings of these names or types of group.

A 'learning group' format is a variety of 'small group' where the members meet regularly over time. It usually refers to a group of people who meet with the common aim of enhancing their personal and/or professional development by learning from each other. If the main purpose is to improve personal development, this might include learning more from each other about boosting self-confidence, self-esteem and personal presentation skills, as well as increasing achievement and career progression. If professional development is the main purpose, the group might be more topic-based around healthcare service management or organisational issues.

Groups that are established for peer support (e.g. Balint groups, where members discuss particular doctor–patient relationship issues on an ongoing basis) are another type of 'learning group' but are not discussed further here.

BOX 10.6 THINGS THAT CAN GO WRONG WITH A LEARNING GROUP

- Members do not prioritise group meetings and send last-minute apologies for their absence.
- The facilitator is not skilled enough to moderate vocal members who inappropriately dominate the quieter ones.
- The group appears purposeless, without a defined purpose.
- Alternatively, the opposite may occur, with the prescriptive curriculum stifling exploratory discussions and development.

- Members have false expectations of what being in the group means and want more direction, networking or support than is on offer.
- Insufficient effort is put into the 'forming' stage of the group to build sound relationships, respect and mutual understanding.
- The facilitator interferes too much in the group's development, and it is unclear whether they are a group member or not.
- There is too much external input and insufficient time to make the most of group members' potential contributions.
- Personalities clash and members don't gel, creating friction and frustration within the group, which boil over and disrupt progress in discussions.

A learning group facilitator has to be especially skilled in group dynamics, as learning groups often consist of those who have already achieved a great deal in their own field and want to develop themselves and their ideas further. Such people may be used to authoritative roles in their workplaces and struggle to leave this position behind, listen attentively to others and consider peers as equals.

Because of the members' backgrounds, little external input should be necessary, as members should be willing to impart their considerable previous experience, knowledge and skills to others.

A learning group should enable participants to develop their own learning needs with regard to their own individual needs and the organisation's needs. It should assist members through varied learning support mechanisms to meet their learning needs. Within a healthcare service, learning groups consisting of a mix of healthcare professionals can be set up to enhance understanding of each others' roles and responsibilities, and to promote respect for the skills and strengths of colleagues from other disciplines.

You may avoid problems with learning groups if you complete the following:

- Issue a learning group charter or contract with the invitation to potential members to join, explaining the purpose and nature of the learning group format.
- Only invite people to join the learning group if they are likely to get on with other members and are at similar stages of their personal and/or professional development.
- Make the establishment of good relationships within the group a priority at the first meeting. This may involve agreeing and owning group rules, encouraging group members to regard each other as peers whatever their professional status or position, and taking time for members to introduce themselves as individuals.
- Clarify the role of the facilitator in relation to being a group member, providing expertise and arranging hospitality and meetings.

- Fix dates for meetings well in advance so that members have the maximum opportunity to attend.
- Hold learning group meetings when the members are most likely to attend and feel relaxed. For example, for a full-day meeting avoid work being squeezed in around them, or late-afternoon meetings can end with a meal to encourage further networking between members.
- Accept that learning group members can gain technical knowledge elsewhere and that the two main purposes of the group are to learn more about the 'softer' aspects of personal and professional development, such as attitudes, feelings, relationships and values, and to give each other peer support.
- Agree some outcomes of the learning group so that members can gauge whether they are making progress and whether their time is being wisely invested.

PROBLEM-BASED LEARNING (PBL)

Problem-based learning (PBL) is a form of group working that can powerfully facilitate active learning. It requires attention to particular aspects of learner study skills, a high degree of learner self-directedness, excellent facilitation skills and an understanding of the process by the teachers (Bate et al. 2013).

PBL can be considered to reverse the traditional approach to teaching and learning. It starts with individual cases or problems, through the consideration of which learners develop general principles and concepts that they can generalise to other situations (see Table 10.1). It is a method that encourages resource investigation and leads to an increase in team working skills as well as content.

PBL can result in:

- Deep learning
- Learners activating prior learning and integrating new knowledge with it
- Lifelong learning skills
- Generic competences (e.g. collaboration)
- Learners assisting each other to find ways to understand and retain knowledge
- The sharing of useful sources of information

HOW TO CREATE EFFECTIVE PBL SCENARIOS

- Learning objectives must be defined in advance to construct the problem/case, but not shared.
- Problems should be appropriate to the stage of the curriculum and the learners' level of understanding.
- Scenarios should be relevant to practice.
- Problems should be presented in context to encourage integration of knowledge.
- Scenarios should present cues to stimulate discussion and encourage learners to seek an explanation.

TABLE 10.1 Seven Steps in the Problem-based Learning Process

1. The group clarifies the text of the problem scenario	*The mother of a 13-year-old girl phones the surgery to ask the receptionist whether her daughter has been seen that day by a doctor.*
2. Learners define the problem	*Isn't that confidential information?*
3. Brainstorming is used to identify possible explanations/solutions	*The girl is under-age, so the mother must be worried.*
	The girl might never come to the doctor again if she thinks we tell her mother everything.
	Should that be something the receptionist deals with or the doctor?
4. Group reaches interim conclusion	*It is an ethical/medico-legal dilemma.*
5. Group formulates learning objectives	*To find out what the law says.*
	To find out what ethicists think.
	To find out what doctors say in real life.
6. Learners go away and work independently to achieve the learning outcomes	*Library visits, internet searches, interviews with practitioners, discussion among peers, friends and family.*
7. Group reconvenes to discuss the knowledge acquired	*Pooling of results and sources. Tutor checks learning, clarifies and corrects if necessary.*

- Each problem should be of sufficient depth to prevent too early resolution.
- Learners should be actively engaged in searching for information.

DISADVANTAGES OF PBL

There are some disadvantages of PBL (Wood 2003):

- Learners may feel 'all at sea' if the process is not managed and introduced well and/or they are unprepared for such self-directedness.
- Facilitators may not have the competences to manage PBL, particularly if they were taught according to a traditional curriculum.
- Facilitators may resent not being able to 'teach' (i.e. transfer their knowledge and understanding).
- The knowledge gained can be disorganised, and important information may not be identified as such. Good tutoring is required to address this during the group discussion of knowledge acquired.
- Learners may fail to identify all of the necessary points from the case, and thus fail to learn parts of the curriculum.

- More staff and resources may be needed to support and facilitate the sessions and the resulting searches.
- Learners may miss out on role modelling from inspirational teachers.

Many of these disadvantages can be addressed through training and preparation of both learners and tutors.

EQUIPMENT AND VISUAL AIDS

During face-to-face teaching you should use any audiovisual aids that will enhance the delivery of your material, reinforce your messages and command the learners' attention. However, if you are totally reliant on audiovisual equipment, consider what you will do if it fails to work.

USING A FLIPCHART

A flipchart allows small groups to identify and record their concerns and ideas as they arise. As the pages are filled, they can be posted around the room so that the learners can refer to earlier suggestions and ideas. The flipchart is a useful interactive educational tool so long as the scribe faces the other learners and doesn't just list their own ideas. They are best used to capture brainstorming with some attempt by the facilitator to organise ideas into themes but not to reject or filter suggestions.

POWERPOINT PRESENTATIONS

We are all very familiar with PowerPoint (and other static visual presentation media such as prezi). This does not mean however that you won't ever go to a conference or attend a lecture where the speaker has clearly struggled to organise either their ideas or the slides. The following tips might seem basic to you, but perhaps reflect back on presentations you have seen (or given!) where these rules were not followed. What was the impact on the teaching?

- Prepare a structured framework for the content. Create a 'storyboard' that takes you logically through the content, from objectives through the main content material, concluding with learning points.
- Choose a format that is appropriate to the theme of your talk. Be alert to the right ratio of illustrative graphs, artwork, and sound and video linked to your presentation as appropriate. Only include such extras if they enhance the educational delivery.
- Use clear, legible text in short phrases or sentences to aid the viewers' understanding and keep their attention.
- Employ a sans-serif font such as Arial, where the letters have no tail, as these are less decorative and therefore more easily read on the screen.

- Match the font size to the size of the lecture room, from a 36 point size text in lecture theatres with more than 200 seats down to a 24 point size in classrooms with less than 50 seats.
- Include a maximum of one idea or point per screen.
- Limit yourself to six or fewer words per line in six or fewer lines per slide.
- Use predominantly lower-case letters, as they are more comprehensible to the reader. Restrict capitals to headings.
- Do not overuse colour. Stick to a maximum of four colours and be consistent with what different colours represent throughout your presentation to signpost learners.
- Make sure that your text is legible against your background. Maximise the contrast between text and background colours.
- Check that colours look the same when projected on to a screen.
- Check that your computer output is compatible with the equipment and software at the venue.
- Always have a back-up in case technology fails you. Perhaps email your presentation to a drop box and take it on a memory stick and consider what you might do if you cannot access your slides.
- Rehearse the presentation to ensure that you keep to time without moving through the slides too quickly. Ensure that you are giving learners enough opportunity to read and digest your slides as well as hear what you are saying.
- Know and plan how you will operate the computer.
- Consider whether to use handouts. Find the *handout* print option that enables you to print the slides on the left-hand side of the sheet of paper, leaving room for notes and questions on the right-hand side.
- Place a logo in the same position on each slide to give the impression of a coherent presentation.

AUDIOVISUAL PRESENTATIONS

Video clips can distract the audience. For example, if the equipment fails to work or causes a delay, it can disrupt the flow of your presentation. If you do show a video, explain the points of interest before you show it, and then expand on what the viewers will have noticed after they have finished watching it. Use short clips to maintain the momentum of the presentation.

You can incorporate the clip into your PowerPoint presentation, but ensure that this works away from the computer on which you created the presentation, as such links sometimes become corrupt.

If you are giving a lecture overseas, make sure that your equipment will be compatible with the audiovisual systems that are provided.

Any patient who appears on an educational video must give informed consent to be filmed and know the context in which you will be using and showing the video.

(See also Chapter 11 on digital teaching and learning for more on recording presentations with voice over, podcasts and creation of reusable learning objects.)

Tips from experienced teachers

When considering which teaching method to use, try asking yourself the following questions.
- What are the learners' objectives?
- What am I trying to achieve? What are my objectives?
- Is this the best way of achieving them?
- What other ways are there of achieving them?
- What are the strengths of the way I have chosen?
- What are the potential weaknesses that I will have to be on guard for as facilitator?
- How will I know that this way is the most appropriate way – for me and my learners?
- How will I assess whether the objectives have been achieved?

WRITING EDUCATIONAL MATERIALS

Writing educational materials is a crucial teaching skill. Providing written information that is easy to use and well-presented shows respect for learners. It is still common to use handouts in small groups or lecture situations.

USES OF HANDOUTS

1. To aid note taking by providing a place for learners to make notes alongside an outline of the session, ensuring that they have all of the important information.
2. To provide extra detail or information that would detract from the flow of the lecture, but which learners need to make sense of what is being presented, such as reports, figures or tables.
3. To provide extra information, such as vignettes for case discussion or small group work.
4. To provide an aide-memoire, perhaps for revision for examinations, of what was said, with personal annotations noting what was interesting or seemed important.
5. To provide a record of what was said, in order to:
   a. Avoid note-taking and thus aid concentration.
   b. Replace missed teaching sessions.

Consider whether you will provide the handouts in electronic form, by email or in the students' e-Portfolio, for example. Materials included in a portfolio can allow preparation or homework, set the scene, allow problems to be identified, and enable learning at the session to build upon a common foundation of knowledge.

Tips from experienced teachers

- Write in clear, simple language.
- Use short sentences.
- Do not use two-syllable words if a one-syllable word will suffice.
- Pitch the content at the right level for the reader.
- Make the layout attractive, with plenty of white space.
- Include boxes for key points.
- Use subheadings to break up the text.
- Add illustrations and diagrams to complement the text.
- Focus on relevant material rather than rambling anecdotes.
- Explain any jargon or abbreviations.

ORGANISING EDUCATIONAL ACTIVITIES

Good organisation and preparation are key to obtaining maximum benefit from any educational activity. You have a duty of care to ensure that learners will not be wasting time or money by attending the activity, especially if clinical duties have been cancelled or postponed to attend. Not only should you aim to facilitate quality education, but you should also ensure that everything runs smoothly and nothing is left to chance. Increasingly, large meetings and conferences are a hybrid model, with elements online for attendees to join from home and minimise travel, but with some face-to-face to encourage networking and sharing of ideas. The logistics of a hybrid conference or meeting range from simple (schedule a Teams meeting) to complex (invest in a virtual events platform such as Virtway™, where delegates create an online avatar to participate in virtual spaces). Online break out discussions, interactivity and even social networking are all possible. It is not quite so easy to carry out skills teaching or updating online, but virtual objective structural clinical examinations have already been tried successfully (Grover et al. 2022). Consider what you are hoping to achieve from the event, and that should dictate the format.

All meetings are better organised by a team. Meet early, identify and delegate tasks, check in with each other frequently and keep a timeline of what should happen when, so you are not caught out as time runs by. If you are too busy to organise an event, you could employ a commercial conference organiser. They may organise the entire event at no cost to you, but will arrange and retain a proportion of sponsorship and delegates' fees. After any educational event, be sure to gather participant feedback and include that in an evaluation of the event to carry any improvements forward.

REFERENCES

Bate E., Hommes J., Duvivier R. and Taylor D. (2013) Problem-based learning (PBL): Getting the most out of your students – Their roles and responsibilities: AMEE Guide No. 84. *Medical Teacher*, 36(1). DOI: 10.3109/0142159X.2014.848269.

Edmunds S. and Brown G. (2010) Effective small group learning AMEE Guide 48. *Medical Teacher*, 32(9): 715–726. DOI: 10.3109/0142159X.2010.505454.

Feltz D.L. and Landers D.M. (1983) The effects of mental practice on motor skill learning and performance: A meta-analysis. *Journal of Sport & Exercise Psychology*, 5: 25–57.

George J.H. and Doto F.X. (2001) A simple five-step method for teaching clinical skills. *Family Medicine*, 33: 577–578.

Gordon K., Meyer B. and Irby D. (1996) *The one minute preceptor: Five microskills for clinical teaching*. Seattle: University of Washington.

Grover S., Pandya M., Ranasinghe C., et al. (2022) Assessing the utility of virtual OSCE sessions as an educational tool: A national pilot study. *BMC Medical Education*, 22: 178. https://doi.org/10.1186/s12909-022-03248-3.

Neill S. (1999) In the stare of ravens. *Times Higher Education*, 11 June. Available at https://www.timeshighereducation.com/news/in-the-stare-of-ravens/146798.article (Accessed 1.12.22).

Simpson E.J. (1972) *The classification of educational objectives in the psychomotor domain*. Washington, DC: Gryphon House.

Tuckman B.W. (1965) Developmental sequence in small groups. *Psychological Bulletin*, 63: 384–399. Available at http://web.mit.edu/curhan/www/docs/Articles/15341_Readings/Group_Dynamics/Tuckman_1965_Developmental_sequence_in_small_groups.pdf (Accessed 10.4.22).

Virtway Events. Avatar based virtual events platform. Available at www.virtwayevents.com.

Walker M. and Peyton J. (1998) *Teaching in theatre. Teaching and learning in medical practice*. Rickmansworth: Manticore Europe Limited, pp. 171–180.

Wood D. (2003) ABC of learning and teaching in medicine: Problem-based learning. *BMJ*, 326: 328–330.

CHAPTER 11

Digital teaching and learning

....

Elaine Swift

INTRODUCTION

The Office for Students has gathered some of the early lessons from online and digital teaching and learning through the pandemic (Barber 2021). As we saw in Chapter 6, some authors have already thought about the complexity of evaluation (Wasfy et al. 2021). This chapter focuses on some of the key concepts that are now pertinent to success with digital learning and teaching and references some of the main digital learning technologies most typically found and supported in higher education.

BLENDED AND ONLINE DIGITAL LEARNING AND TEACHING

The term 'e-learning' is less common now in reference to the use of technology for learning and teaching. While reference to Technology Enhanced Learning can still be found across the education sector, more often you will see this referred to as either Digital Education, Digital Learning or Digital Learning and Teaching. The change in terminology reflects the growing use of digital technologies in both campus and online educational settings either using physical technologies such as virtual reality headsets, classroom audio-visual and media technologies or through employing a range of web-based technologies within a classroom setting.

Online learning refers to the delivery of learning and teaching that is dependent on web-based technologies and an internet connection to deliver the learning and teaching. The term 'blended learning' has been open to more interpretation. The Quality Assurance Agency (QAA) recently defined 'blended' learning as that used 'to describe different models of delivery and/or student engagement' (QAA 2020). The QAA also notes that the term 'hybrid' has also emerged where there may be more flexibility and choice by students about how they wish to engage with their studies. However, for most of this chapter we will be using the more commonly known 'blended learning' term.

DOI: 10.1201/9781003352532-13

DIGITAL CAPABILITIES

Jisc defines digital capabilities as 'the skills and attitudes that individuals and organisations need if they are to thrive in today's world' (Jisc 2022a). This recognises how the use of technology has grown and extended in many aspects of our lives beyond just learning and teaching. This umbrella term captures a variety of different digital practices that are relevant to both staff and students and which to a greater or lesser extent are dependent on the topic of study. The Jisc Digital Capabilities Framework (Jisc 2022a) articulates the range of digital competencies that most higher education (HE) educators and their learners need to consider either within or beyond the curriculum. The NHS has integrated digital literacy and the Jisc Framework to support the Digital Readiness programme (Health Education England 2020).

It is tempting to agree with the narrative of 'digital natives' (Prensky 2010), but educators need to be cautious in making assumptions regarding students' competence in using digital technologies for learning and their studies. An alternative model allows educators to challenge preconceptions about the use of technology and students' confidence when starting courses (White and Le Cornu 2011).

The reliance on the digital skills and associated technologies was starkly highlighted during the pandemic, and issues such as digital poverty clearly became one of the factors in how well students were able to continue their studies in a purely online format. Whenever considering digital learning and teaching, issues such as availability of information and communication technology equipment and internet access need to be factored in, and this is particularly important internationally or when teaching in resource poor environments.

Determining which digital capabilities should be included within digital learning and teaching will be dependent on the subject matter and might be different for different health professions.

DESIGNING FOR BLENDED AND ONLINE LEARNING AND TEACHING

Designing learning and teaching, whether for campus-based, blended or online, is an iterative process. In this section, we will consider the approaches that aid those key decisions.

Factors to be taken into account include the following:

- Learning outcomes – what needs to be learnt?
- Cohort make-up and size – who, and how confident with digital learning, are the learners?
- Availability of technology – what are our resources?
- How confident and competent are the teaching team in using technologies and supporting students?

Box 11.1 lists some sources of design support.

BOX 11.1 SOURCES OF DESIGN SUPPORT

- Conole's 7 Cs' Framework (2015) draws upon Gilly Salmon's Carpe Diem approach (Salmon and Wright 2014) and the Open University's Learning Design Initiative (OU 2008).
- The University of Northampton's Active Blended Learning framework draws upon some of the same foundational methods (UoN 2022).
- University College London's ABC Learning Design Method (UCL 2015) builds upon the concepts articulated in Diana Laurillard's Conversational Framework and Jisc's Viewpoints, originally developed by the University of Ulster.

Key elements for success:

- Bring together the course and modules teams to create a shared vision and understanding of the core aims, purpose and approaches being adopted.
- Involve learning design experts (who often have significant experience in the use of digital learning and teaching technologies either at a subject or general level), e.g. learning technologists and educational developers.
- Involve current students in the co-creation process to input and act as critical friends to the design process.

This process can be beneficial to overall success of the design of new courses and modules in that it provides a clear roadmap for the agreed design. Often it can highlight, at an early stage of the process, where potential challenges, opportunities and resourcing needs in terms of expertise or technologies will be encountered. If your institution provides such a design service as part of course or programme approval, it is recommended to consider using it. Institutional experts will also be able to advise on aspects of data protection and cyber security.

HOSTING DIGITAL LEARNING AND TEACHING

The most common virtual learning environments (VLE) are now more than 20 years old. In the UK, Moodle and Blackboard are still the top VLEs employed (Ucisa 2020).

These environments are now integrated with student record systems and provide a range of integrated services, including video capture, reading list software, tools that facilitate collaborative groupwork, online quizzes and surveys, e-Portfolios, electronic management of assessment, including rubrics and feedback, as well as the ability to present synchronously online through webinar technologies such as Zoom, Blackboard Collaborate or Microsoft Teams.

Whichever system is used, good clear design and presentation of the range of learning materials and learning activities employed within the curriculum helps all students. The principles of inclusive design apply equally to the virtual learning environment as they do to the design of the learning and teaching itself.

LEARNING MATERIALS

The opportunities for presenting key concepts and knowledge have expanded as multimedia presentations have become increasingly easier to develop. Many practitioners still utilise slides to deliver on-campus lectures, often having these lectures recorded using systems such as Echo360 or Panopto to provide students, especially those with specific learning differences or English as a second language, an opportunity to review sessions and review ahead of assessments.

Pre-recorded video content such as narrated PowerPoints are often used to set the scene, illustrate key concepts or procedures, or prepare students around a topic for a seminar or groupwork session.

Interactive content that learners can work through as part of their self-directed learning can be created, sometime using specialist software such as Articulate Storyline or through the integration of interactive content tools within the VLE itself; H5P and Xerte being two.

Open Educational Resources provide copyright free resources that can be employed alongside an educator's own resources. Academic Liaison Librarians are always a useful contact in terms of both copyrighted and open educational resources and can advise on the best resources available. They can also often support resource or reading list software such as Talis Aspire. These systems provide the ability to link students directly with library copies of recommended reading lists, with many of those now available as e-books.

ACCESSIBILITY

The UK Public Sector Web Accessibility Regulations (Gov.uk 2018) put additional emphasis on all public sector bodies to ensure that digital technologies and the content hosted on them are digitally accessible. For educators, this means that presentations and learning materials need to consider a range of accessibility needs.

While not completely comprehensive, Microsoft provides support through their accessibility checker in the Office 365 products, and some institutions have brought in an equivalent for their VLEs – often Blackboard Ally (the add-on is available for four of the main VLEs available). Both these systems give educators the ability to identify where their learning materials may need accessibility improvements and also provide advice on how to make changes (see also Chapter 17).

LEARNING ACTIVITIES

As with all learning, it is the combination of learning content and relevant learning activities with aligned assessments that provide pathways for students to make sense of their course of study.

Salmon's (2020) five stage model (see Box 11.2) outlines an approach which considers the stages of readiness for students, and paying attention to these stages can help ensure learners grow in confidence to take on more complex activities:

BOX 11.2 SALMON'S FIVE STAGE MODEL

- Access and motivation: How comfortable are your learners already with using technology in everyday life?
- Online socialisation: What can you as moderator or facilitator do to encourage a 'micro-community of e-learners' to develop online?
- Information exchange: Have you included online activities and interactive activities that can improve time management and enhance learner experience.
- Knowledge construction: Do you know when to step back as learners develop independence and start to construct their own learning?
- Development: What can you do to support experienced learners now transitioning to implement their learning in their workplace?

DISCUSSIONS AND COLLABORATION

Having space to discuss ideas and concepts with peers provides students with a chance to explore their understanding of core knowledge or concepts. Whether on-campus or online, these types of learning activities provide opportunities for students to develop their communications skills as well as their abilities in negotiating with peers, especially when engaging in collaborative activities.

Often, as part of designing activities, there are decisions to be made about whether activities are being delivered either synchronously or asynchronously.

Synchronous discussions online can be facilitated through various webinar technologies such as Zoom, Teams and Blackboard Collaborate. When designing synchronous activities, aim to consider the amount of time students need to spend online as part of their digital wellbeing. Being able to design in breaks from screens (either to conduct an offline individual activity or just take a break) is important both from wellbeing and learning perspectives.

Groupwork in synchronous sessions can be facilitated using breakout groups, which all the main webinar systems mentioned previously provide, with the smaller group sessions tasked to discuss a topic or to produce a collective piece of work.

For asynchronous discussions VLE discussion boards still have a place, though they are by no means the only tool to facilitate discussions. Other systems such as Microsoft Teams or dedicated tools such as Discord can also provide those spaces for discussion. While there will often be good reasons for providing such 'walled garden' spaces where students can express opinions in safe spaces (Beetham and Sharpe 2020), social media can also be utilised to good effect, allowing for the opportunity for a wider audience to be brought into the conversation. The Social Media in Higher Education Conference outputs has many examples of where this has been used effectively (SocMedHE 2021).

Other collaborative technologies allow groups of students to collectively pool ideas or produce artefacts together. While shared Office 365 documents and VLE wikis are some of the simpler tools available, tools such as Padlet or Miro bring the chance for students to refine their teamworking skills and to develop new digital capabilities in blended and online working.

REFLECTION ON PRACTICE

Over the last ten years there has been significant growth in e-Portfolio systems that provide individual students with personal spaces to capture their reflections or evidence of their development and share with peers, tutors, or placement colleagues. PebblePad and Mahara are two of the main e-Portfolios often integrated with virtual learning environments. Others such as OneFile, which is often used with apprenticeships, are also common, and if you are a UK-based health professions educator, you will be familiar with others such as Horus in the Foundation Programme or fourteenfish for training and appraisal.

ASSESSMENT AND FEEDBACK

The Principles of Good Assessment and Feedback Guide (Jisc 2022b) draws on research from across the sector with respect to digital assessment and feedback, and there is an ever-growing range of tools available for assessment.

Multiple choice formats may be the following:

- Integral to most VLEs as part of the standard package
- Stand alone, e.g. Questionmark, Perception and Respondus
- Some e-books also come with banks of questions that can be uploaded into the systems question bank or used online.

It is recommended to talk to a learning technology specialist if this is something you are considering.

Online submission through a VLE of a range of assessments, including video submissions, is common, and academic integrity of written submissions can be facilitated through the integration of originality software, e.g. Turnitin Software. This produces 'originality reports' providing guidance of the potential level of plagiarism with other submissions or online materials. Online 'essay mills' where one might commission someone to complete an assignment, or buy a readily available version, and other issues of student academic integrity is an ongoing area of concern.

Feedback and **feedforward** are a critical piece of student success. Feedback Studio, part of the Turnitin suite, provides the chance to give individual and model answers and feedback to students. Most VLEs also provide the opportunity to provide audio feedback.

Online exams, including proctored exams facilitated by systems such as Proctorio, were an area of significant growth during the pandemic. There are a range of issues to consider about online exams, especially in relation to inclusion and, with proctored exams, ethical issues about their suitability (Coghlan et al. 2021).

EMERGING AREAS OF INNOVATION

The pandemic accelerated and necessitated a significant amount of innovation in online and digital learning and teaching. Some areas of research and exploration were already underway; other have emerged as a response to the challenge.

STUDENT ENGAGEMENT

Research into areas such as learning analytics started well before the pandemic, but with the shift to online learning and teaching, the use of digital learning and teaching student data as a proxy for engagement with their studies took on more importance. Some institutions have dedicated teams who use dedicated systems to identify students at risk of disengagement and then work with the student to put in place extra support to address the student's needs, be they related to welfare or academic study. Jisc provides ethical guidance on the use of learning analytics and also provides a learning analytics service (Jisc 2022c). SolutionPath is one of the other providers in the UK, though some of the main VLEs do provide analytics solutions as well.

ARTIFICIAL INTELLIGENCE

The use of data combined with artificial intelligence is growing. From simple chatbots that can support student basic enquiries to digital assistants supporting disabled students, this is an area of experimentation, again with a range of ethical considerations that run alongside.

HYPERFLEX/HYBRID LEARNING

This is an emerging area of learning and teaching that has been implemented in situations where students have not been in a position to attend physical sessions due to restrictions on travel (international students, for example) or being restricted due to an enforced period of staying at home. Sessions are taught to students physically in the classroom at the same time as students join the session remotely. There are several factors to consider when deciding whether to utilise hyperflex or dual teaching: the provision of technology that can allow remote students to interact with students and the tutor in the room, the design of the sessions that allows both remote and physical students to be equally involved in the sessions, the additional workload considerations for a tutor(s) in delivering a session and monitoring the interactions and questions from both the physical students and remote students. Often this involves a combination of audio-visual equipment, webinar technologies and potentially additional resources to ensure a smooth session. This is an area of ongoing research and experimentation in some institutions.

Tips from expert teachers

Like any other learning and teaching modality, digital technologies should be used where they are the best modality to support the learning outcomes.

Using learning design methodologies with advice and support from learning technologists/digital learning developers can help with ensuring a quality learning experience for students aligned with the most appropriate pedagogies.

The range of digital technologies that can be applied in learning and teaching is broad, but effective virtual learning environments are still the main element for hosting and linking to materials, activities and assessments.

Scaffolding the introduction of digital technologies with students needs to be part of any blended design. It is important not to make any assumptions about students' digital capabilities when considering digital technologies as part of learning and teaching.

REFERENCES

Barber M. (2021) *Gravity assist: Propelling higher education towards a brighter future.* London; Office for Students. Available at www.officeforstudents.org.uk/publications/gravity-assist-propelling-higher-education-towards-a-brighter-future (Accessed 8.4.22).

Beetham H. and Sharpe R. (2020) *Rethinking pedagogy for a digital age: Principles and practices of design.* 3rd edn. New York: Routledge, 2019.

Coghlan S., Miller T. and Paterson J. (2021) Good proctor or 'big brother'? Ethics of online examination supervision technologies. *Philosophy & Technology,* 34: 1581–1606. https://doi.org/10.1007/s13347-021-00476-1.

Conole, C. (2015) The 7C's of learning design. In Dalziel J. (ed) *Learning design: Conceptualizing a framework for teaching and learning online.* 1st edn. New York: Routledge. https://doi.org/10.4324/9781315693101.

Gov.uk (2018) *Understanding accessibility.* London: Gov.uk. Available at www.gov.uk/guidance/accessibility-requirements-for-public-sector-websites-and-apps (Accessed 8.4.22).

Health Education England (2020) *Digital readiness education programme.* London: HEE. Available at www.hee.nhs.uk/our-work/digital-readiness.

Jisc (2022a) *What is digital capability?* Bristol: Jisc. Available at https://digitalcapability.jisc.ac.uk/what-is-digital-capability/ (Accessed 8.4.22).

Jisc (2022b) *Principles of good assessment and feedback guide.* Bristol: Jisc. Available at www.jisc.ac.uk/guides/principles-of-good-assessment-and-feedback.

Jisc (2022c) *Code of practice for learning analytics.* Bristol: Jisc. Available at www.jisc.ac.uk/guides/code-of-practice-for-learning-analytics.

Open University (2008) Learning design initiative. Available at www.open.ac.uk/blogs/archiveOULDI/

Prensky M. (2010) *Teaching digital natives, partnering for real learning.* Thousand Oaks, CA: Sage.

Quality Assurance Agency (2020) *Building a taxonomy for digital learning.* London: QAA. Available at www.qaa.ac.uk/docs/qaa/guidance/building-a-taxonomy-for-digital-learning.pdf (Accessed 8.4.22).

Salmon G. (2020) The five stage model. Available at www.gillysalmon.com/five-stage-model.html (Accessed 8.4.22).

Salmon G. and Wright P. (2014) Transforming future teaching through 'carpe diem' learning design. *Education Sciences*, 4(1): 52–63. Available at www.mdpi.com/2227-7102/4/1/52.

Social media in higher education conference (2021) Available at https://blogs.shu.ac.uk/socmedhe/.

Ucisa (2020) 2020 survey of technology enhanced learning for higher education in the UK. Available at www.ucisa.ac.uk/TEL2020.

University College London (2015) ABC learning design method. Available at https://abc-ld.org.

University of Northampton (2022) Active blended learning handbook. Available at https://mypad.northampton.ac.uk/lte/2021/10/29/active-blended-learning-abl.

Wasfy N.F., Abouzeid E., Nasser A.A., Ahmed S.A., Youssry I., Hegazy N.N., Shehata M.H.K., Kamal D. and Atwa H. (2021) A guide for evaluation of online learning in medical education: A qualitative reflective analysis. *BMC Medical Education* 21, Article 339. Available at https://bmcmededuc.biomedcentral.com/articles/10.1186/s12909-021-02752-2 (Accessed 21.5.22).

White D.S. and Le Cornu A. (2011) Visitors and residents: A new typology for online engagement. *First Monday*, 16: 9. Available at http://firstmonday.org/ojs/index.php/fm/article/view/3171/3049 (Accessed 8.4.22).

CHAPTER 12

Teaching in ambulatory care settings

....

Helen Batty

It is easier for learners to remember knowledge, skills and attitudes when they are recalled in the same context as that in which they were learned. It is therefore important that all health professions learners experience a variety of teaching and learning settings. Opportunities for learners to work in a setting away from the wards, starting early in their professional training, also helps them to understand the variety of career options and styles of practice available to them in their own futures. In the UK, and other countries where general practice is an established discipline, it is probably universal for all undergraduates to spend a varying amount of time in primary care and for postgraduate doctors to rotate through general practice in the Foundation Programme, or internship, whether that is their final career intention or not (see Dent 2005).

LONGITUDINAL INTEGRATED CLERKSHIPS (LICS)

For undergraduates, the longitudinal integrated clerkship (LIC) sets the scene for such rotational posts by facilitating long periods based in primary care. These can lead to learners becoming embedded as part of the community. Typically, when these are included in the undergraduate curriculum, students will be based in a general practice, but learning takes place in settings such as community hospitals, secondary care outreach clinics as well as the practice. Students from different disciplines will often learn together in peer-to-peer teaching or peer assisted learning (PAL). Clinical teaching might be opportunistic, following patients who make appointments with the GP for example, but can also be arranged, with expert patients being brought in specially for teaching. Experiences in community hospitals may be lower acuity such as podiatry or tissue viability (wound care) clinics but might also include day case surgery, outpatient investigations such as endoscopy, or treatments such as dialysis. The advantage for the learner is that the patients being seen in these settings may be known to them, and the chance of continuity of care is increased.

DOI: 10.1201/9781003352532-14

The early literature around LICs tended to focus on community-based immersion programmes; more recently this has broadened to include specialist ambulatory care in community settings. In rural areas community-based healthcare has often developed quickly to overcome issues of distance and access to secondary care. It might also include settings such as hospices, prisons or homeless shelters. 'Longitudinal' might refer to the location such as one town, or patient base such as one practice, or it might refer to supervision which is based in one centre with students travelling around a variety of local settings. Placements might vary one half day per week for six months through to full time immersion for more than 12 months (Thistlethwaite et al. 2013).

Success and participant satisfaction depends on the preparation of both students and clinical supervisors. The effectiveness of the learning is said to arise from the focus on *continuity* – of patient care, supervision or mentorship, or location, with peers or systems of care (Hudson et al. 2015).

TEAMWORK

Teamwork is crucial for effective, safe and cost-efficient healthcare outside the hospital, especially for patients with complex or chronic serious illnesses. Preparing learners to practise in teams and in these difficult ambulatory situations by introducing them early and supporting their growing involvement is essential for building their confidence and competence.

The *communities of practice* theory (see also Chapter 9) suggests that well-functioning teams grow together over time and develop new knowledge, protocols and supportive networks. This allows teams to improve the care of their specific community of patients. Therefore, it is very important that team function is understood and valued by teachers and learners. Informally, learners can be 'legitimate peripheral observers' watching from the edge of a team function or meeting. As the learners' time and experience with the team increase, teachers should highlight opportunities when learners can take a more active role within the team and in team meetings (e.g. making a case presentation for team discussion, or undertaking a literature search for information required by the team; Wenger and Wenger-Trayne 2015).

Learning the manners, etiquette, courtesies and nuances of team cooperation and communication are vital competences for healthcare professionals. Helping learners to appreciate teamwork and to feel supported to participate in healthcare teams is a major role for teachers.

Teamwork takes time. Teachers and learners need protected time away from direct patient care to discuss cases with other team members informally or at formal team meetings. Initially this may feel as if the patients are being disadvantaged. However, in the long run, patients who are being cared for by a well-functioning team will have a greater proportion of their care attended to more efficiently, particularly if they have complex or chronic illnesses.

When learners are at an early stage of developing confidence in patient interviewing and physical examination, the teacher needs to balance this important practice time with their need to also learn about being part of a team.

TECHNOLOGY IN THE AMBULATORY CARE SETTING

Increasingly, and particularly following the changes of the COVID-19 pandemic, technology is playing an important role in community-based care. Video meetings via Teams or Zoom enable care-at-a-distance. Applications such as Accuryx enable documents to be sent to patients and from patients, for example, photographs of lesions or rashes (see also Chapter 14).

APPLICATIONS OF TECHNOLOGY

Technology can be used for

- Communication – between and among healthcare professionals and patients
- Health information:
  - Storage and management of patient records (in electronic medical records).
  - Quality of care assurance (audits, service evaluations).
- Knowledge acquisition by
  - Health practitioners.
  - Patients and families.

Learners should not spend all of their time undertaking direct patient contact. They will benefit from spending some time on project work and in multidisciplinary meetings. Supervise this activity to help learners to become time-efficient, follow appropriate professional protocols and display appropriate attitudes.

GETTING YOURSELF READY

With the increasing involvement of new ambulatory settings in education and training for a variety of learners, including paramedics, physician's associates, nurses, midwives, therapists and pharmacists as well as medical students, many clinical teams may be welcoming learners for the first time. The following tips are drawn largely from general practice experts, which is perhaps the site with the longest experience, but not all of what follows will be relevant to your site.

If you or your setting are a teaching site for the first time, or if the curriculum has been newly revised, make sure that you read all of the available documentation, learning objectives, outlines, forms requiring completion, etc., well in advance. Check to see whether the programme has any faculty development sessions available to acquaint you with their expectations and usual teaching methods. If you have questions or concerns, discuss them with the programme director ahead of time.

BEFORE THE LEARNER ARRIVES

Identify where the learner will be able to:

- Securely leave their personal belongings
- Observe and talk with team members

- Take a break or use toilet facilities
- Interview and examine patients privately
- Discuss quick questions with you
- Sit with you for a full case discussion
- Write information in the patient's notes

Also decide where you can observe the learner.

Your team members must be involved in discussions before you agree to accept a learner into your clinical setting. This discussion should include issues relating to the following:

- Who is responsible for the learner's clinical work?
- Who will supervise the learner?
- Who is providing informal feedback and formal assessment?
- Have you acknowledged that the presence of a learner will add complexity and reduce efficiency for the whole team?
- Is any remuneration or reward available to the team as a whole in some form, or to individual team members?

Some teams may also want to ensure that no one health profession is favoured. Without clear and appropriate reasons, there should be no prioritisation of learners from one health profession over acceptance of learners from other health professions.

PATIENTS AND THEIR FAMILIES

There must be full awareness and disclosure when a clinical setting or healthcare team is part of an educational programme with careful preparation for the clients or patients. Giving advance notice by verbal explanation and/or by posting signs in waiting-room areas works well. Patients and their families must always, whenever appropriate, be allowed to refuse to have a learner present during their care. Talking to patients in advance may help to introduce the idea of including a learner, or actually introducing the learner in person may win agreement for the learner to be involved.

Patients and families can often feel that they are making a significant contribution to improving the healthcare system for themselves and others in the future when they allow a learner to be part of their encounter and ongoing relationship with the healthcare team. Such patients may even agree to schedule sessions at times when teaching is required.

Tips from experienced teachers

- Patients who are healthcare professionals, teachers in other topic areas or whose families have benefited from effective healthcare (or occasionally suffered unfortunate adverse experiences in the healthcare system) may be eager to help you and your team in training future healthcare professionals. Never be afraid to ask patients to volunteer to be included in your teaching team.

- The more time you spend appropriately orientating a learner, the more efficient your subsequent teaching and their clinical work will be.
- You can learn a lot from your learners, sometimes in unexpected ways.

APPROPRIATE LEARNING RESOURCES

Everything that the learner sees, hears, smells, touches and feels in your clinical setting adds to their education experience. Capitalise on these opportunities by taking a broad view of what is happening from minute to minute. Introduce this concept to the learner at the beginning of your orientation, and ask the learner to communicate what they are noticing or wondering about while they are with you. Help them to reflect on it.

Learners benefit from many of the information sources that are available in any healthcare setting. Encourage them to review whatever paperwork is completed or given to patients and their families. Similarly, make sure that they are aware of the forms, guidelines, brochures, booklets and other hard copies that team members share. Show them whatever reference resources you use, and suggest that they begin to build their own selection of resources. Watch to see what they are using to solve clinical problems while they are with you.

ORIENTATION: INTRODUCING THE LEARNER

Once your clinical setting and team are ready to receive learners, plan how you will orientate them.

Introduce all learning resources to the learner as early as possible. Useful information could be written in a letter or memo to be given to the learner on the first day or sent in advance. Generally, the longer you expect a learner to be with you, the more extensive an orientation you should organise. For example, you might spend two weeks orientating a learner who will be training with you for two years.

You can select appropriate patients and clinical tasks by checking in advance the list of cases scheduled for a teaching session. 'Prime' the learner about patients before they see them. Provide a quick synopsis and advise them of the task or area on which to focus. Also prepare learners if you anticipate any difficulties.

During your first sessions with a new learner, consider allowing them to observe you. Role modelling is an efficient way to show what is possible, appropriate and expected from them. Demonstrate a variety of activities to provide a full picture – interviewing and examining patients, discussions with the team, and managing paperwork and telephone calls. For novice learners, start by highlighting basic aspects of what you are doing. For more advanced learners, use this as an opportunity to share subtle techniques and fine points and receive helpful comments from them.

APPROPRIATE MONITORING OF LEARNERS' ACTIVITIES

Direct observation

You may be supervising a situation where neither the learner nor the patient is known to you. This can be stressful, as you hold full responsibility for the clinical care of the patient. If you are in doubt about the learner's level of competence, directly observe the clinical encounter. Once you are confident in the learner's growing abilities, you can reduce the amount and intensity of direct supervision. Watching the learner work while you are in the room, or remotely using video/web cams and microphones, is the most accurate way to gauge their confidence and competence. With novice learners, focus on only one aspect of the clinical encounter – perhaps the part that seems most appropriate or the main priority (e.g. physical examination, the closing summary). Discuss and agree with the learner in advance what you plan to focus on. Avoid overloading yourself, the learner or the patient. In all cases, the camera is focused primarily on the learner. Cameras should be turned off when a patient disrobes or is in the room without the learner. You must have appropriate patient consent prior to activating any such system.

Generally, you should try not to interrupt the learner once they have started. However, occasionally you may be concerned enough to take over and finish the patient encounter. If this happens you could do any of the following:

- Consider moving away from the patient briefly to discuss the case, and advise the learner that you will take charge of the situation when you both return.
- Make a gentle but direct comment to the learner suggesting that, given the available time, you recommend switching places so that the patient can be appropriately accommodated.
- Suggest that the learner moves to another task, such as looking up laboratory results, taking a message to another team member or consulting the literature, while you expeditiously proceed with the care of the patient.

INDIRECT SUPERVISION

Depending on your setting and the level of your learner, you may wish to regularly review what the learner is doing during a session and before the patient leaves. With novice learners, you can request that they come to you after interviewing a patient to discuss the information that they have acquired, before and after any physical examination, before finalising a treatment plan and before sending the patient away or finishing the visit. For senior learners, you may be happy that they work at an efficient pace throughout the whole session and come to you only with occasional urgent questions. At the end of either situation discuss the highlights of the cases that they have seen, and arrange a final sign-off.

Tips from experienced teachers

- If you are simultaneously trying to undertake clinical work of your own while teaching others, you must clearly give learners permission to interrupt your work at any time if they need your advice. You should remain close at hand.
- Many teachers in the ambulatory clinical session find the 'One Minute Preceptor' a helpful framework for time-effective teaching and giving feedback (see Chapter 10).
- If you are short of time to give feedback to learners, share the positive feedback publicly and write any specific suggestions for change in a private hard-copy message, with an invitation to the learner to contact you later for further discussion if they wish.

Keeping alert to cues that a learner might be struggling is an important skill for a teacher in an ambulatory care setting to develop.

Signs that the learner is struggling include the following:

- Taking an unusually long time with the patient.
- Coming to you with unexpected concerns about a patient.
- Behaviour that is out of character for that particular learner (they may be mimicking the patient's behaviour unconsciously – confusion or hypomania can be contagious).
- Bringing a disorganised description of the history or examination that they have just completed.
- The learner discussing the case with another health professional when you are available to review the clinical work.

CONCLUDING A TEACHING SESSION

Arrange a final summative 'sit-down' group review of all the cases seen in the session before everyone leaves. Involving learners at a variety of levels and other team members can be very beneficial.

Ask the members of the group to take turns to summarise and highlight each case individually to stimulate reflection, or discuss the most interesting or unusual cases or a particular clinical theme that has emerged. For example, you may have noticed that a number of similar cases seem to be related to a particular virus. You could facilitate a shared discussion about the aspects and implications of this infection currently prevalent in your community.

FEEDBACK: FORMATIVE DISCUSSION

Learners highly value constructive comments about their work. They may not feel confident about asking you directly, so consciously plan to offer generous, honest, positive reinforcement of their correct actions and strong qualities. Suggestions for improvement may be given in small, careful doses throughout any teaching session (see Chapter 15 for information on providing effective feedback).

In an ambulatory care setting you may only be working with learners briefly, so provide succinct feedback with every case, at the halfway point of any teaching session and before you part each day. If you have the opportunity to work with a learner for more than one session, arrange with them in advance how any topics that have been discussed will be monitored in future sessions. You must have some follow-up on actions agreed to or discussed.

FOSTERING INDEPENDENCE

Encouraging increasingly independent practice, self-directed learning and team-based continuing professional development are all valuable lessons for learners in an ambulatory care setting. Learners must experience taking responsibility, problem solving and working with other healthcare team members. The longer you are working with a learner, the easier it will be for you to judge how much independence they can be granted. Initially, assign learners very specific small tasks to determine how much they can handle. Ask them what they feel they are prepared for and what they would like to do in each case. Obtain the opinions of other members of your healthcare team about learners' levels of competence.

If you have several learners simultaneously, encourage them to interact, teach and help each other. Advanced learners can share your supervision of a novice learner. In return, you should provide extra stimulation and intellectual challenge to the senior learners.

ASSESSMENT: SUMMATIVE EVALUATION REPORTS

You may be required to assess learners (see Chapter 17). Ambulatory teaching provides the opportunity for workplace-based assessment to make a particularly accurate assessment of a learner's capabilities, as it is a realistic setting. Often learners have not previously had a chance to build an ongoing relationship with a teacher who can assess them as individually as this.

Tips from experienced teachers

- Keep brief 'field notes' for each teaching session, just as you would for clinical case work.
- If unexpected difficulties arise, you might:

  ask a team member or senior learner to work with or directly teach the learner

  tell the learner to continue with you at their side for support

> speak privately with the person to obtain more understanding of the situation
> take over and model appropriate actions
> - A teaching session with too few patients can provide the opportunity to role model making good use of time in your management of paperwork, attending to other team responsibilities, and following up unanswered questions or interesting cases.
> - A session in which you are feeling overwhelmed with patient problems is an excellent time to teach about maintaining professional composure, setting priorities, delegating responsibility and working with patients' and families' prime concerns.

As assessments can be major turning points in a learner's career, you must find out *before* the learner arrives exactly what kind of assessment is expected. Clarify any uncertainties about programme expectations or assessments with the authorities who are responsible for the learner well in advance.

DEVELOPING TEACHING STRATEGIES FOR UNEXPECTED SITUATIONS AND ADAPTING TO AMBULATORY SETTINGS

Boxes 12.1 and 12.2 list the advantages and disadvantages of teaching in ambulatory settings.

BOX 12.1 ADVANTAGES OF AMBULATORY TEACHING

- Builds a meaningful one-to-one relationship with learners.
- Enables clinical experience to be tailored to individual learner needs.
- Stimulating for the team.
- Educational for the teacher.
- Patients derive satisfaction from contributing to education of healthcare professionals.
- Perceptive learners bring new ideas to the clinical setting on many levels.
- The learner's experience is aligned with the needs of their own real-world future practice.

BOX 12.2 DISADVANTAGES OF AMBULATORY TEACHING

- Adds another layer of unpredictability for the clinical team.
- Results in extra responsibility and work for the clinician teacher.

- Time-stressed environment.
- Potentially chaotic clinical setting.
- Unhappy patients and families.
- Reduced efficiency of care.

Things to do

By their very nature, you cannot specifically prepare for unexpected events. However, you can prepare to manage unexpected circumstances to the best of your abilities.

- Expect the unexpected.
- Take a moment to consider the situation.
- Trust your first instinct.
- Ask the learner for ideas.
- Ask your team for ideas.
- Ask the patient and their family for ideas.
- Limit yourself to only highlighting one teaching point per case.
- Focus on a positive aspect of the situation.
- Debrief afterwards with the learners, discussing your reflections on aspects of the process or content that surprised you.
- Explore what other teachers do by attending education conferences, reading about teaching, and encouraging discussion among your colleagues.

Things that can go wrong

- No patients are available: this might be an opportunity to model effective use of time, use as a teachable moment or reflect back on a previous patient.
- Patients refuse to see or speak with a learner: this is their right, accept it and explain to the learner that there will be other opportunities. However, in the face of active racism or other discriminatory behaviour towards your trainee or learner, the good educational supervisor acts as an active ally and does not tolerate such behaviour.
- A patient requires emergency treatment and urgent transfer to a hospital setting: perhaps the learner can follow on after the ambulance and follow the patient journey?
- Too many patients have been booked for the number of learners scheduled: this is difficult; can some see patients, in turn, and then discuss in pairs or small groups in between patients?
- The learner refuses to see a particular patient or follow your treatment recommendations: this is highly unusual behaviour and could have a variety of causes. You might decide to stop this learner seeing patients whilst you work to uncover the issue. Suggestions in Chapter 20 might help.

SPECIAL THINGS TO REMIND LEARNERS ABOUT HOME/COMMUNITY VISITS

- You are guests in the setting.
- It will take extra time initially to acknowledge the people present and their context.
- Be prepared to leave at any time if requested to do so.
- Social conventions may require you to drink, eat, look at photographs, admire special objects and otherwise become involved with your patient and their life. Take advantage of the opportunity to make observations about aspects of the patient and the situation which you have not previously considered.
- Establishing appropriate professional boundaries can be challenging, but this is an ideal opportunity for learners to gain practice in doing so.

Travelling together may give you and the learners an excellent opportunity for conversation about the particular case, general education issues or broad philosophical ideas.

TIME MANAGEMENT

The challenge is to find an efficient balance of good patient care with meaningful contributions to learners' education experience. In ambulatory care settings you might be with your learner for long periods of time when they accompany you on home visits or you supervise their time in clinic. There are a number of things you can do to manage time effectively (see also Irby and Bowen 2004):

- Accomplish your most difficult teaching task at the beginning of any session.
- Focus on the learners' identified interests.
- Choose one small but significant teaching point per case.
- Avoid 'over-teaching'. Conserve your strength and don't talk too much.
- Check with the learner halfway through the session for adjustments of your initial time management plan.
- Rescue any learner who appears to be flagging – offer them a break or change of activity.
- Find opportunities to enable senior learners to become part of your teaching team.
- Listen to any immediate scheduling concerns that team members bring to you.
- Encourage all team members to watch for and act upon ways to improve educational efficiencies minute by minute.
- Monitor your own energy level and plan accordingly.
- Advise the learners and team of any unusual time constraints at the beginning of the session.
- Plan to end the session with a teaching activity which you and the learners look forward to.

REFERENCES

Dent J.A. (2005) AMEE guide no 26. Clinical teaching in ambulatory care settings: Making the most of learning opportunities with outpatients. *Medical Teacher*, 27: 302–315.

Hudson J.N., Poncelet A., Weston K., Bushnell J. and Farmer E. (2015) Longitudinal integrated clerkships (AMEE guide 110). *Medical Teacher*, 39(1): 7–13. DOI: 10.1080/0142159X.2017.1245855.

Irby D.M. and Bowen J.L. (2004) Time-efficient strategies for learning and performance. *Clinical Teacher*, 1: 23–28.

Thistlethwaite J.E., Bartle E., Chong A.A., Dick M.L., King D., Mahoney S., Papinczak T. and Tucker G. (2013) A review of longitudinal community and hospital placements in medical education (BEME guide 26). *Medical Teacher*, 35: 8.

Wenger E. and Wenger-Trayne B. (2015) *Communities of practice: A brief introduction.* Available at https://wenger-trayner.com/introduction-to-communities-of-practice (Accessed 9.4.22).

CHAPTER 13

Involving patients and the public and simulation in teaching

....

Janina Iwaszko

Patient and public involvement (PPI) is now widely considered to be an integral part of the teaching and training of healthcare professionals (GMC 2009; DoH 2010). Although for a long time there has been passive involvement of patients in clinical learning, especially at the bedside, a more active pattern of involvement is now thought to have further beneficial effects. The benefits of patient involvement include encouraging and enabling learners to develop high levels of communication skills, a patient-centred approach and shared decision-making skills (Gordon et al. 2019).

These are vital but complex skills that need to be developed over time, therefore it is now believed that early opportunities to learn these skills are core to modern clinical training. The achievement of these skills can result in an improvement of the patient experience, but this can also have a positive effect on the quality of patient care, patient safety and the management of chronic clinical conditions. Successful introduction into curricula requires several factors to be taken into account. Although learning for these skills can occur through a variety of teaching modalities, including didactic lectures, small and large group tutorials and simulation sessions, studies show interactions with real patients have the potential to be more effective, authentic and diverse (Jha et al. 2009).

DESIGN AND DELIVERY – HOW TO INVOLVE PATIENTS AS CLINICAL TRAINERS

Patients with a long-term condition, and those who attend clinics on a regular basis (sometimes known as 'expert patients') often have an extensive knowledge of their condition and are able to offer real-life insights concerning their health, and insights into aspects of continuity of care and interdisciplinary working. There is a consensus that the 'patient as teacher' role is most effective when patients have been trained and integrated into the healthcare teaching in a manner that makes clear the links

DOI: 10.1201/9781003352532-15

of their involvement to clear expected objectives (Wykurz 2002; GMC 2009; DoH 2010). The patient experience can be seen as an illustration of healthcare theory in practice, thus enhancing student understanding and recall of the teaching session. Patient input brings a far more complex contextual learning environment to healthcare education, creating an environment similar to that of the healthcare workplace (Bell, K et al. 2009).

EQUITY, DIVERSITY AND TRAINING

It is important to be both flexible and inclusive about which patients are involved in teaching, and there should be an appropriate diversity of age, culture, ethnicity, gender and social or economic status. Patient recruitment can be through patient support groups, community agencies or through general practices or outpatient clinics. The dignity and confidentiality of the patient must always be respected, therefore it is important that before patients support the training of learners that they understand and are comfortable with their role. Training of patients beforehand can help to reduce any anxiety, and due attention should be given to patient sensitivities and the possibility of distress caused by sharing painful experiences or undergoing repeated examinations. This reduction in anxiety can also be achieved by ensuring that patients know the planned learning outcomes and that time is taken to clarify the expectations of their involvement. It can also be helpful if the choice of the information offered is guided by the preferences of the patient. Although teaching sessions will be well defined, if they are also designed to cover several areas of the patient's condition, this can then create a very informative framework that the learners can take into the clinical setting to enrich their understanding of the patient journey.

The vast majority of patient involvement is very positive, but patients should be supported to know that they can stop at any time and who to contact if they find it difficult to continue. It is important to avoid specialty-specific language and terminology during the training and to use inclusive communication. It is also important to plan for appropriate comfort breaks. Further personal support, such as remuneration and transport, should always be considered for patients, especially if they are involved with student training for significant lengths of time, and this should be agreed in advance.

If patients are to be more formally involved with learners, for example, in either formative or summative assessment, they may require more wide-ranging and structured preparation and training for the role. In addition to guidance on general communication, a clarification of the concept of shared decision making and information on the delivery of feedback following the encounter increases expert patient confidence in their role.

GIVING FEEDBACK

The process of giving and receiving feedback is a skill that can be acquired only with practice and may take time to develop. Feedback is integral to high quality healthcare education as it encourages and enhances the learners' knowledge, skills and professional performance. The fact that feedback will be given should be signposted at the beginning of a session, and before feedback is to be delivered, it should be clearly announced. Patients need to know that feedback should focus on the performance and not on the individual, and that it should be clear and specific. To be effective, feedback needs to be delivered in non-judgemental language, emphasise the positive aspects of the encounter and suggest actions for improvement.

PATIENTS' INVOLVEMENT IN CURRICULUM DEVELOPMENT, EVALUATION AND ASSESSMENT

Patients are often involved in healthcare training briefly and in an ad hoc manner, but if they are involved over a significant period of time, they have been shown to be effective co-designers of the healthcare curriculum (Wykurz 2002). They can also offer significant input when consulted on the strategic development of new medical schools and can identify relevant competencies for graduates.

If part of the aim of assessment is to assess preparedness for practice, then the reality of patient involvement, including potential variability, can be regarded as an opportunity to enhance assessment authenticity, increasing the validity of assessments.

Patients can be effectively involved in the assessment of the theoretical knowledge of healthcare students during the early stages of learning, through contributions to question content. Patients can also contribute during the implementation of practical clinical assessment, both through suggestions for authentic scenarios and as patients in OSCE (Objective Standardised Clinical Examination) stations. The involvement of patients in OSCEs can add an increased level of reality to the clinical examination station.

Sufficient resources do however need to be allocated to enable sustainable, active patient involvement in curriculum development and theoretical and practical assessments, due to the physical and psychological impact on the patient of this involvement. This should be taken into account and appropriate support incorporated.

VALUE FOR PATIENTS AS TEACHERS

There can be a demonstrable benefit for patients from their involvement in the training of healthcare professionals, and patients appreciate sharing their knowledge. From the patient perspective, involvement in teaching or training is a mainly positive process. It may be regarded as both enjoyable and rewarding, with perceived benefits, including feelings of enhanced self-esteem, companionship and acknowledgement as partners in the healthcare process.

The active involvement of patients in teaching not only utilises their knowledge and experience, but it may go on to increase their knowledge of their own condition and also cause them to consider their condition in a more positive light. The process of patient involvement in training healthcare students acknowledges their expertise and may go on to engender a sense of empowerment. Furthermore, patients may feel that this activity could help future patients, and there may also be satisfaction knowing that they are contributing to the education of future doctors. Patients' motives can range from the wish to improve student training to 'giving something back' with respect to the management of their condition.

Occasionally negative effects occur, with some patients reporting anxiety and concerns over recalling previous negative experiences; they may feel that they are being judged or superficially viewed as just a disease rather than a person. Thus care must be taken to prevent these occurrences to minimise harms and maximise the benefits.

To benefit from being involved as teachers, patients need to be adequately trained, supported and remunerated. For some people, this involvement may provide a starting point towards ongoing future employment.

THE BENEFIT TO STUDENTS OF PATIENT INVOLVEMENT

The benefits to students who engage with and learn from patients early in their medical education has a considerable evidence base in the literature. This includes acclimatisation to clinical environments, support with professional development, increased confidence and reduced stress when interacting with patients. It also extends to aspects of development of a professional identity and how they are becoming members of a medical community of practice (Rees et al. 2006). Contact with real patients has the potential to increase learner engagement in theoretical aspects of learning, and the importance of authenticity for strengthening adult learning has been described well in Knowles's adult learning theory (Koons 2004). Early interaction with patients also has been shown to strengthen student learning and focus that learning to become relevant to clinical practice (Littlewood et al. 2005).

Patients contribute a unique and invaluable perspective to the teaching of clinical learners with respect to the patient journey and contribute to learners' knowledge of how patients experience their health conditions. This strengthens the concept of a patient-centred approach, which has been shown to not only improve the patient experience, but also improve levels of patient safety (Dykes et al. 2017; Guastello and Jay 2019). Direct patient interaction can also enhance the development of the core clinical skills of obtaining a medical history, performing a comprehensive physical examination and using clinical reasoning to reach a diagnosis and management plan.

Involvement of patients in feedback that can then influence the attitudes and behaviour of the learners in clinical settings encourages reflection and can aid professional identity development. The wider use of a reflective approach, with more insightful questions, fosters the development of problem solving and clinical reasoning skills (Towle et al. 2016).

Through being involved in individual patient narratives, learners are enabled to improve communication skills, understand the importance of advocacy, develop cultural humility, and apply ethical concepts. Other issues such as dignity and cross-cultural awareness are often best conveyed through direct patient contact and exposure to, and experience of, interacting with a variety of individuals, including those with disabilities or from vulnerable groups. Done in an integrated and structured manner, this can then further assist in the breakdown of hierarchical barriers by focussing on patient needs and patient safety.

Following patient contact, the learners will be in a position to place their scientific and pharmacological learning into context, whilst improving their acquisition of wider clinical skills. The opportunity to apply basic science concepts to the authentic clinical material encountered helps learners to better understand the disease processes described and enhances awareness of the complexity of patient care. In addition, learners may gain an altered perspective, an enriched context and an appreciation of the complexity of clinical encounters (Rieffestahl et al. 2020).

As contact with real patients offers learners opportunities to experience authentic and engaging experiences, transformative learning often results. Transformative learning occurs if it involves a learner in fundamental critical analysis of an event that results in a reordering of how they think and the acquisition of an alternative perspective. Thus, learning that occurs with real patients is often more meaningful, more durable than lectures and supports students to acquire a wide range of complex clinical skills and knowledge and an increased preparedness for practice (Taylor 2007; Van Schalkwyk et al. 2019).

Evidence is mounting that there is great added value of linking patients and healthcare students for longer periods of time (Dijk et al. 2020). Through linking learners with patients, their families and communities, the awareness of the importance of longitudinal relationships is increased, it improves students' social interaction and communication skills and facilitates learning how patients are able to cope with conditions over a period of time in the real world.

BENEFITS FOR COURSES OF INVOLVING PATIENTS AS TEACHERS

In summary, if patients, patient groups and lay people are involved in a medical curriculum from the outset, they can not only add authentic highlights garnered from their specific experience of coping with illness, thus making the curriculum more relevant and current, but also help to identify competencies and outcomes for students and offer a new perspective on the emphasis and importance of the patient-facing aspects of the curriculum (GMC 2009; Dijk et al. 2020). Patients also act as an additional teaching resource, which has been shown to improve student motivation to learn. This integrated method of teaching with authentic patient input can also improve the depth of student learning, together with a more accurate understanding of the complexity of healthcare.

SIMULATION, AUGMENTED (AR) AND VIRTUAL REALITY (VR)

Simulation with manikins or simulated patients (SPs), augmented and virtual reality are modalities that can also offer all healthcare students a patient's perspective of coping with a condition. In addition, they have the ability to provide realistic, repeatable and standardised experiences for learners in a controlled environment without exposing patients to harm and can facilitate teaching clinical and non-clinical skills simultaneously. They offer a different experience to those encounters with real life patients and may not have the same level of authenticity. However, the range of mental health problems or range of personality changes in the acute settings can be greater than those which would be appropriate with real patients. Simulation also offers students access to events that otherwise cannot be readily observed, in a safe and controlled environment with the benefit of feedback. Simulation can also be tailored to specific learning outcomes and altered to match the study needs and level of the learners.

Therefore, the aims and learning objectives with reference to these modalities should take a different perspective. The emphasis should be placed on the opportunity to experience deliberate practice, critical thinking, clinical reasoning, problem solving and team-working skills in a safe environment.

Design of the simulation or AR/VR activity should always come after the first step of analysing the specific needs and level of the learners. These scenarios could include aspects of interpersonal communication, professionalism, and non-technical or human factors that are all core to clinical competence. Simulated experiences with SPs, AR and VR give learners the opportunity to practise each of these skills in a controlled, often low-stress setting. Receiving immediate and constructive feedback gives information to the learner through a detailed description of their performance in the observed situation. After observation and constructive feedback on their performance, the students are better prepared to interact with actual patients.

However, simulation has some drawbacks when it is required to replicate clinical cases that require pathological signs in the patients, as the signs and symptoms of these cases cannot always be easily simulated. The recent development of a wide range of new technologies, such as augmented and virtual reality, now means that pathophysiological signs can be replicated. Signs can also be added with equipment such as interactive stethoscopes, and augmented reality details can be projected onto manikins, as well as added into fully immersive virtual reality simulation. Furthermore, the use of virtual reality either in the form of flat screen 'serious games' or fully immersive VR with headsets can now add further dimensions to clinical simulation, thus widening the learning objectives that can be met.

Augmented reality has been demonstrated to be particularly effective in helping learners extend their anatomical knowledge, and when this modality is used within clinical scenarios, anatomy can be learnt in appropriate clinical context.

STANDARDISED OR SIMULATED PATIENTS, ACTORS OR ROLE-PLAYERS IN SIMULATION

Standardised patients are actors or role-players, and they need to be trained in the same way that expert patients need to be trained. This includes not only how to portray the characteristics of a patient, to give learners opportunities to learn, but also on how to offer timely and constructive feedback.

SPs are evaluated differently to patients by medical students who appreciate the authenticity and realism of working with real or expert patients, but feel that SPs enable access to a differing variety of clinical scenarios and an alternative type of feedback. The scenarios more suitably portrayed by SPs would be emergency scenarios, trauma, acute/severe mental health or scenarios that are time critical, such as birth, or maybe those conditions that have very few outward signs or symptoms, but where a history is core to diagnosis.

Furthermore it is possible, by the careful design of scenarios with SPs, to include a higher level of emotion, and learners are able to develop the skills required, for example, to manage acute mental health and psychotic patients in a safe environment. Learning to distinguish between hypoglycaemia and alcohol intoxication in a verbally or physically aggressive patient, for instance, would be challenging to engineer with an expert patient but can be modelled by simulation.

TRAINING SPS

SPs act as a proxy, representing the type of patient they have been assigned, and they often do not have a health professional background. Their training should enable them to respond to how a learner is communicating. This includes training on nonverbal communication and how to monitor and relay how they are feeling as the patient, back to the learner. Initially they need to be given the patient story of signs and symptoms and why they have sought healthcare. This should also include a detailed back story so that the SP can react in a natural manner to the learner's consultation. It is then imperative to the success of the simulation encounter for the learner that the SP develops an appropriate level of skill to offer accurate and constructive feedback.

The next level of training for an SP should involve the recognition of cognitive bias and how it can be reduced and how poor human factor skills can also be improved. The training of SPs should enable them, in a formative simulation, to develop responsiveness in individual learners that allows the scenario to go in the direction that would have been most likely for the patient. However, in summative simulation settings, the SPs need to be trained to be as consistent as possible so each student has a comparable experience.

VIRTUAL PATIENTS

Virtual patients (VPs) are interactive computer-based avatars of an SP that allow for even greater flexibility of clinical topics than role player SPs, together with the added benefit of opportunities for deliberate practice at a time suiting the learner. The learner takes the role of a healthcare professional and, by working through a VP scenario, can develop clinical skills such as clinical examination, making diagnoses and developing management decisions. VPs require less human resource than

SPs, they can be developed to be more standardised and they can be programmed to contain a large library of cases. However, they may not be able to react to learners with the same level of flexibility as SPs. Patients are often involved in developing the scenarios to increase authenticity.

The use of VP technology also enables the collection of large amounts of data on student performance, which can clarify which educational strategies are most effective and adapt accordingly. While technology-enhanced learning can never substitute for interaction with and learning from a patient, it is a safe, innovative and accessible way of putting theory in the context of a clinical encounter.

CONCLUSION

Undergraduate medical education is a complex, dynamic and changing field where a range of pedagogical philosophies, educational practices and conceptual paradigms meet. Much of medical education is planned and organised, but a substantial amount remains opportunistic and patchy. The ultimate aim of medical education is to train a range of safe, competent, skilled, healthcare professionals who put patients at the centre of their care, and who have the skills and expertise to undertake their core clinical competencies, but can also maintain and extend their expertise over the course of a long career.

Involving patients in medical education can be beneficial to learners: not only does it facilitate acquisition of skills such as communication, but it can also change professional attitudes positively and develop empathy and clinical reasoning. It provides context to theoretical material and motivates learners. Patient feedback on encounters with students, if carefully designed and used formatively, is largely welcomed by students and appears to improve their performance and depth of learning, as measured by examination results. Some learners prefer the teaching they receive from trained patients to that from healthcare professionals. Many students comment on gaining new insights and confidence when practising examination skills on patients who can offer constructive feedback, and claim that such training increases their respect for patients and deepens their understanding of the experience of disease.

The use of simulation and technologically enhanced learning can also add differing perspectives, the opportunity for deliberate practice and the exposure to rarely encountered clinical scenarios. All of these modalities offer learners the opportunity to learn in a wide range of cognitive, affective and experiential levels and enable learners to develop a clinical perspective that is more open, reflective and capable of change.

REFERENCES

Bell K., Boshuizen H.P.A., Scherpbier A. and Dornan T. (2009) When only the real thing will do: Junior medical students' learning from real patients. *Medical Education*, 43(11): 1036–1043. DOI: 10.1111/j.1365-2923.2009.03508.x.

Department of Health (DoH) (2010) *Equity and excellence: Liberating the NHS: Presented to parliament by the secretary of state for health by command of Her Majesty July 2010*. Norwich: TSO.

Dijk S.W., Duijzer E.J. and Wienold M. (2020) Role of active patient involvement in undergraduate medical education: A systematic review. *BMJ Open*, [online] 10(7): e037217. DOI: 10.1136/bmjopen-2020-037217.

Dykes P.C., Rozenblum R., Dalal A., Massaro A., Chang F., Clements M., Collins S., Donze J., Fagan M., Gazarian P., Hanna J., Lehmann L., Leone K., Lipsitz S., McNally K., Morrison C., Samal L., Mlaver E., Schnock K. and Stade D. (2017) Prospective evaluation of a multifaceted intervention to improve outcomes in intensive care. *Critical Care Medicine*, [online] 45(8): e806–e813. DOI: 10.1097/ccm.0000000000002449.

General Medical Council (GMC) (2011) *Patient and public involvement in undergraduate medical education. advice supplementary to tomorrow's doctors (2009). General medical council*. Great Britain: GMC.

Gordon M., Gupta S., Thornton D., Reid M., Mallen E. and Melling A. (2019) Patient/service user involvement in medical education: A best evidence medical education (BEME) systematic review: BEME guide no. 58. *Medical Teacher*: 1–13. DOI: 10.1080/0142159x.2019.1652731.

Guastello S. and Jay K. (2019) Improving the patient experience through a comprehensive performance framework to evaluate excellence in person-centred care. *BMJ Open Quality*, [online] 8(4): e000737. DOI: 10.1136/bmjoq-2019-000737.

Jha V., Quinton N.D., Bekker H.L. and Roberts T.E. (2009) What educators and students really think about using patients as teachers in medical education: A qualitative study. *Medical Education*, 43(5): 449–456. DOI: 10.1111/j.1365-2923.2009.03355.x.

Koons D. (2004) *Applying adult learning theory to improve medical education*. UCHC Graduate School Masters Theses 2003–2010. [online] Available at https://opencommons.uconn.edu/uchcgs_masters/51 (Accessed 11.6.22).

Littlewood S., Ypinazar V., Margolis S.A., Scherpbier A., Spencer J. and Dornan T. (2005) Early practical experience and the social responsiveness of clinical education: Systematic review. *BMJ*, 331(7513): 387–391. DOI:10.1136/bmj.331.7513.387.

Rees C.E., Knight L.V. and Wilkinson C.E. (2006) 'User involvement is a sine qua non, almost, in medical education': Learning with rather than just about health and social care service users. *Advances in Health Sciences Education*, 12(3): 359–390. DOI: 10.1007/s10459-006-9007-5.

Rieffestahl A.M., Risør T., Mogensen H.O., Reventlow S. and Morcke A.M. (2021) Ignitions of empathy. Medical students feel touched and shaken by interacting with patients with chronic conditions in communication skills training. *Patient Education and Counseling*, 104(7): 1668–1673. DOI: 10.1016/j.pec.2020.12.015.

Taylor E.W. (2007) An update of transformative learning theory: A critical review of the empirical research (1999–2005). *International Journal of Lifelong Education*, 26(2): 173–191. DOI: 10.1080/02601370701219475.

Towle A., Farrell C., Gaines M.E., Godolphin W., John G., Kline C., Lown B., Morris P., Symons J. and Thistlethwaite J. (2016) The patient's voice in health and social care professional education. *International Journal of Health Governance*, 21(1): 18–25. DOI: 10.1108/ijhg-01-2016-0003.

Van Schalkwyk S.C., Hafler J., Brewer T.F., Maley M.A., Margolis C., McNamee L., Meyer I., Peluso M.J., Schmutz A.M., Spak J.M. and Davies D. (2019) Transformative learning as pedagogy for the health professions: A scoping review. *Medical Education*, 53(6): 547–558. DOI: 10.1111/medu.13804.

Wykurz G. (2002) Developing the role of patients as teachers: Literature review. *BMJ*, 325(7368): 818–821. DOI: 10.1136/bmj.325.7368.818.

CHAPTER 14

Teaching technology supported healthcare

....

It is becoming normal to use and recommend digital technology to promote people's health and social wellbeing, matching their needs with digital solutions. This might be for the prevention of deterioration of long-term conditions (e.g. technological reminders to take medication regularly), aiding their treatment (e.g. wearable technology measuring blood sugar levels or someone's heart rate) and supporting their safety and independence at home (e.g. with light sensors or a personal digital assistant). Over recent times there has been a rapid shift to remote consultations between a patient and a healthcare professional.

But for those patients who are not digitally savvy, many of whom are older people who are more likely to have multiple health conditions, this risks creating more health inequalities from their lack of ready access to primary care, and their lack of digital skills in the use of apps, online interactions or video-consultation. For our learners there is a risk that they make assumptions about the digital literacy of patients, based on their own situation or understanding, that further widen these inequalities.

RISK OF 'DIGITAL MISMATCH'

- Learners may make assumptions about prior knowledge, without checking a patient's understanding about their use of technology.
- They may over- or under-estimate an individual patient's skill level or ability to engage. They need to be reminded to observe how the patient uses a device.
- They may not take into account whether the patient can afford or trusts healthcare technology; they need to practise a form of words that enables them to tactfully explore this.

DOI: 10.1201/9781003352532-16

Role play and the use of simulated patients can help learners address these areas. Patients as educators can be a very powerful way to explore barriers to understanding and raise awareness in our learners of how to involve patients in their own care and discussions about digital technology.

The Topol Review covered how:

> Technological and other developments (including genomics, artificial intelligence, digital medicine and robotics) are likely to change the roles and functions of clinical staff in all professions over the next two decades to ensure safer, more productive, more effective and more personal care for patients.
>
> *(Topol 2019)*

It looked at the implications of these changes for the skills, training, development and lifelong learning of current and future staff in the NHS.

Preparing the healthcare workforce to deliver the digital future will require that such adoption of technology enabled care services:

- Is patient-centred
- Has clinical validation
- Enables and empowers a patient to choose to opt in
- Retains the elements of trust, clinical presence, empathy and communication in virtual delivery of clinical care
- Cultivates a cross-disciplinary approach in the delivery of digitally enabled care

SUPPORTING LEARNERS TO BECOME COMPETENT IN DIGITAL DELIVERY OF CARE

To be digitally ready a practitioner needs to be willing and able to use, and have ready access to, suitable technology devices underpinned by their organisation's up to date technology support and service delivery (Chambers et al. 2018). For example, each practitioner conducting a non-face-to-face consultation with a service user is responsible for ensuring that the mode and quality of the digital delivery for that consultation is of sufficient standard and scope for safe practice in relation to the patient's health and care needs. If not, they should discontinue the consultation and arrange an appropriate mode of clinical consultation to be delivered by themselves or another practitioner in a safe timescale.

All practitioners delivering digital modes of health and care need to have the 7Cs to be able to apply and implement their knowledge of digital delivery of care in their frontline setting (see Box 14.1).

BOX 14.1 THE 7 'CS' RELATING TO TECHNOLOGY-ENABLED DELIVERY OF CARE

1. **Competence:** personal ability to use a range of digital delivery modes for agreed purposes, including feeding-in information/acting on advice, adhering to information and clinical governance requirements.

2. **Capability:** adopt best practice in the use of a range of digital delivery modes for agreed purposes.

3. **Capacity:** have protected and prioritised time for initiating and participating in remote delivery of care that is regarded as a key element of the workrole, and the IT infrastructure and equipment is available and easily accessed by all service providers and users.

4. **Confidence:** confident that organisational infrastructure is in place in line with code of practice, including reliability and validity of equipment and its outputs. Patient/carer/citizen confident that usage of technology is an integral part of clinical best practice as agreed with clinician, and that their responsible practitioner will access/act on relay of online messages or interchanges.

5. **Creativity:** able to adopt and adapt agreed modes of digital delivery of care for different purpose or patient/carer group in line with their code of practice.

6. **Communication:** sharing and dissemination of digital modes of delivery and associated clinical protocols; evaluation of applications/outcomes/challenges, etc. with a team or organisation; working together and sharing what has worked well and what has not worked so well.

7. **Continuity:** is able to interact via a selected digital mode of delivery along one pathway for management of specific long-term condition(s)/lifestyle habit(s) in line with the agreed shared care management plan with the patient.

Source: Chambers et al. (2018).

There are a variety of digital learning platforms, including several endorsed by the health service such as eLearning For Health (eLFH), where free, online learning can be accessed 24 hours a day for updating and upskilling by individual health professionals (HEE, e-Learning for Healthcare 2022).

Social media

The use of social media is now a fact of life, but it is not without risk. A good example of the use of social media by a clinician is the creation of a closed Facebook group set up for patients with a long term condition by the practitioner, or their organisation.

The clinician must understand that no confidential information about any individual patient(s) should be uploaded on any social media site set up that is managed by a health professional; this includes identity, personal life, health or circumstances. Any educational material posted on such a site should be generic and in the best interests of service users with no commercial component.

Learners should be reminded that posting about patients on social media is effectively the same as discussing them in a public place: 'You are still a doctor or a medical student on social media' (BMA 2018). The BMA has published a series of guidance documents for doctors and medical students on the use of social media (BMA 2021).

Remote consulting

Telephone consultations

The learner needs to ensure that a reliable clinical assessment of a patient can be made via the telephone when the patient or their carer describes their health problem or concern. If there is any doubt after taking a full history, the patient needs to be brought in for a face-to-face review and examination.

Tips for an effective telephone conversation between a health or care professional and patient are given in Table 14.1.

Potential benefits: immediate access to care, easier and more convenient access, opportunities to empower patients to self care and improve their compliance with treatment, may avoid need for face-to-face consultation, which has cost savings (e.g. savings on travel time and costs for patient/carer/clinician), allows prioritisation of delivery of care.

TABLE 14.1 Steps to Take for Conducting a Successful Telephone Consultation

Before consultation	*Make sure that you are aware of the case background, including the patient's current medications and ongoing care.*
During consultation	*Confirm the patient's identity. Introduce yourself clearly.* *Check this is a good time, that you cannot be overheard by a third party.* *Set a time limit (e.g. ten minutes).* *Discuss the patient's current condition(s), their concerns, take a careful history and follow this by clear direct questions that address the purpose of the consultation.* *Agree and confirm the management plan(s); check patient understands and agrees with plan.* *Agree an appropriate follow-up arrangement.*
After the consultation	*Write up the notes of the consultation in the patient's medical file in the same was as usual.* *Ensure you record it was a telephone consultation.*

Potential risks: a telephone consultation may not allow a full assessment of the patient and thus miss the real problem. The clinician might make assumptions – for instance, that the patient understands the information that they relay; lack of visual clues, facial expressions and postures might lead to clinician uncertainty or inappropriate outcomes; reliance on the telephone caller (their comprehension of their symptoms and signs/memory/communication skills). The clinician has to use 'active listening' skills, and concentrate on the conversation to appreciate the patient's tone of voice, their inferences used, and what information is emphasised. They might not appreciate the hesitancy or agitation, for example, at the patient's end.

Telephone contact can also be used as initial contact to triage or prioritise patient contact. Depending on an initial history, the consultation can be handed on to the appropriate member of the multidisciplinary team to enhance service provision and optimal use of resources.

Running a video consultation

The video consultation provides additional visual aids to gauge a patient's signs and discuss their symptoms (Greenhalgh et al. 2022).

Written explicit patient consent is no longer required – their consent is implied by them accepting the invite and entering the consultation. The clinician must safeguard personal or confidential patient information as they would for any other type of consultation. If a practitioner is running the video consultation from home, they can use their own device for video consultations and mobile messaging. They should be able to access the electronic patient record on a password protected device, using secure channels that use encryption, and not storing personal or confidential patient information on the device unless absolutely necessary. All data must be transferred from the remote consultation to the patient's medical record as soon as is practicable.

The video consultation must still be conducted with usual delivery by a trusted clinician, in a private location with a good professional approach – dressed for work with no distractions in the background. You need to check the identity of the patient and run the consultation from greeting to wrapping up as you'd usually do if sitting in your practice or other healthcare setting with a face-to-face consultation. If the video consultation is between a clinician and patient in a nursing or residential home, the carer may have been able to take biometric measurements of the patient prior to the video call, or during it, by arrangement: e.g. BP, temperature, weight, oxygen saturation, pulse rate, blood glucose, sputum colour, peak flow.

Some example selection criteria for appropriate and safe mode of clinical consultation

The following list identifies inclusion and exclusion criteria proposed for patients who might consult remotely via a video link between doctor/nurse and a patient in their own home or chosen setting, or Nursing/Care Home:

Inclusion criteria:

- Children aged between 13–15 years with parental consent
- 16 years of age and above
- Routine review by practice nurse or GP of any chronic health condition or adverse lifestyle habit, e.g. smoking
- Medication review
- Low risk patients requesting a consultation for any symptom

Exclusion criteria:

- Children aged 12 years and under (unless has responsible parental consent and presence)
- Acute deterioration of chronic health conditions or a person's wellbeing
- Any condition requiring face-to-face, hands on clinical assessment or clinical examination
- Intermediate to high risk patients for specific symptoms
- Someone who is distinctly unwell, has raised temperature (and for instance will need clinical assessment of heart/lungs)
- High risk patients where it is not possible to monitor vital signs

So video consultations for clinical delivery of care should focus on situations where this mode of care has clear advantages – such as strong patient or clinician preference, remote locality so travel difficult, out-of-hours services and nursing or care homes. Despite the national policy enthusiasm for digital healthcare, the number of general practice appointments conducted via video consultation has remained low at fewer than 0.5% of general practice consultations as of December 2021 (Greenhalgh et al. 2022). In this review, the majority of clinicians and patients considered that telephone was adequate for most remote consultations, and if a hands-on physical examination was required, they would prefer it to be in-person. Staff attitudes are often affected by their own lack of technical competence and confidence, experience and knowledge of technology-enabled care, their perceptions of quality and risk and lack of role models.

Distinguishing between high and low risk patients for online consulting (risk based on potential significance of the presenting complaint given their past medical history or description of their symptoms):

TABLE 14.2 Exclusion and inclusion criteria when consulting remotely

Low risk	Intermediate risk	High risk
0–2 comorbidities; comorbidities that are present must be of low significance in terms of patient longevity, e.g. osteoarthritis, acne	≥ 3 comorbidities of any significance Comorbidities present should not be directly related to presenting complaint	≥ 3 comorbidities of any significance Comorbidities that could be related to presenting complaint Current or previous diagnosis of cancer Age >90 years Poor mobility Dementia

DIGITAL MATURITY IN THE HOSPITAL TRUST, GENERAL PRACTICE, CARE ORGANISATION

Following advances made through the requirements of the COVID-19 pandemic, there is increasing connectivity of technology-enabled care services in the wider health and social care services. There is still a way to go to completely enable all health and care services in the wider health economy to be linked, for example, via integrated care records. However, joint working empowering patients to take more responsibility for own care, with agreed shared management plans, is increasing. Training may be needed to ensure all healthcare professionals are aware of local protocols and are familiar with the new digital infrastructure. It is particularly important to ensure induction programmes and mandatory online learning cover these aspects.

Nowadays GP practices must offer their registered patients (and their carers if appropriate) a range of modes of digital consultation as a standard service. Consultations should be matched to patient preferences and clinical need. They must also have an accessible online presence, such as a website, that links to an online consultation system and other online services such as to request prescriptions or book online appointments, signposting to a validated symptom checker and self-care health information and shared medical record access.

ENHANCING PATIENT SELF-CARE VIA DIGITAL MEANS

Wearable technology

Wearable devices integrate sensors that gather data about a person's activity or other aspects of their health into a device that they carry or wear. Some products display data for that person on their device; others send the information elsewhere as a form of telecare, for analysis centrally.

If you are teaching a patient about wearable technology, chances are you will need to teach yourself first. The reliability of a device, its limitations as well as benefits will vary from one machine to another.

Assistive technology

Assistive technology includes any device or system that allows a person to perform a task that they would otherwise be unable to do, or increases the ease and safety with which they can perform the task. So this might include substantial equipment like stair lifts or clever technology like exit sensors that can detect if a vulnerable person leaves their home. This presents a good opportunity for inter-disciplinary learning; workshops with occupational therapists and physiotherapists can help learners to become familiar with what is available and which patients might benefit.

GUIDANCE FROM NATIONAL ORGANISATIONS

General Medical Council (GMC)

The GMC expects that all doctors who are delivering telemedicine or other remote modes of delivery of care meet recognised UK standards of practice. The standards expected of doctors communicating with patients via social media, telephone or email are no different than those applied to face-to-face consultations (e.g. confidentiality, maintaining professional boundaries) (GMC 2022).

Nursing and Midwifery Council (NMC)

Nurses must use all forms of spoken, written and digital communication responsibly – so that includes social media and networking sites. The NMC instructs nurses to stay objective and have clear professional boundaries at all times with people in their care, especially with the use of social media (NMC 2022).

CONCLUSION

The rapid pace of change in technology-enabled care means that we as educational supervisors or mentors are likely to be just as new to the field as our learners (if not lagging far behind!). Demonstrating that we don't always know the answers, and jointly engaging with learning with our learners, or suggesting they teach us, is a very positive opportunity for role modelling the importance of life-long learning.

REFERENCES

British Medical Association (BMA) (2018) Social media, ethics and professionalism. Available at www.bma.org.uk/media/1851/bma-ethics-guidance-on-social-media-2018.pdf (Accessed 10.5.22).

British Medical Association (BMA) (2021) Ethics of social media use. Available at www.bma.org.uk/advice-and-support/ethics/personal-ethics/ethics-of-social-media-use (Accessed 10.5.22).

Chambers R., Schmid M., and Al Jabbouri A. (2018) *Making digital healthcare happen in practice. A practical handbook*. Oxford: Otmoor Publishing.

General Medical Council (GMC) (2022) Available at www.gmc-uk.org/ethical-guidance/ethical-hub/remote-consultations (Accessed 11.5.22).

Greenhalgh T., Ladds E., Hughes G., et al. (2022) Why do GPs rarely do video consultations? *British Journal of General Practice*. https://doi.org/10.3399/BJGP.2021.0658.

Health Education for England (HEE), e-Learning for Healthcare (2022) Available at https://portal.e-lfh.org.uk.

Nursing & Midwifery Council (NMC) (2022) Available at www.nmc.org.uk/standards/code/ (Accessed 11.5.22).

Topol E. (2019) *The topol review. Preparing the healthcare workforce to deliver the digital future*. Health Education England. Available at https://topol.hee.nhs.uk.

SECTION 3

For healthcare educators making
and reporting judgements that
capture, guide and make decisions
about the achievement of learners,
and the feedback required

CHAPTER 15

Feedback

....

Feedback is a very important concept in education, and has long been recognised to make or break any educational activity: 'Feedback, or knowledge of results, is the lifeblood of learning' (Rowntree 1982). It is considered 'constructive' when suggestions for improvement are given without damaging morale.

Concern about the standard of clinical teaching across UK, American and Australian hospitals in the past led to a review of clinical teaching (SCOPME 1992). Claims had been made that teaching included humiliation and ritual sarcasm, was variable, unpredictable and gave virtually no feedback; assessment was haphazard and supervision was poor.

Subsequently, nursing and midwifery research throughout the 1990s, similarly, also showed that feedback was handled poorly or, worse, was not carried out at all. Consider the following quote from a nursing assessor:

> I shy away from having to give criticism. I'll always go to great lengths not to give criticism. . . . I'll always highlight the positive aspects and tend not to go into many details if the student isn't doing terribly well in certain areas.
>
> *(Bailey 1998)*

Research has highlighted the importance of feedback being perceived as constructive. 'Giving feedback constructively' was the top theme chosen by 441 junior and senior doctors when asked what they thought should be the key content of 'Teaching the Teachers' courses (Wall and McAleer 2000).

GIVING CONSTRUCTIVE FEEDBACK: SOME EVIDENCE THAT IT WORKS

Does it work? Is there evidence that giving constructive feedback improves learning? In short, the answer has been known for some time to be yes. Constructive feedback

DOI: 10.1201/9781003352532-18

can improve learning outcomes and enable learners to develop a deep (rather than superficial) approach to their learning with the active pursuit of understanding and application of knowledge. It can improve competence at least in the short term (Rolfe and McPherson 1995). Giving constructive feedback does produce significantly better learning outcomes.

WHAT TO AVOID IN FEEDBACK

Some teachers struggle to find the balance between giving 'feedback with teeth' – that is, feedback containing enough specific examples of where performance needs to be improved (sometimes, confusingly, called negative feedback), and doing it in a negative or unhelpful way. You may hear teachers say that in a situation where time is short, it is better just to focus on aspects that the learner needs to improve on, without seeming to realise that this approach, and being encouraging in tone, are not mutually exclusive. The risk of not using feedback to highlight aspects that are going well however is that these are lost to the learner, who may not realise she has these positive aspects to her practice, which they can build on. A positive, supportive tone enables the supervisor to engage with the learner to continue the educational conversation, and the identification of areas of good practice promotes morale and focus on good practice.

Many well-trained teachers know the principles of giving constructive feedback. However, they may slip back into giving negative feedback when time is short or they themselves feel under pressure, with potentially disastrous results on learner wellbeing and performance.

It is also important to highlight the benefit of timely feedback at 'teachable moments':

> performance cannot improve without knowledge of what was wrong, and there will come a time when it may be too late to give critical feedback – the learning opportunity may be lost and the behaviour entrenched.
>
> *(Stuart 2003)*

There is also some evidence that the particular characteristics of learners that are highlighted in feedback can also impact their future learning. An individual's perception of their own ability can play a key role in their motivation and achievement, so if feedback focuses on the potential for development and improvement, achievement can be boosted. Dweck and colleagues have shown that learners who believed their intelligence could be developed (a growth mindset) outperformed those who believed their intelligence was fixed (a fixed mindset) (Dweck 2006).

CONSTRUCTIVE FEEDBACK

Having realised the potential in a teachable moment, when an opportunity to pause and enhance learning presents itself, educational supervisors and mentors need to

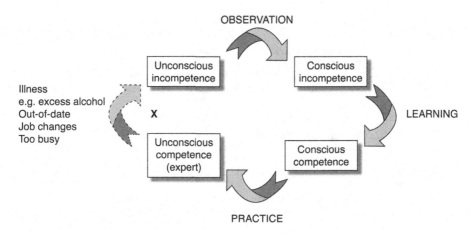

FIGURE 15.1 Development of competence.

find the balance: as well as being positive in tone, there should be a balance between comment on areas where improvement is needed and feedback that is positive in content. You should give feedback about both deficiencies and strengths to assist your learners to develop expertise (see Figure 15.1).

Starting in the top left-hand quadrant in Figure 15.1, learners are blissfully unaware of their shortcomings until something happens to highlight them. It could be a patient complaint or an adverse incident, or it could be feedback from a teacher.

This realisation is painful, and is often referred to as cognitive dissonance – the gap between how you understood things to be and the reality. However, until learners are aware, they cannot start the process of learning. You might inform learners that often when they feel most uncomfortable, they are just about to learn something.

However, too much discomfort can be demotivating, and some learners might give up at this stage if they feel that there is too much to learn or that they will never be good enough. Providing feedback about their strengths will undoubtedly be supportive at this stage.

The process of learning can then proceed to master the new understanding, knowledge or task. The learner reaches a stage where they know something new or know how to do something and can competently perform it, so long as circumstances remain constant (see the bottom right quadrant of Figure 15.1). With practice and experience, learners become expert and can apply and modify their knowledge and skills in new situations. At this stage (bottom left quadrant), learners can teach others. It is also the stage when, through familiarity, learners can lose sight of their strengths, as skills become automatic. Feedback on performance at this stage must include strengths so that learners do not accept them as commonplace, and so that they reflect on them, keep them up to date and highlight them. In some ways, feedback should take learners from left to right across the bottom of the competency cycle to ensure that they are aware of their expertise so that they can effectively teach others.

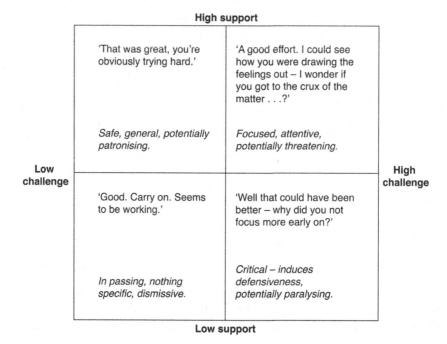

FIGURE 15.2 Support and challenge in feedback.

It is possible to move back to unconscious incompetence from the position of expertise, in the direction of arrow X, through, for example, dementing illness, degenerative disease without insight, and failure to keep up to date. Feedback in this position is difficult, which is another good reason to include a reminder of remaining skills and positive attributes. (This model has some similarities with the Johari window, which describes balanced communication between feedback seeking and self-disclosure to minimise either the areas of hidden information in a relationship or lack of insight; see Chapter 19.)

This model provides a theoretical reason why constructive feedback must contain a commentary on strengths as well as areas for improvement. It also reinforces the imperative for feedback to 'have teeth'. The skill of the effective teacher is to find the balance between support and challenge (see Figure 15.2). The best feedback is high in both.

METHODS OF GIVING CONSTRUCTIVE FEEDBACK

Good feedback focuses on descriptions, not judgements, and Table 15.1 shows some examples of giving feedback that distinguishes between the two:

TABLE 15.1 Examples of Feedback

Evaluative, interpretive or judgemental	Descriptive, sensory-based
The beginning was awful, you just seemed to ignore her.	*At the start you were looking at the notes, which prevented eye contact.*
The beginning was excellent, great stuff.	*At the beginning you gave her your full attention and never lost eye contact – your facial expression registered interest in what she was saying.*
It's no good getting embarrassed when patients talk about their sexual history.	*I noticed you were very flushed when she spoke about her husband's impotence, and you lost eye contact.*

Here are some rules to consider and some models of feedback that will help you to do this in a structured way. Four examples are given, but you will be able to find or devise more. Just remember one golden rule – give positive praise for things that have been done well first. The four examples are:

- Pendleton's rules
- The SCOPME model for giving feedback
- The Chicago model
- The six-step problem-solving model

PENDLETON'S RULES

This model provides a useful set of general principles to be used in giving feedback after all kinds of activities, including practical skills, consultations, case presentations, etc. It is a step-by-step model, in which each step is important and should be performed sequentially (Pendleton et al. 1984).

1. The learner performs the activity.
2. Questions are allowed only on points of clarification of fact.
3. The learner says what they thought was done well.
4. The teacher says what they thought was done well.
5. The learner says what was not done so well and could be improved upon.
6. The teacher says what was not done so well and makes suggestions for improvement with discussion in a supportive manner.

This is useful for formal situations, with learners who do not like feedback (e.g. those who are nervous), when the learner lacks insight and to encourage learners to identify the good points of their performance.

THE SCOPME MODEL

This model is not the most simple or clear cut, but it does follow the same principles in order to give constructive feedback (SCOPME 1996):

1. Listen to the learner.
2. Reflect back – for further clarification.
3. Support.
4. Counsel.
5. Treat information in confidence.
6. Inform – without censuring.
7. Judge constructively.
8. Identify educational needs.
9. Construct and negotiate achievable learning plans.

The Chicago model

The 'Chicago' model is similar to the other models but has the great advantage of starting with a reminder of the aims and objectives that the learner is supposed to be addressing. It has six steps (Brukner et al. 1999).

1. Review the aims and objectives of the job at the start.
2. Give interim feedback of a positive nature.
3. Ask the learner to give their self-appraisal of their performance to you.
4. Give feedback focusing on behaviour rather than on personality (e.g. what actually happened, sticking to the facts, not your opinions).
5. Give specific examples to illustrate your views.
6. Suggest specific strategies for the learner to improve their performance.

A six-step problem-solving model

This model seeks agreement between two individuals to solve problems, agree goals, aims and objectives, and so on. It depends on negotiations between two people who come to an agreement at two stages in the model. The six steps are as follows:

1. Problem is presented.
2. Problem is discussed.
3. Problem is agreed.
4. Solution is proposed.
5. Solution is discussed.
6. Solution is agreed.

As well as agreeing educational aims at the beginning of a job, you may find other uses for this model. For example, when things have gone wrong it can help you to decide exactly why this happened and where the difficulty lies.

Feedback about unacceptable behaviour

If you need to give feedback to someone whose behaviour is completely unacceptable, there are ways of delivering the information and still maintaining a relationship that will enable you to continue to work together and support that learner. Consider the following tips:

- Make sure that the person is in the right frame of mind to receive feedback (e.g. not tired after a night on-call) before you start.
- Use a 'wake-up', warning phrase.
- State very simply what is not right.
- Give an example, if necessary.
- Relax the tone to allow for a positive response (usually an offer to improve ensues).
- Respond to the offer positively, but define specific measurable outcomes.
- Do not be drawn into discussion on justification of behaviour or your right to judge.
- If there is complete rejection, seek help (e.g. from your peers or line manager).

The conversation might sound something like this one:

> Morning John, I hope the on-call was not too busy? I saw Mrs Smith yesterday, she said to thank you for those new tablets, and they've done her the world of good. . . . John, there is something very serious that I have to bring up in our session today . . . I am worried that you are drinking alcohol too heavily and I would like to talk about why that is. . . . Yesterday when we spoke after evening surgery I could smell alcohol on your breath, and you were slurring your words. I had the same impression at lunchtime the day before, but was not sure. . . . Is this something I can help you with? . . . I am glad you plan to cut down, how about if we agree that you will not drink during the working day, and not at all if you are on call? . . . I am afraid we cannot debate this, you need to address it or you will not be able to work here. . . . Then I must ask you to take a fortnight's leave until I can take advice from the deanery about this.

Or:

> I am afraid we cannot debate this, you need to address it or you will not be able to work here. . . . Excellent, let's have another chat about it on Thursday and we can see how it's going. In the mean time, shall we meet at lunchtime to look at that audit? It's coming on really well.

There is also the need to consider professional help here. This should be the general practitioner of the doctor concerned, and possibly a consultant in occupational medicine. You must not become your learners' medical practitioner.

MULTI-SOURCE FEEDBACK (MSF OR 360 DEGREE ASSESSMENT)

MSF is a structured way of gathering feedback from people with different perspectives about a learner or a colleague. Several team members will be asked to complete an anonymous feedback form, and the educational supervisor is usually the one to sit down and handover the findings personally. Chapter 17 looks at the use and research behind MSF in more depth, but here we focus on its use to give feedback.

ACTING ON MSF RESULTS

Be positive and constructive. For most people, even those with problems, there will be some good comments. Box 15.2 gives an example set of comments from a real MSF, organised under headings from the UK NHS appraisal format.

BOX 15.2 MAINTAINING TRUST/PROFESSIONAL RELATIONSHIPS WITH PATIENTS

- He needs to take time to develop a good rapport with patients.
- Always polite and listens to patients.
- Poor listener – gives the impression he is not listening at times.
- Takes time to communicate with patients' relatives, but often uses jargon few can understand.
- Always polite and caring.
- He has gained in confidence in recent months and has become more aware of the patients' needs, and spends time talking to them and trying hard to understand what the patients want – to understand the problem in simple terms.
- Always polite, and treats both staff and patients with dignity. I have been *****'s consultant for the last six months; I have tried hard to get him to interact with patients with a more caring attitude and behaviour. He is trying hard I think!
- Good with patients, but some find the accent difficult. One patient commented that she needed an interpreter.

Verbal communication skills

- Speaks with a heavy accent – difficult for some to understand.
- Good English sometimes – but speaks very quickly at times and difficult to understand.
- Good communication skills at times – but not consistently.
- Good English always – understandable when giving information.
- Problems speaking to patients' relatives; speaks in tone and pace they find difficult to understand, and uses jargon.

The comments in Box 15.2 reveal problems both with communication with patients and in terms of being a poor listener, using jargon and speaking too quickly. However, there are good comments as well, and this learner seems to be trying hard to improve. This reinforces the fact that a 360-degree feedback will take views from people with a variety of experiences with this learner and from different perspectives.

When giving feedback, sit down in private with your learner and show them the results. Use one of the models mentioned for giving constructive feedback.

Using the example in Box 15.2, we might start with being a polite and caring doctor and making improvements. There are still areas to be improved on, however, including speaking too quickly, using jargon, and the learner's accent. When discussing these areas, emphasise that much of this can be improved upon with good communication skills training and feedback. Explain how this may be accessed and how you will reassess the learner to measure their progress. You need to jointly negotiate a clear action plan and be sure to follow it up.

In another individual, accessibility was one of the problems (see Box 15.3). Comments included statements about being late and being difficult to find when on call.

BOX 15.3 ACCESSIBILITY

- Sometimes difficult to find when on call.
- Takes proper responsibility. Always willing to help when asked.
- Always attentive to his job, responds when called.
- Responds when called, but is often too willing to make decisions on his own without asking advice.
- No problems – some difficulties with other supervising consultants, but I have always found him to be accessible and well organised.
- Often late for clinics.

Again, the comments in Box 15.3 highlight some good points, but there are also serious problems which need to be fed back unambiguously so the learner understands clearly where the issues have been identified. Perhaps underlying difficulties account for these problems, and just as in clinical practice, any intervention can only follow an accurate diagnosis (see Chapter 17).

Your feedback must then highlight exactly what you expect, in terms of accessibility and turning up on time, and the sanctions for not following these expectations. You may set ground rules, such as the following:

1. Ground rule
   E.g. Punctuality and accessibility are very important when working here.

2. Spell out what you expect.
   - *We start at 8 am with the first patient booked.*
   - *When you are the on-call doctor, you must be available and here in the building and contactable.*
   - *You need to be here by 7.50 am and ready to start for the 8 am appointment.*
3. Monitor what actually happens.
4. If your expectations are not met, spell out the sanctions.
5. Measurement and feedback are the key strategies here.

Create and agree a plan with the learner. Explain the improvements required and the reasons underlying these. Highlight your standards, outline what you expect and write it all down. It is essential to check what is happening – to measure it and to feed it back to the learner.

TEACHING TEACHERS HOW TO GIVE CONSTRUCTIVE FEEDBACK

You can best learn how to give effective feedback through practice. Sometimes structured models feel artificial and unhelpful until you develop a language and series of phrases to help. It is also useful to seek and then reflect on feedback given to you by others, and to think about helpful aspects of what was said and the aspects that hindered you from improving your performance.

You could do this in several ways. Training courses that focus on developing feedback skills sometimes require participants to bring a practical skill to teach to another colleague, to give a five-minute lecture on a non-medical subject, or to appraise a trainee in a role-play situation using a prepared case scenario. In all of these settings, the teachers are watched by their colleagues and feedback is given at the end of the activity. It is especially useful for the person who is role-playing the trainee to give feedback. Sometimes colleagues launch straight into criticism of faults and need to be reminded that they must state good points first, and only later discuss points which need to be improved, in a helpful and constructive way. One drawback of these exercises is that participants can get lost in the content and forget to talk about the process. Facilitators need to draw the discussion back to how the teaching was done so that observers can hone their feedback skills.

FEED-FORWARD

One fundamental principle of good feedback is that it should also feed-forward so that it can be used to inform future work. Phrases in your feedback to learners such as 'what can you take from this to improve things next time?' are feeding forward. The truly formative aspect of feedback is enhanced when (after sufficient comment on what *has* happened) we turn our attention to what *could* happen.

An increased understanding of the importance of including feedback on people's strengths and how to give feedback constructively using one of the models available will improve the educational climate in your organisation. This can improve the learning outcomes, as well as the competence and motivation of your learners.

REFERENCES

Bailey J. (1998) The supervisor's story: From expert to novice. In Johns C. and Freshwater D. (eds) *Transforming nursing through reflective practice*. London: Blackwell Science.

Brukner H., Altkorn D.L., Cook S., et al. (1999) Giving effective feedback to medical students: A workshop for faculty and house staff. *Medical Teacher*, 21: 161–165.

Coles C. (1993) Developing medical education. *Postgraduate Medical Journal*, 69: 57–63.

Dweck C.S. (2006) *Mindset: The new psychology of success*. New York: Random House.

Pendleton D., Schofield T., Tate P., et al. (1984) *The consultation: An approach to teaching and learning*. Oxford: Oxford Medical Publications.

Rolfe I. and McPherson J. (1995) Formative assessment: How am I doing? *Lancet*, 345: 37–39.

Rowntree D. (1982) *Educational technology in curriculum development*. 2nd edn. London: Paul Chapman Publishing.

Standing Committee on Postgraduate Medical and Dental Education (SCOPME) (1992) *Teaching hospital doctors and dentists to teach: Its role in creating a better learning environment*. London: Standing Committee on Postgraduate Medical and Dental Education.

Standing Committee on Postgraduate Medical and Dental Education (SCOPME) (1996) *Appraising doctors and dentists in training*. London: Standing Committee on Postgraduate Medical and Dental Education.

Stuart C. (2003) *Assessment, supervision and support in clinical practice: A guide for nurses, midwives and other health professionals*. Edinburgh: Churchill Livingstone.

Wall D. and McAleer S. (2000) Teaching the consultant teachers – Identifying the core content. *Medical Education*, 34: 131–138.

CHAPTER 16

Assessment

....

Assessment can be a hurdle to be passed in order to allow the learner to progress to the next stage. This pass or fail assessment is known as summative assessment, in that it sums up achievement from a period of learning. This is distinguished from formative assessment, which informs the learner of their achievements as they go along, giving feedback, highlighting progress and identifying areas for further development, while there is time for further development and learning.

The ideal assessment or gold standard is probably not achievable in real life, but certain principles can help to make assessments as fair as possible. The 'ideal' assessment should be:

- *Valid:* it measures what it is supposed to measure (if it has face validity as well, it also appears to the learner as if it is measuring what it purports to measure)
- *Reliable:* it measures it with essentially the same result each time (learners with the same level of performance will be judged equally regardless of who administers the assessment)
- *Practicable:* it is easy to perform in terms of cost, time and skills of the assessors
- *Fair to the learners and the teachers:* for example, differences between learners which are irrelevant to the subject that is being assessed do not affect the result; marking is not unnecessarily burdensome for teachers
- *Useful to the learners and the teachers:* for example, it discriminates between good and poor candidates
- *Acceptable:* in terms of, for example, cultural and gender issues
- *Appropriate:* to what has been taught and learned on the programme

DOI: 10.1201/9781003352532-19

ASSESSMENT IN THE EDUCATIONAL CYCLE

The educational cycle (see Chapter 7) reminds us of the importance of alignment in setting assessments mapped to learning objectives. A four-step model may be useful:

1. Identify needs
2. Set objectives
3. Decide methods
4. Design assessment

Having identified learning needs, objectives and methods of teaching are set and assessment tool(s) are designed early on. In this way both you and your learner will be clear about what you are working towards and what to expect. You will then have an aligned way to test the learner at the end to establish whether they have achieved the objectives.

LINKING AIMS AND OBJECTIVES WITH ASSESSMENT

Curriculum development (see Chapter 5) is an essential first step in designing an assessment tool. From the curriculum, the aims and objectives, as well as teaching and learning methods should flow.

In day to day language, 'aims' and 'objectives' are synonymous – they are 'those things that we work towards'. However, in education these have specific and different meanings.

Aims are broad statements of intent. For example, you might aim to produce a competent nurse or an effective healthcare teacher. Aims specify the broad direction in which you want your learner to go, but they do not specify how far they have to go, how they will get there, or how they will know when they are there.

Objectives are outcome measures and are specific statements addressed at aspects of the aim. They are usually written in terms of what the learner will be able to do at the end of the course of study. For example, 'At the end of this post the nurse will be able to apply a dressing using a sterile technique' or 'at the end of this course the learner will be able to put the examination results into the statistics programme SPSS and calculate Cronbach's alpha' (see Section 16.19).

Objectives usually specifically describe desirable outcomes, so we can see clearly what our assessment tool needs to be able to measure. They may be subdivided even further into highly specific steps in each of the activities to be learned. Writing objectives is crucial to the effectiveness of the teaching process to help to focus your curriculum design as well as for assessing learners. It is not uncommon for people to set out to teach without having a clear idea in mind of exactly what they are hoping to achieve.

Consider, for example, a decision to run a tutorial on Lyme disease. Without clear objectives it is impossible to choose the most appropriate teaching method, to know what content can be omitted, to be sure whether the teaching has worked or to know how to evaluate it. From the learner's perspective, clear objectives, framed as learning outcomes, help them to decide whether a course of study is for them and will suit their learning needs, help plan their study, choose what aspects to go into in depth and how to prepare for assessments. A tutorial on Lyme disease might focus on the clinical presentations, the importance of early diagnosis and the NICE guidance on Lyme disease. Or it might focus on the incidence and epidemiology of the condition and control of insect vectors; a very different tutorial.

Objectives are usually written in behavioural terms – that is, a statement of what the satisfactory learner will be able to do at the end of the period of study. These outcomes need to be as specific as we can make them, and one way to do that is to pay attention to the verbs you use. If you set a behavioural task in the objective such as to be able to list (testing recall), categorise (testing ability to differentiate) and rank (testing ability to prioritise), you are testing learners' understanding. But the choice of specific verbs is also guiding them on how to demonstrate it and helping you to assess it.

THE DOMAINS OF LEARNING

In one of the earliest attempts to produce a systematic classification of the types of learning, Bloom led a team of educationalists to devise Bloom's taxonomy (Bloom 1956). He divided the three areas of learning into the following:

- The cognitive domain (pertaining to intellectual processes)
- The psychomotor domain (processes of physical skills)
- The affective domain (attitudinal and emotional processes)

More simply this may be thought of as knowledge, skills and attitudes.

A taxonomy is a hierarchical and orderly classification in which each stage builds on the one below. For example, each domain, proceeding from the simple to the complex, can be subdivided and the levels specifically described.

To be clear about what you are asking your learners to do, you need to consider which domain you are assessing and at which level – hence the importance of the wording of the objectives.

The knowledge domain

- Knowledge
- Comprehension
- Application
- Analysis
- Synthesis
- Evaluation

The skills domain

- Observation
- Imitation
- Practising
- Mastering
- Adapting

The attitudes domain

- Receiving (listening)
- Responding
- Valuing (advocating, defending)
- Organisation
- Characterisation (judging)

In Bloom's taxonomy of the cognitive domain, each of the six levels has been described in greater detail:

Knowledge: the remembering (recalling) of appropriate previously learned information.

Comprehension: grasping (understanding) the meaning of informational materials.

Application: the use of previously learned information in new and concrete situations to solve problems that have single or best answers.

Analysis: breaking down informational materials into their component parts, examining (and trying to understand the organisational structure of) such information to develop divergent conclusions by identifying motives or causes, making inferences and/or finding evidence to support generalisations.

Synthesis: creatively or divergently applying prior knowledge and skills to produce a new or original whole.

Evaluation: judging the value of material based on personal values/opinions, resulting in an end product with a given purpose, without real right or wrong answers.

MILLER'S PYRAMID

George Miller described a pyramid of outcomes that help categorise methods of assessment in healthcare (Miller 1990). These are:

- Knowledge (knows)
- Understanding (knows how)
- Competence (shows how)
- Performance (does)

Assessments based on observation in the work setting are represented by competence and performance assessments at the highest level of Miller's Pyramid: 'does'. Miller differentiated between an assessment in an artificial situation (such as in a clinical skills lab) 'shows how', and being assessed in real life clinical situations.

A common mistake is to mismatch the domain or the level and the assessment tool to be used. For example, assessment of practical resuscitation skills (competence) will be less successful if learners are asked to write an essay (declarative knowledge) than if a mock scenario is arranged. Similarly, asking candidates at interview to give a lecture presentation on a specific topic (declarative knowledge) is not the best way to assess communication skills (performance) with patients and colleagues.

As a guide, one way of aligning assessment choices with level of learning might be as follows:

Knowledge (Knows)	Multiple choice questions
Understanding (Knows How)	Case scenarios
Competence (Shows How)	Simulations
Performance (Does)	Workplace based assessments, multi-source feedback

A typical simulation to test competence is an OSCE – an objective structured clinical examination which usually consists of a series of tasks to be completed in a circuit of stations.

PROGRESSION FROM NOVICE TO EXPERT

Dreyfus and Dreyfus's (2005) levels of competence are important here as a theoretical framework.

Level 1 – Novice: Rigid following of taught rules and plans, little situational perception and no discretionary judgement.

Level 2 – Advanced beginner: Guidelines for action used, but only after some prior experience. Situational perceptions are still limited. All attributes are treated separately and given equal weighting.

Level 3 – Competent: Able to cope with numbers of patients, and pieces of information and activities which compete for attention. There is some conscious deliberate planning. Able to use standardised and routine procedures.

Level 4 – Proficient: Able to see situations holistically. Can see and focus on what is most important in a situation. Able to see deviations from the normal presentation of situations. Decision making is more skilful and less laboured.

Level 5 – Expert: No longer relies entirely on rules, guidelines and protocols. Can grasp a situation intuitively based on deep understanding. Uses an analytical approach only in novel or unusual situations when problems arise. Has a grasp of what is possible.

The goal of all teachers is to help learners progress from novice to expert. The challenge is that some trainees seem to get stuck at level 2 – the advanced beginner. Whether from lack of confidence or fear of repercussions, there can be too great a reliance on 'following the protocol', whether the patient fits the protocol or not. Unusual presentations might not be recognised. Patients with more than one diagnosis at the same time also seem to be less well accommodated. Skilful selection and use of assessments can help with this transition, particularly in the use of formative assessment.

FORMATIVE ASSESSMENT

Formative assessment describes any assessment process which is specifically used to give feedback (Wood 2014). It has been defined as encompassing all those activities undertaken by teachers and/or learners which provide information to modify the teaching and learning processes. Formative assessment in healthcare education should be an active process. It should be ongoing, frequent, non-judgemental and informal. Importantly, formative assessment does not result in a pass or fail judgment. It should be a positive experience for both teachers and learners.

DOES FORMATIVE ASSESSMENT HELP THE LEARNERS? YES.

It gives specific feedback on learning, promotes self-directed learning and encourages a deeper learning and understanding. It can motivate the learner. Difficulties can be identified, and help offered in terms of remediation, whilst there is still time to improve outcomes, in terms of examination success for example. And formative assessment does improve examination performance as was shown in a large review of 250 studies by Black and Wiliam (1998). Many studies show that improved formative assessment helps the (so-called) low attainers more than the rest, and so reduces the spread of attainment whilst also raising it overall.

DOES FORMATIVE ASSESSMENT HELP THE TEACHERS? YES.

It facilitates specific feedback. It promotes self-directed learning and can help develop interactive teaching and learning methods and encourages a variety of teaching methods. It can develop teaching skills and support curriculum design and improvement.

Coaching and mentoring can be important parts of formative assessment. Coaching is training or development in which the coach supports a learner in achieving a specific personal or professional goal – so the activity lasts a short time. Mentoring is a relationship in which a more experienced colleague uses their greater knowledge and understanding of the work or workplace to support the development of a more junior or inexperienced member of staff. The relationship continues over time, sometimes for some years.

SUMMATIVE ASSESSMENT

Summative assessment is designed to discover if the learner has learned what has been intended, as a way of gatekeeping entry to the next stage of learning. It is a pass or fail assessment. Passing allows progress to the next stage, while failing means that further learning and re-assessment needs to take place. Examples in everyday life include the GCSE and A Level school exams, and the driving test. In medicine and dentistry these include examinations for degrees such as MB ChB, BDS, MD, PhD and postgraduate training qualifications such as MRCP, MRCS and MRCOG. Also end-of-year examinations and end-of-training programme examinations are summative assessments.

These are all pass or fail and indicate whether the learner is competent to be awarded the qualification, move on in the training programme or enter independent clinical practice.

REFERENCING

In order to make such judgements, summative assessments need to be referenced to a standard. A raw score is meaningless otherwise. For example, Dr A scored a mean of 2.7 for team working skills in their recent multi-source feedback. This is impossible to interpret unless we know whether 2.7 is a good score (is it out of 3, for example, where the average result is 2.5, or is it out of 10 where the average score is 7?).

Scores themselves need to refer to a standard of performance – such as a percentage of correct answers or a percentile standing in a class – or a range of marks from the top to the bottom. If we now say that the team working is based on a 1 to 7 scale where 1 is hopeless, 4 is acceptable through to 7 is excellent, then from this we can make some judgement about Dr A's performance in scoring a mean of 2.7. We may now say that the performance is not good enough. We can make a summative judgement, but we would need to know the descriptions of all the points 1 to 7 in order to help the doctor to improve.

There are two methods of referencing: norm and criterion referencing.

NORM REFERENCING

Norm referencing is when we describe the individual's performance in terms of their position in the group. The individual is judged by comparison of the marks achieved by colleagues all taking the same test. It is a common method of referencing, which ranks the students, and allows students to be compared with each other.

However, it fails to show what the student can or cannot do. It does not pinpoint strengths and weaknesses – so feedback cannot be focused on helping the student. It encourages competition rather than cooperation. This might be problematic in healthcare where fostering competition could be counter-productive in relation to working as a team.

There can also be big problems in setting a pass mark. For example, in an examination in surgery for final year medical students, all students take a ten-station OSCE. The OSCE is marked, and the marks are added up. The total marks for each student are ranked in order, with the highest marks at the top. The top 80% of students pass, and the bottom 20% fail. This is repeated each year for each cohort. What might be the problems with this? Cohorts of students vary from year to year. So in a strong year, some will fail who would pass in another year. In a poor year, some who should fail will pass, with consequences for the future.

Nevertheless, there are some situations where norm referencing is appropriate. Selection of candidates for appointment to medical school, or a training scheme – with a limited number of places – are examples where this holds true. Candidates will be ranked, and the top ones offered places. In addition, many organisations give prizes for the best performance in an examination. Some medical schools and Royal Colleges award a gold medal for the top performing individual in their examinations each year.

CRITERION REFERENCING

Criterion referencing sets out to measure a learner's abilities by placing them along a continuum. Standards of performance are set by experts using minimum levels of competence before the test is applied. Following the test there is no attempt to control the percentage passing or failing as the standards of performance are based on uncompromising pre-set objectives. Set criteria are established against which the student is judged. Assessors set the level of performance which is required. It may be minimal acceptable level or complete mastery of the task. For example, the level of performance in a paediatrics examination defined and required for a medical student will be very different than for a year eight specialty registrar (almost at consultant level).

IN CONCLUSION, WHAT SHOULD WE USE IN REFERENCING?

In the vast majority of medical education assessments, criterion referenced methods are more appropriate than their norm-referenced counterparts, as the former are based on expert judgement as to what constitutes minimal competency. Norm referenced standards *are defensible for selection decisions only.*

(De Champlain 2014)

RELIABILITY AND VALIDITY

Reliability

An assessment which is reliable is one you have faith in – one that you can trust. Reliability is *the degree to which a test consistently measures whatever it measures.* So, if you measure it again you will get essentially the same results. This is usually not a problem when measuring physical properties, such as weight (mass), speed and temperature. However, there can be a problem in relation to measuring psychological and educational characteristics.

Reliability *is a way to reflect the amount of error, both random and systematic inherent in any measurement* (Streiner and Norman 2003a).

A test result has two components, true score and error. For example, with weather, the outside temperature may have a plus/minus 1 degree Celsius error of measurement. This does not matter much if, as in the UK, outside temperatures may vary between minus 10 in the winter and plus 30 degrees Celsius in the summer. So, 1 degree Celsius variation may not matter much. Minus 10 degrees and minus 9 degrees are both very cold! But with body temperature, with a much narrower range of 37 to 40 degrees Celsius, a plus/minus 1 degree error is much more significant.

We carry out lots of tests on our students and trainees in the healthcare professions. We need to reduce errors to the minimum and ensure we are using the true score which an examinee achieves. So, we need to know how reliable our tests are. Reliability is expressed as a coefficient (0 to 1). A zero indicates no reliability at all through to 1 indicating perfect reliability. High reliability indicates that the effect of measurement errors has been reduced.

Errors in an examination come from many places, including the examination method itself, different examiners, consistency within one examiner, the candidates, interactions between examiners and candidates, the questions, and random errors for which no explanation seems to be apparent.

RATER RELIABILITY

Inter-examiner reliability refers to how well the marks of different assessors correlate with each other.

Intra-examiner reliability refers to how well the several scorings of an individual judge correlate.

This is very important in terms of marking examinations as, ideally, we would want examiners to be consistent.

Recently we held a clay shooting competition to raise money for the Army Benevolent Fund. Shooters in teams of five shot at a flush of 80 clays. Four of us with click counters noted the number of misses. Our individual scores for one group were very close, 25, 26, 27 and 24 misses. This is an illustration of inter-rater reliability.

We wish to minimise the impact of hawks and doves. Some examiners are hard markers and give low marks. These are the hawks. Some examiners are soft markers who give high marks. These are the doves.

TEST RE-TEST RELIABILITY

This is one way to test the reliability of an assessment, by issuing the same test to the same candidates and comparing their scores statistically. How long should you wait between the two tests? Too soon and people will remember the answers, while too long may enable the learner to benefit from further learning and give a higher score. In practice, a two week gap between the first and the second administrations of the test is reasonable.

EQUIVALENT FORMS RELIABILITY

This is defined as the consistency of measurement based on the correlation between scores on two similar forms of the same test taken by the same subjects. A difficulty is getting two forms that are essentially equivalent.

SPLIT HALF RELIABILITY

This is a measure of the internal consistency of a test. The test is divided into two equal parts. Scores for both parts are calculated, and scores for both parts of the test are then correlated.

However, if the test has sub-domains that measure very different constructs (communicating with patients and time keeping for example) this may not be possible to get true results.

INTERNAL CONSISTENCY USING CRONBACH'S ALPHA

Internal consistency is a measure of how homogeneous the question items in a test are in terms of measuring one dimension only. Cronbach's alpha is an estimate of reliability based on all possible correlations between all the items within the test. As a general rule of thumb, 0.7 is the minimum level of reliability, and 0.8 is regarded as acceptable for a high stakes test situation.

TEST LENGTH

The longer the test the better is the reliability. A 20 station OSCE has a better reliability than a five station OSCE, as will be demonstrated later in this chapter. There is better sampling of content, and reduction in the effects of guessing the answers. More frequent tests are a substitute for longer tests.

NUMBER OF EXAMINERS

Having more examiners improves the reliability. Two examiners per station in an OSCE is better than one and improves the reliability.

GENERALIZABILITY THEORY (G THEORY)

Generalizability theory is an extension of the concepts described earlier – of true score and error (Streiner and Norman 2003b). A detailed account of generalizability theory is really well beyond the scope of this chapter, but you should have heard about it! It will come up in research papers and books you will read on assessment.

G theory uses the true score and error variances for all aspects of an assessment (candidates, examiners and questions). In addition, there are interactions (say between candidates and stations, and candidates and examiners) – and these have error variances as well. All these contribute to the reliability.

G theory can calculate the reliability of an examination from the data presented. This Generalizability Coefficient may range from zero to one, where 0.7 is the minimum level of reliability, and 0.8 is regarded as acceptable for a high stakes test situation. This is called a Generalizability Study or G study for short.

Also, error variances for examiners, candidates and questions can be calculated. We should expect smaller error variances for questions and examiners, and perhaps a somewhat larger one for candidates (because candidates differ in their abilities in the exam). If we find that examiners present the largest error variance, then we have work to do with examiner briefings and examiner training!

In addition, using the examination data we already have we can find out the effects of changing the numbers of observations on the reliability. So, if we had a five station OSCE, we could ask what would happen to the reliability if there were 10 stations, 15 stations or any number. This is called a Decision Study or D Study for short.

Consider a final year surgical OSCE with five stations. From the results of all 112 students who did this OSCE, the reliability was low at G = 0.508. This was unacceptably low for a final year pass or fail examination. Using generalizability theory, we could calculate how the reliability would change if the numbers of stations were increased. Here are the results of this Decision Study:

5 stations   G = 0.508 (what we got)
6 stations   G = 0.554 (calculated)
8 stations   G = 0.623 (calculated)
10 stations G = 0.673 (calculated)
14 stations G = 0.713 (calculated)
20 stations G = 0.805 (calculated)

So, in order to achieve a reliable OSCE examination, we need at least 15, if not 20 stations, not 5.

VALIDITY – TYPES OF VALIDITY

Validity of a test is when it measures what it is supposed to measure (Streiner and Norman 2003c).

Here is an illustration. If you make jam or marmalade, you need the ingredients to reach the setting point. A jam thermometer should accurately measure the boiling point of jam – about 105 degrees Celsius. If the temperature repeatedly reads 80 degrees Celsius when the jam is obviously boiling vigorously (a rolling boil), then the thermometer is not giving valid readings. So, throw your old jam thermometer away and buy a new electronic one, or use other traditional methods of achieving the setting point!

There are various forms of validity. Types of validity include:

- **Content** – measures the intended content
- **Concurrent** – test scores correlate with an established test
- **Predictive** – can predict future performance
- **Construct** – measures a hypothetical construct – empathy, wisdom or professionalism for example
- **Face** – does it appear to measure what it is supposed to?

Evidence to support procedural validity needs to be clearly documented and might include:

- Overview of examination and its purpose
- Clear description of the standard setting method used with reasons
- Process used to select the panel of experts – their qualifications and the extent to which they represent the profession as a whole
- Outline of all phases of the exercise, including training, definition of performance standard and how data were collected
- Evaluation of staff training and understanding

EVIDENCE TO SUPPORT THE INTERNAL VALIDITY

These include:

- Item response theory results
- Reliability – Cronbach's alpha
- Generalizability theory – items, stations, examiners as sources of measurement error

EVIDENCE TO SUPPORT EXTERNAL VALIDITY

These include:

- Assessing the reasonableness of the pass mark (referred to as the cut score) in light of the pass and failure rates for the exam
- Compare this examination with other exams taken by the same cohort

For example, a final year medical school OSCE in surgery has a failure rate of between 8% and 10% each year. If this year the failure rate is 55% following a standard setting exercise, we would need to look carefully at the cut-score and its appropriateness.

STANDARD SETTING IN ASSESSMENT

All assessments are relative, in that they are (or should be) referenced to some standard (De Champlain 2014).

The standard: a qualitative description of an acceptable level of knowledge and performance in practice. For example, for a final year OSCE, the standard might be entry into supervised medical practice as a foundation year one doctor.

The cut score: a number along a scale which reflects having attained that standard. For example, the cut score in the OSCE above might be an OSCE mark of 71%.

STANDARDS AND THE CUT SCORE – THE BORDERLINE CANDIDATE

Most standard setting methods aim to set the pass mark around the borderline candidate.

Is this the minimally competent (just scraping a pass) candidate? Or is this the candidate who is neither qualified nor unqualified to pass (an on-the-fence candidate)? Often in health professions education, the borderline candidate is someone who '*just passes*' the examination.

STANDARD SETTING METHODS – SETTING THE PASS MARK

There are many methods in use to set the standards used in assessments. These are divided into two main types, Examiner Centred Methods and Examinee-Centred Methods. Despite differences, both depend on the concept of the borderline or minimally competent candidate.

EXAMINER-CENTRED METHODS

Examiners (experts) visualise the theoretical minimally competent candidate and how many items they would answer correctly. Examiner-centred methods include the following:

- Jaegar
- Bookmark
- Angoff
- Modified Ebel

THE JAEGER METHOD

A group of examiners are asked to decide yes or no whether a *just passes* candidate will be able to answer the question correctly. The results of each examiner are then discussed with other group members. The scoring is then repeated. The total number of yes scores out of the total scores is the standard.

	Examiner 1	Examiner 2	Examiner 3
Q1.	No	Yes	Yes
Q2.	Yes	No	Yes
Q3.	Yes	No	Yes
Q4.	Yes	Yes	Yes
Q5.	Yes	No	No
Pass	4/5	2/5	4/5

Final yes scores are 4 + 2 + 4 out of 15 which is 10 out of 15 which is 67% rounded up. So, the pass mark is 67%.

THE BOOKMARK METHOD

Again, using a group of examiners, each examiner is asked to consider the questions and place them in order, from easy to difficult. Then each examiner is asked to place a 'bookmark' to separate the questions that a minimally competent candidate would get right from those the candidate would get wrong.

Examiner 1	Examiner 2	Examiner 3
Q4	Q4	Q4
Q3	Q1	Q3
Q2	Q2	Q1
Q5 Wrong	Q5 Wrong	Q2
Q1 Wrong	Q3 Wrong	Q5 Wrong

Pass   3/5   3/5   4/5

Correct marks are 3 + 3 + 4 out of 15 which is 10 out of 15, which is 67% rounded up. So, the pass mark is 67%.

THE ANGOFF METHOD

The Angoff method is one of the most used and most researched set of procedures for producing a cut score in an examination. The examiners are asked to discuss in their group the characteristics of a borderline (minimally competent) candidate. Then for each question each examiner decides the probability of a minimally competent candidate getting the answer correct – on a 0 to 1 scale. Proportions are summed up for each examiner.

Modifications of the Angoff Method include group discussion of scores – once made individually, and providing item difficulty and item discrimination results after the initial round of scoring.

Advantages of the Angoff Method include it being a well-established method, used extensively. There is a host of published literature available. It has an intuitive appeal as judgement is made by experts on knowledge of the material and the candidates. It is used widely for multiple choice question (MCQ) papers and OSCE assessments in many situations and many countries.

Disadvantages include criticism of two main tasks required of the expert panel. These are spelling out what constitutes minimal competency and estimating consistently the proportions of items a minimally competent candidate would answer correctly. De Champlain (2014) suggested that staff training, item performance information and feedback to members of the expert panel as being helpful in achieving valid and reliable results.

THE MODIFIED EBEL PROCEDURE

Examiners are asked to categorise each of the test items into various categories before the examination takes place. These are:

1. Essential to know   2. Important to know   3. Questionable to know

The examiners are then asked to decide the proportion in each of the three groups that a group of borderline candidates should score correctly. The number of items in each category multiplied by the proportion is calculated, and the sum of these three is the pass mark.

For example:

Essential to know	10 items examiners decide 6 out of 10	10 x 6/10
Important to know	5 items examiners decide 3 out of 5	5 x 3/5
Questionable to know	5 items examiners decide 1 out of 5	5 x 1/5

Pass mark is 6 + 3 + 1 = 10 out of 20 items

EXAMINEE-CENTRED METHODS

Examiners (experts) observe and mark candidates and also give a global rating of pass, fail and borderline pass. Calculations using the marks of the candidates and their global ratings then achieve a pass mark. Examinee-centred methods include the borderline group, Contrasting Group and Cohen methods and are commonly used in performance assessment such as OSCEs.

THE BORDERLINE GROUP METHOD

This method does not need an examiner to visualise a hypothetical borderline candidate. Instead, examiners work from their direct observations at the time of the examination taking place. Examiners must be expert judges of the candidates. Both an itemised checklist and a global rating scale are used. Candidates are assessed as pass, borderline pass and fail on the global scale. Borderline candidates are identified by the global rating scale for each test item, and the mean checklist mark for all those borderline candidates is then calculated. This sum of the mean score (plus one SEM – the standard error of measurement) is the pass mark for each question in the exam.

For example, marks (out of 10) for the five borderline registrars on given OSCE question might be as follows:

- Candidate 1   5
- Candidate 2   5
- Candidate 3   6
- Candidate 4   6
- Candidate 5   5

Using the statistical programme SPSS, mean is 5.4 and standard deviation (SD) is 0.55. The statistical package will also calculate the standard error of measurement using the formula:

$SEM = SD \times \sqrt{(1 - R)}$ where R is the reliability (Reliability is 0.81 here – Cronbach's alpha)
$SEM = 0.55 \times \sqrt{(1 - 0.81)} = 0.55 \times \sqrt{(0.19)}$
$SEM = 0.55 \times 0.44 \qquad = 0.24$

Pass mark is mean score plus 1 SEM
Pass mark is $5.4 + 0.24 = 5.64$ rounded up to 6 to nearest whole number

So going back to the five borderline candidates above, candidates 3 and 4 have passed, while the others have failed this question, or this station.

Why do we add on one standard error of measurement?

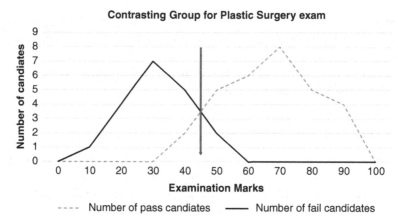

FIGURE 16.1 Contrasting group method to set a pass mark.

Remember that the score is composed of true score and error. It incorporates the error variance and the variance between subjects (the other examinees). Using an SEM allows us to draw a confidence interval around a score. So, if you achieve the pass mark – it allows for these errors.

THE CONTRASTING GROUP METHOD

In this method, examiners as a group choose a random sample of candidates (De Champlain 2014). They categorise each candidate into a 'pass' or a 'fail' group based on the candidates' answers to all test items in the examination. The examination scores for the two groups (pass and fail) are plotted on the same graph (as two curves). The numbers of candidates on y axis, and the number of questions correct on x axis are plotted. The fail candidates' scores go on the right, and the pass candidates' on the left (see Figure 16.1).

The point of least overlap which provides the maximum discrimination between the two groups – in the above case between pass candidates and fail candidates – is the pass mark.

Consider this worked example. Here, in Table 16.1, are the marks for 49 candidates in a fictitious plastic surgery examination.

Thirty candidates passed, and 19 candidates failed, according to the examiners' global assessments.

The perpendicular arrow at the point of intersection of the two graphs will be the pass mark, where the arrow crosses the x axis of the graph. In this example the pass mark would be about 45 marks out of 100.

THE COHEN METHOD

This is a simple user friendly low cost method of setting the pass mark (Cohen-Schotanus and van der Vleuten 2010). The top performing students are used as a point of reference

TABLE 16.1 Cohen method for setting the pass mark

Marks	No. of pass candidates	No. of fail candidates
0	0	0
10	0	1
20	0	4
30	0	7
40	2	5
50	5	2
60	6	0
70	8	0
80	5	0
90	4	0
100	0	0
Totals	30	19

to set the pass mark. The performance of the students on 95% centile are used as a benchmark. Pass is set at 65% of the benchmark. So, the 95% mark is multiplied by 65% to give the pass mark (see Figure 16.2). Entering all candidates' marks into an Excel spreadsheet and using the centile function will calculate these scores fairly easily.

However, remember that this is a norm referenced method, with the provisos described earlier.

Consider this worked example. Here are 20 fictitious candidates and their plastic surgery marks for (a different!) examination (out of 100).

Joseph Walker	49
John Smith	74
Dawn Jones	67
David Brown	59
Jane Evans	62
Bill Williams	58
Fred Walker	56
Pippa French	80
Baldev Singh	83
Gurpreet Kaur	67

Vinit Kumar	*81*
Khalid Khan	*87*
Taruna Sharma	*76*
Jay Gupta	*66*
Mustafa Shah	*78*
Tariq Arafat	*54*
Ben Jacobs	*54*
Grace Lucas	*79*
Elizabeth Hunter	*63*
Fiona Charlton	*90*

METHOD

Put all of these names and their scores into an Excel spreadsheet.

- Column A for each name.
- Column B for each corresponding score.
- You can copy and paste from a Word document using the Paste as 'text' function.
- In Column B, B1 is the heading (score) so the results of all 20 candidates lie in the column B2 to B21.
- In the **function box** type in the text = PERCENTILE(B2:B21, 0.95) which gives the 95th centile as 87.15.
- Pass mark is set at say 65% of the benchmark 95th centile.
- So pass mark is 87.15 x 65 divided by 100 which equals 56.6.
- Rounded up to nearest whole number the **pass mark is 57**.

THE HOFSTEE METHOD

Sometimes a criterion-based method of setting the pass mark may lead to an unacceptable result in terms of the number of candidates who either pass or fail an examination.

For example, an OSCE in paediatrics for senior paediatric trainees may have a failure rate of around 10% of candidates year on year. This rate may be fairly stable, as the candidate population is comparable year on year in terms of ability and training. If the cut score from a borderline group method this year gives a failure rate of 50% of candidates, then this is unrealistic and will no doubt be unacceptable from an educational policy and political viewpoint.

To give a 'reality check', Hofstee (1983) suggested a compromise method which asks examiners two questions (with two answers in each one). These are:

1. Overall, what are the maximum and minimum tolerable cut scores?
2. Overall, what are the maximum and minimum failure rates?

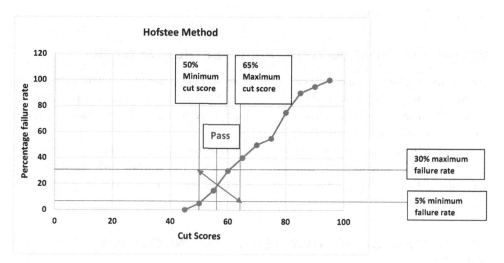

FIGURE 16.2 The Hofstee calculation.

These scores are discussed by the examiners and may be changed to achieve a consensus before a final version is agreed.

A graph is constructed with total cut score along the x axis and percentage failure rate along the y axis (see Figure 16.2). Candidates' scores are plotted on the graph, and a curve drawn through the points. Next, two vertical lines for maximum and minimum tolerable cut scores, and two horizontal lines for maximum and minimum failure rates. These four lines will (hopefully) produce a box through which the curve of candidates' scores will cross. Finally a straight line is ruled between the top left corner of the box and the bottom right corner of the box. Where the line crosses the candidates' score line, a perpendicular is dropped to the x axis. This will give the acceptable cut score for this examination.

The Hofstee method is not generally regarded as a primary standard setting method, but instead it is a reality check to support other standard setting approaches (whether examiner-based or examinee-based methods). So, it should not be used as a stand-alone measure, but as a check on another accepted method.

HOW TO CHOOSE WHICH METHOD OF SETTING THE PASS MARK TO USE

Examiner-centred methods (Jaegar, Bookmark, Angoff, modified Ebel) are well suited to setting a pass mark on knowledge assessments – such as MCQs. The Angoff and Bookmark are most commonly used as they are simpler to do. Other methods are more difficult to do.

Examinee-centred methods (borderline group, contrasting group, Cohen and Hofstee) are well suited to OSCE and Workplace-Based Assessments of performance

– as these are multi-dimensional integrated examinations. Of these the Borderline Group method is commonly used.

FOR WHAT PURPOSE DO YOU NEED TO SET THE PASS MARK?

For the vast majority of medical education assessments, criterion referenced methods are more appropriate than their norm referenced counterparts (De Champlain 2014). This is because criterion referenced assessments are based on expert judgements of what is minimal competency.

Norm referenced assessments are defensible for selection decisions only. So these are used for competitive appointments to a programme where places are limited, or for awarding the gold medal for the best performing student in the final examinations.

POST TEST ANALYSIS OF ITEMS (E.G. QUESTIONS OR OSCE STATIONS)

After an item has been used in a test, we will wish to know whether it performed well and we can have confidence using it in future assessments (Jolly 2014).

For example:

- Did the item cover its own knowledge territory appropriately?
- How did the item perform in relation to the test as a whole?
- Did the item discriminate between good and poor examinees?
- Are there errors in the items set which examiners have made or have not spotted?

HOW MAY ITEM ANALYSIS BE DONE?

Simply, we can read every question again. Using item analysis, we can work out the statistics. How many candidates got the question correct (Item Facility or Item Difficulty)? Which options were selected most often? Which options were chosen by high, medium and low scoring candidates on the test as a whole (Item Discrimination)? How did success on an item correlate with performance of the test as a whole? What were the inter-item correlations?

ITEM DIFFICULTY

Item Difficulty (or facility) (represented by P) is the percentage of candidates who answer the question correctly. So really when talking about *facility* we should be talking about easiness rather than difficulty! Remember that the Latin *facilis* meaning *easy to do*. So, the higher the score – the easier it is.

Item difficulty has a range from 0–1. If no one answers correctly the value is 0.00, but if everyone answers correctly the value is 1.00. The optimum level for an acceptable value depends on the number of options per item. The formula is 1.0 + G / 2 where G is the level of chance. G for 4 options is 0.25, and for 5 options is 0.20.

ITEM DISCRIMINATION

Item Discrimination measures how performance on one item correlates with performance in the test as a whole. We would not want a test item where most of the good performers get the question wrong and most of the poor candidates get the question right. Discrimination Power is a measure of this. Value expected will range from 0.2 to 1.0.

SOME EXAMPLES OF ASSESSMENT TOOLS AND THEIR USES

Multiple choice questions (MCQs)

MCQs are widely used in the healthcare professions. They can be used to examine knowledge, application of knowledge and understanding.

MCQs include the True/False, Single Best Answer or One from N options (often 5) and the extended matching question (EMQ).

Scores are 1 for a correct answer and 0 for an incorrect answer. Negative marking where marks are subtracted for incorrect answers is now rarely used.

TRUE/FALSE QUESTIONS

A statement is followed by several options (between three and six). Each option needs to be absolutely true or absolutely false. As a result, these questions may be difficult to write. The advantage is that these questions can be machine marked.

In astronomy:

1. The Earth is the fourth planet from the sun   True/False
2. Jupiter is a planet composed mainly of iron   True/False
3. The Geminids are a regular annual meteor shower   True/False
4. A lunar eclipse is caused by the Earth's shadow   True/False
5. A coronal mass ejection comes from Mars   True/False

Items 3 and 4 are correct.

SINGLE BEST ANSWER OR ONE FROM N OPTIONS

A statement is followed by three to six options. Only one of these options is correct. Candidates choose the option which is the best fit. These are easier to write and to check the answers. These questions can be machine marked.

The capital of Scotland is:

1. Glasgow.
2. Dundee.
3. Inverness.
4. Edinburgh.
5. Aberdeen.

Edinburgh is the correct answer.

EXTENDED MATCHING QUESTIONS (EMQs)

A topic (often a clinical symptom) is followed by many options, linked to a clinical group, such as a diagnosis. The linked question is to choose the most likely diagnosis. EMQs do have some fidelity to real life medical practice. They are more reliable than the True/False or one best answer type of MCQs.

The structure of an EMQ consists of four parts:

• Theme.
• Options.
• Lead in.
• Scenario or Vignettes.

Theme: Abdominal Pain – diagnosis
Options:

a. Acute appendicitis.
b. Ruptured ectopic pregnancy.
c. Kidney stone.
d. Cholecyctitis.
e. Pancreatitis.
f. Perforated peptic ulcer.
g. Ruptured abdominal aortic aneurism.

Lead in: For each of the case scenarios described below, select the most likely diagnosis.

Scenario 1: A 30-year-old woman has sudden onset of central abdominal pain, with nausea. Pain moves to the right lower abdomen, where it persists. Bowel movement was normal two hours before the pain started. She is not pregnant. Examination reveals tenderness and guarding in the right lower abdomen. Bowel sounds are normal. Temperature is 37.3 degrees C. Serum amylase is normal. Urine analysis is normal.

Answer: A: Acute appendicitis

Scenario 2: A 78-year-old man with known ischaemic heart disease is sitting having his breakfast when he starts to have abdominal pain that spreads to his lower back. He complains of feeling dizzy and his partner notes that he is sweaty, pale and has clammy skin. When he arrives in the emergency department his blood pressure is 90/60 mmHg, pulse 120/minute, his legs are mottled and blue.

Answer G: Ruptured abdominal aortic aneurysm

OBJECTIVE STRUCTURED CLINICAL EXAMINATION (OSCE)

Since the late 1970s, OSCEs have become a reliable way to assess basic clinical skills (Dent and Harden 2013). In terms of Miller's pyramid, an OSCE assesses competence (*shows how*), although this might not reflect what the health professional really does in the workplace (*does*). It consists of a circuit of stations where candidates interact with materials, equipment or standardised patients. They can also be used as teaching or practice opportunities. As a rough rule of thumb, 20 stations or 100 minutes of OSCE time may be needed to achieve an acceptable level of reliability. (See our generalizability calculation earlier in this chapter.) The number of stations needs to be balanced. Too few stations will result in unreliable scores, whereas too many will give unmanageable numbers of marks and organisational headaches.

Each station requires three components:

> *The stem*: this sets the scene for the learner and clearly states the task and the time available.
> *The checklist*: for the assessor to score the performance, as detailed and specific as necessary to ensure reliability.
> *The background to the station*: e.g. instructions to simulated patients, model answers, information to be revealed in response to learners' observations.

Factors that affect reliability include the following:

- Too few stations or too little testing time
- Checklists or items that do not discriminate (too easy or too hard)
- Inconsistent performance by simulated patients
- Examiners who score idiosyncratically, who are poorly trained
- Administrative problems (e.g. poor organisation, noise)

Factors that affect validity include the following:

- Whether the problems are relevant and important; whether they are aligned with programme outcomes

- Whether the stations will assess skills that have been taught
- Whether content experts have reviewed the stations

PORTFOLIOS

Portfolios are now widely used in UK education and training in medicine and other health professions. For example, the e-Portfolio for the Foundation Programme (years one and two after qualification as a doctor) is a record of core procedures, Foundation Programme capabilities, curriculum mapping, and supervised learning events (UK Foundation Programme Curriculum 2022b).

Portfolios are personal collections of evidence from practice, demonstrating that a learner has met the learning outcomes or performance indicators. They are increasingly being used in clinical practice to demonstrate competence, and they work well as a formative assessment tool. As summative assessment tools, portfolios generally have reasonably high levels of validity, because learners construct them to demonstrate particular learning outcomes that matter to them. They may be less reliable, due to their variation and the time taken to assess them. A specified structure and a clear assessment policy can help to make them fairer.

Criteria for assessment might include minimum and maximum word counts, time limits on items that remain valid for inclusion, required items for inclusion or required numbers of types of material, and the presence and quality of reflective self-evaluative documentary evidence. Portfolios tend to be rated in terms of satisfactory completion or referral (requiring resubmission), as it is very difficult to make finer judgements about performance.

REFERENCES

Black P. and Wiliam D. (1998) Assessment and classroom learning. *Assessment in Education*, 5: 7–74.

Bloom B.S. (1956) *Taxonomy of educational objectives. 1. Cognitive domain.* New York: David McKay.

Cohen-Schotanus J. and van der Vleuten C.P.M. (2010) A standard setting method with the best performing students as point of reference: Practical and affordable. *Medical Teacher*, 32(2): 154–160. DOI: 10.3109/01421590903196979.

De Champlain A. (2014) Chapter 22, Standard setting methods in medical education. In Swanwick T. (ed) *Understanding medical education: Evidence, theory and practice.* 2nd edn. Oxford: Wiley Blackwell, pp. 305–316.

Dent J.A. and Harden R.M. (2013) Objective structured clinical examination. In *A practical guide for medical teachers.* 4th edn. London: Churchill Livingstone, Elsevier, pp. 308–310.

Dreyfus H.L. and Dreyfus S.E. (2005) Expertise in real world contexts. *Organisational Studies*, 26: 779–792.

Hofstee W.K.B. (1983) The case for compromise in educational selection and grading. In Anderson S.B. and Helminck J.S. (eds) *On educational testing.* San Francisco, CA: Jossey-Bass, pp. 107–122.

Jolly B. (2014) Written assessment – item analysis. In *Programme evaluation: Improving practice, influencing policy and decision making.* In Swanwick T. (ed) *Understanding medical education: Evidence, theory and practice.* 2nd edn. Oxford: Wiley Blackwell, pp. 272–274.

Miller G.E. (1990) The assessment of clinical skills/competence/performance. *Academic Medicine*, 65(9): s63–s67.

Streiner D.L. and Norman G.R. (2003a) Reliability. In *Health measurement scales – a practical guide to their development and use.* 3rd edn. Oxford: Oxford University Press, pp. 126–152.

Streiner D.L. and Norman G.R. (2003b) Generalizability theory. In *Health measurement scales – a practical guide to their development and use.* 3rd edn. Oxford: Oxford University Press, pp. 153–171.

Streiner D.L. and Norman G.R. (2003c) Validity. In *Health measurement scales – a practical guide to their development and use.* 3rd edn. Oxford: Oxford University Press, pp. 172–193.

UK Foundation Programme Curriculum (2022b) E portfolio. Available at https://foundationprogramme.nhs.uk/curriculum/e-portfolio/ (Accessed 12.5.22).

Wood D.F. (2014) Formative assessment. In Swanwick T. (ed) *Understanding medical education: Evidence, theory and practice.* 2nd edn. Oxford: Wiley Blackwell, pp. 317–328.

CHAPTER 17

Workplace-based assessment

....

OBSERVATION OF PRACTICE

Look back at Chapter 16 on assessment and consider Miller's Pyramid. Workplace-based assessment tools look at the top of the pyramid, what the practitioner does in real life settings (Miller 1990). Norcini and Burch (2007) described workplace-based assessment as an 'educational tool'.

When assessing the competent clinical practice of healthcare professionals, direct observation of real-life practice samples performance and makes an inference about competence. This is based on the concept that competence is not directly observable but can be inferred from successful behaviour. Assessors must position themselves to be able to accumulate enough evidence to make a judgement, since not all practice can be observed of course. The assessment may be of practical skills, behaviours and behaviour patterns, but these may also indicate the underlying attitudes and values held by the learner.

An ability to perform is only one aspect of competence, and questioning frequently complements observation to gain further, indirect evidence of competence that is 'hidden' and not available to observation.

Guidelines from the Nursing and Midwifery Council (2022) state that each practice assessor is responsible for the assessment and confirmation of the achievement of proficiencies and outcomes for the student(s) they are assigned to, for the period they are assigned to them. Assessment should be continuous throughout the time in which a practice assessor is assigned to a student. The practice assessor should be up to date on the progress of the student, and collation of information on a student's performance should be managed in a way that enables this. Feedback to the student about their achievement and collaborating with them to review possible areas for improvement also forms a fundamental part of the assessment process.

DOI: 10.1201/9781003352532-20

Advantages of observation

- Observation of practice can provide a high level of integrated assessments, testing several competences at the same time.
- It allows assessment of attitudes and interpersonal skills.
- It offers realistic evidence of competence.
- It allows assessment of problem-solving skills.

Disadvantages of observation

- The circumstances of observation may be too specific.
- It is lengthy and costly if reliability is to be assured.
- Only indirect evidence of knowledge and understanding is obtained.
- It does not assess ability to learn through practice and transfer skills to another setting.
- It is subject to observer bias and observer effect.

For some of these reasons, as well as others such as the huge cost implications, direct observation of actual practice does not occur widely in undergraduate training, although it does have a place. Postgraduate assessment processes however include several observed competences and video recordings of consultations for external assessment – an extension of observation of practice.

In 2009, the first Guide to Postgraduate Dental Training (The 'Gold Guide') called for assessments utilising direct observation of clinical work to minimise criticism that the assessments are not well related to patient care, and this guidance has continued in each revision (COPDEND 2021). The other main findings were that attention needed to be given to aspects of the following:

- Assessment that supports an integrated period of general professional training.
- Training and inspection of trainers, to minimise variation in assessment.
- More authentic assessments, to enhance the predictive value of the tests for future success.

MINI-CLINICAL EVALUATION EXERCISE (MINI-CEX)

The mini-CEX assesses history taking, examination, communication skills, clinical judgement, professionalism, organisation and overall clinical care. A supervisor watches the doctor carrying out the interaction with the patient and assesses the doctor on these domains on a numerical scale. After the assessment there is a period of feedback (hopefully constructive) lasting five to ten minutes.

The original mini-CEX was developed with a nine-point scale where 1–3 is unsatisfactory, 4 is marginal, 5 and 6 is satisfactory and 7–9 is superior. In the UK Foundation Programme (for doctors in their first two years after qualification as a doctor) and in many UK medical specialty training programmes, a six-point scale has been adopted, with 1–2 being unsatisfactory, 3 being borderline, 4 being satisfactory and 5–6 being superior. As far as we are aware, the mini-CEX tool has not been re-validated from using the nine-point scale to the six-point scale.

Norcini et al. (1995) and the American Board of Internal Medicine (ABIM) developed the mini-CEX to assess short, specific tasks within a patient encounter (e.g. history taking, examination of the cardiovascular system). The mini-CEX replaced the CEX (Clinical Evaluation Exercise), which assessed an entire patient encounter (e.g. both history taking and physical examination). The main reason for this change was to enhance sampling of the assessment material, i.e. patients with different conditions and to increase the number of examiners or raters. Originally developed for formative assessment, it has also been used for summative assessment – as in the UK Foundation Programme, and in many specialty training programmes where trainees may be asked to provide several assessments per year in their e-portfolio. Although initially developed for postgraduate assessment, it has also been successfully adopted in undergraduate assessment. A patient encounter in the undergraduate version, however, is reported to take much longer (30–45 minutes) than the original 15 to 20-minute postgraduate mini-CEX.

Holmboe et al. (2004) found that mini-CEX ratings for videoed patient encounters could differentiate levels of candidate ability. Twelve to 14 patient encounters are sufficient to achieve a reliability of 0.8 (Norcini et al. 1995; Holmboe et al. 2003). For doctors in the Foundation Programme in the UK, Jackson and Wall (2010) found that eight encounters gave an acceptable reliability of 0.8. If, however, results with variability of one rating point or less on the rating scale with 95% confidence are acceptable, approximately four encounters are sufficient. In this case, additional encounters may only be needed for borderline candidates (Norcini and Burch 2007).

In real life there are problems with the use of the mini-CEX. There are no descriptors for the various domains being assessed. Reliability is a major problem (Holmboe and Hawkins 2008), with variations between raters, variability from patient to patient, and the scores being completed by raters without observing the actual encounter. In Jackson and Wall's 2010 study, up to 38% of encounters were not observed directly. Trainees were not happy with the tool and scored only 3.8 out of 10 on a satisfaction scale. Only 28% had found it useful to gain feedback, but when feedback was given, this was highly valued by trainees. Many complain about the tool being merely a 'tick box exercise' and not being motivated to improve.

Most recently a review of the utility of the mini-CEX concluded that the mini-CEX had reasonable validity, reliability and educational impact (Hejri et al. 2020). Studies of reliability showed that numbers of assessments in the range of four to ten tests gave acceptable reliability. The statistical method of factor analysis revealed that a single dimension was being assessed – namely global clinical performance leading to the conclusion that as a workplace-based assessment teachers 'can opt for the mini-CEX as an assessment tool with positive educational consequences'.

DIRECT OBSERVATION OF PROCEDURAL SKILLS (DOPS)

Direct observation of procedural skills (DOPS) is an assessment designed for the assessment of clinical procedures or investigations such as lumbar puncture, suturing, joint injection, insertion of a chest-drain and excision biopsy. A supervisor watches the doctor carrying out the procedure with the patient and assesses the doctor on these domains on a numerical scale. After the assessment there should be a period of feedback lasting five to ten minutes.

DOPS is used in the UK in the Foundation Programme and for specialty registrar training and assessment. The original assessment used a nine-point rating scale somewhat similar to the mini-CEX. In many situations in the UK postgraduate training system, the nine-point scale has been altered to a six-point scale that identifies, with regard to foundation year completion, whether the trainee is below expectations (scores 1 and 2), is borderline (score of 3), meets expectations (score of 4), or is above expectations (scores of 5 and 6).

Happy et al. (2019) calculated the reliability of DOPS and compared the tool with a conventional method of skill assessment in dental students. DOPS was 80–90% reliable, compared with 50–70% reliable for a conventional method of assessment.

DOPS is designed to assess:

- Understanding of indications for the procedure/investigation, relevant anatomy and technique
- Obtaining informed consent
- Preparation pre-procedure
- Appropriate use of sedation or analgesia
- Technical ability
- Aseptic technique
- Seeks help where appropriate
- Post procedure management including complications
- Communication skills
- Consideration for the patient
- Interpretation of results
- Overall ability to perform the procedure

Again, there are problems of using the DOPS in real life. In a study of DOPS in the specialty of anaesthesia, surveying consultants and senior trainees (specialty registrars) Bindal et al. (2013) found that reassuringly 100% of consultants had been trained in the use of DOPS. However, only 5% of DOPS assessments were done in a pre-planned fashion, 50% were done ad hoc, and worryingly, 44% of DOPS were filled in retrospectively. Additionally, 19% of consultants said they were too busy and refused to do a DOPS assessment, feedback to trainees was poor, and both consultants and trainees thought that DOPS was not a useful learning tool.

Top tips: If you are going to use the DOPS, it is essential that you make time to observe the encounter yourself, make the scores, and then spend time immediately afterwards while the encounter is still fresh in giving constructive and helpful feedback. With practical procedures, it is useful to pass on 'tricks of the trade' you have learned yourself over many years in terms of the ease, safety and success of the procedure.

CASE-BASED DISCUSSION (CBD)

In the USA the assessment tool known as the Chart Stimulated Recall (CSR) has been developed and used to assess clinical decision making and the application and use of medical knowledge in real cases managed by the trainee. The format is usually a two-hour, standardised oral examination with each case taking five to ten minutes to assess. Reported reliabilities vary from 0.65–0.88 (in the USA).

The method has been adopted in the UK for the assessment of doctors in training in both foundation training and specialty training where it is called case-based discussion (CBD). Here, the trainee selects two sets of patient case notes, for which the trainee has recently seen the patients, and in which the trainee has made notes, and provides the case notes to an assessor (a more senior trainee or a consultant or general practitioner trainer). The assessor then questions the trainee on one of the cases and rates the trainee on the following:

- Medical record keeping
- Clinical assessment
- Investigation and referrals
- Treatment
- Follow-up and future planning
- Professionalism
- Overall clinical judgement

A six-point rating scale is used that identifies, with regard to completion of training, whether the trainee is below expectations (scores 1 and 2), is borderline (score of 3), meets expectations (score of 4), or is above expectations (scores of 5 and 6). There is also an opportunity to flag up an 'unable to comment' box where a specific competence has not been observed in the case. The discussion is expected to last no more than 20 minutes including 5 minutes for feedback.

In terms of reliability Brown et al. (2011) stated that probably eight cases were needed to achieve an acceptable level of reliability.

Again, there are problems with case-based discussion. The record may not adequately reflect what occurred in the clinical encounter. The record may have left out important information. Vital information such as diagnosis, consent, procedures and investigations done – may not be documented in over 50% of case records (Nagurney et al. 2005). Reliability among reviewers may be low.

Top tips: If you are going to use the CBD, it is essential that you make time to meet with the trainee yourself, look at the records they have made, make the scores, and then spend time immediately afterwards while the encounter is still fresh in giving constructive and helpful feedback. With medical records, it is useful to pass on lessons which you have learned yourself over many years in terms of the use of records for research and audit, and medico-legal aspects such as appearing in the coroner's court, where good accurate records are absolutely essential. Also, it is useful to give advice on what not to put, such as comments which are derogatory to patients and/ or colleagues. These can be a disaster for the doctor concerned when read out in open court.

PROCEDURE-BASED ASSESSMENT (PBA)

For the management of more major surgical procedures, however, the Procedure-Based Assessment (PBA) has been developed by the Royal College of Surgeons in the UK.

For orthopaedic surgery, examples of procedures for which specific PBAs are available include ankle fracture fixation, fixation of an extra capsular fracture and hemi arthroplasty of the hip.

For oral surgery, examples of procedures for which PBAs are available include surgical removal of lower third molar, removal of root from antrum, implant placement and removal of mandibular cyst.

The agreement of both trainer and trainee is necessary to trigger a PBA, and it is the trainer's responsibility to provide the level of supervision appropriate for the individual trainee. The PBA rating form includes six aspects:

- Consent
- Pre-operative planning
- Pre-operative preparation
- Exposure and closure
- Intra-operative technique
- Post-operative management

The trainer rates the trainee on each of the six aspects as one of:

- N – not observed or not appropriate for the trainee level of training and ability
- U – unsatisfactory or needs improvement
- S – satisfactory

The PBA form contains areas for written comments, and trainers are required to identify what needs to be done to improve when a U rating is given. There is an additional global rating for each procedure that the trainer is required to give:

- Level 0 – Insufficient evidence observed to support a judgement
- Level 1 – Unable to perform the entire procedure under supervision

- Level 2 – Able to perform the procedure under supervision
- Level 3 – Does not usually require supervision but may need help occasionally
- Level 4 – Competent to perform the procedure unsupervised and can deal with complications

Reliability is key, as with all the workplace-based assessment tools. Marriott et al. (2011) studied the reliability and acceptability of PBAs. They evaluated 81 trainees in 6 surgical specialties and assessed 749 PBAs across 348 operations by 57 clinical supervisors and 4 independent assessors. So how many PBAs did they find were needed to give an acceptability reliability (i.e. above 0.8 G coefficient)? The reliability for the total item score was acceptable using four assessments, and the reliability for the global summary score was acceptable for using three assessments.

MULTI-SOURCE FEEDBACK (MSF)

Multi-source feedback (MSF; or 360-degree assessment as it is often called) is a way of collecting evidence from people who know you and asking them to rate certain defined behaviours and attitudes. Such people may include senior colleagues, junior colleagues, peers, nurses, other healthcare workers and patients. Some MSF assessments also include a self-assessment as well (see also Chapter 15).

It is an important assessment method as it can assess communication skills, attitudes and behaviours, especially in relation to patients and to other team members and colleagues. Different people have different views, as they make observations from their own perspective. In the medical environment, a senior ward sister or charge nurse, with whom a student or trainee is in contact several times a day, will possibly have a different view than a consultant who might only see them twice a week.

QUESTIONS TO CONSIDER ABOUT MULTI-SOURCE FEEDBACK (ANSWERS BELOW!)

- How many raters do you think you need for a valid and reliable answer?
- Who should the raters be?
- Who should select the raters?
- Can you rate yourself in a valid and reliable way?
- How do you feed back the results?
- Do you need descriptions of behaviours – or just numerical scores?

MSF can be used for both summative and formative assessment. Though more widely used in postgraduate medical education settings (Whitehouse et al. 2002), it has been used also in undergraduate medical education (Norcini and Burch 2007). Its use is now accepted as a valid and reliable method of assessing professional behaviours and attitudes, rather than clinical knowledge or clinical skills. So, in terms of assessing knowledge, skills and attitudes, think of multi-source feedback as an attitudes assessment method.

The purposes of MSF include identification of those with problems in terms of communication (communicating with patients, communicating with colleagues and working and communicating within a team) and with unacceptable attitudes to work (dishonesty, turning up late, leaving early and being difficult to contact when on duty). It is also useful to reward good performance in terms of communication, attitudes and behaviours. In practice the process usually results in gratifying, descriptive praise for doctors from their co-workers.

How does it work? An example using Team Assessment of Behaviours (TAB) will illustrate this process. TAB continues to be the accepted MSF tool for assessing professional behaviours in the UK (UK Foundation Programme Curriculum 2022). It was developed and validated in the West Midlands Deanery in the UK and is reliable and has face and content validity (Whitehouse et al. 2005). It is regarded as fair, valuable and practical by trainees (Whitehouse et al. 2007). TAB was the preferred MSF tool in a comparative study with the mini-peer assessment tool (Burford et al. 2010).

TAB has four domains, based on the General Medical Council's guidance on professional behaviour. These are:

- Maintaining trust and professional relationships with patients
- Verbal communication skills
- Team working and working with colleagues
- Accessibility

The UK Foundation Curriculum (2022) document requires a minimum of ten returns for a valid, reliable assessment. The recommended mix of raters is specified, since ratings vary significantly by staff group (Bullock et al. 2009).

Instructions for doctors from the Foundation Programme 2022 are as follows:
Your assessors must include:

- At least two doctors (including your designated clinical supervisor), but none may be other foundation doctors
- At least two nurses (band 5 or senior)
- Two or more allied health professionals (physiotherapists, occupational therapists, etc.)
- At least two others (e.g. ward clerks, postgraduate programme administrators, secretaries, auxiliary staff)

You should nominate at least 15 assessors. A minimum of ten completed TAB forms are essential for a valid assessment. In addition, you must also complete your own assessment using self-TAB. You will not be able to nominate assessors until you complete self-TAB.

Forms are sent out electronically to the raters, and they are asked to complete the scores for the four domains and add comments in the text boxes about the assessed doctor. If a concern is raised in the scores, then the assessor must make comments in the text box for that domain before returning the form. Scores are collated, and a summary of scores and anonymised verbatim comments for each domain are sent to the trainee's educational supervisor. A valid assessment must include ten returns.

Research on self-assessment using Team Assessment of Behaviours (called self-TAB) has been published (Wall et al. 2012). Self-TAB scores for 834 Foundation doctors were compared with other raters' scores in terms of descriptive statistics, concerns, correlations and a multivariate linear regression analysis. Foundation doctors self-scored far fewer concerns than did raters (12 doctors as having some concern, compared with 73 doctors with some concern and 23 doctors with major concern rated by others). The correlations between self-TAB and TAB were positive, but not high, although significant. Of Foundation doctors, 42% correctly identified concerns confirmed by other raters. In conclusion, foundation doctors in this study had a limited ability to self-assess which supports the studies referred to previously. This is a useful finding as it indicates the important need for constructive feedback at appraisal.

SOME ANSWERS ABOUT MULTI-SOURCE FEEDBACK: WHAT DOES THE RESEARCH SHOW?

How many forms need to be returned?

Ten forms need to be returned for a valid result – as this gives an acceptable level of reliability with a Generalizability Coefficient of 0.8 or above (Whitehouse et al. 2005, 2007).

Who should fill in the forms?

Comparisons of raters have been made after detailed 'Hawks and Doves' research work (Bullock et al. 2009). Consultants and senior nurses are harder markers than peers and junior nurses.

How many 'non-passes' makes a fail or a problem?

Two minor concerns or one major concern in any one domain is statistically significant and should be followed up (Whitehouse et al. 2005, 2007).

How many scoring items on the scale?

'TAB 3, 4, 6 or 9 items' research shows that, interestingly, the more items on the scale, the fewer poor performers are detected (Hassell et al. 2012). The TAB form in general use has only three scoring items. When it had greater numbers on the scale, more doctors with concerns were missed. So, the greater number on the scale, the less able is the tool to detect poor performance. Reasons for this are unclear, but it might be related to a more diffused grade being possible with more points on the scale.

What about self-assessment? Can this replace rater assessment?

Self-assessment brings up far fewer concerns than does rater assessment, and only 42% of foundation doctors correctly identified concerns made by other raters (Wall et al. 2012).

Whitehouse and colleagues studied the implementation of the Team Assessment of Behaviours (TAB) in the West Midlands Foundation Programme (Whitehouse et al. 2015). They audited all invalid TAB assessments in the three years 2010, 2011 and 2012. In 2010 large numbers of assessments were invalid owing to an incorrect selection of assessors or insufficient numbers of assessors. After the introduction of a validity checking campaign before signing off there was a great improvement in 2011, which was partly sustained in 2012. The figures for the three years are as follows:

- In 2010 valid assessment by TAB was 437 FY1 (69%) and 380 FY2 (64%).
- In 2011 valid assessment by TAB was 609 FY1 (95%) and 606 FY2 (95%).
- In 2012 valid assessment by TAB was 463 FY1 (73%) and 467 FY2 (75%).

The main reasons for an invalid assessment were less than the specified ten assessors, no senior doctors as assessors and too many foundation doctors as assessors (Whitehouse et al. 2015).

Tips for developing and using MSF

- Develop a positive culture.
- Be clear about its purpose.
- Express clearly what to expect as desirable behaviours.
- Keep the number of items to be scored few in number.
- Keep the rating scale simple and fit for purpose.
- Use ten or more raters.
- Compare the results with self-assessment (but remember reservations here – see above).
- Train those who will give the feedback to involve those who are being assessed.
- Incorporate research, evaluation and development into the process.

WHAT DO TRAINEES THINK OF WORKPLACE-BASED ASSESSMENTS?

In a study of 130 doctors in training in paediatrics (Bindal et al. 2011), trainees were ambivalent about workplace-based assessments being a true reflection of their abilities. A common problem was finding assessors, with 40% of trainees stating that staff had refused to do assessments. Almost half of the assessments were done retrospectively. Trainees did receive feedback, but advice on future improvement was not always given.

The authors concluded that a cultural change is needed for trainees to feel that workplace-based assessments are not just a superficial exercise, but a useful educational tool for learning. Ongoing work on implementation needs to include additional training, especially on the value of these assessments for formative assessment and consultants having protected time in their job plans for training.

Cheston et al. (2021) studied changes in medical trainees' perceptions of workplace-based assessments across ten years, in 2008 and again in 2018. Trainees did not think that WBAs were a true reflection of their abilities or competencies. Again, the phrase 'tick-box exercise' was used. Again, the plea was for educator training, protected time and the need for appropriate useful feedback.

CONCLUSION

A great deal of care has gone into various assessments used in the health professions. These are generally valid and reliable if used correctly. But if not, then these assessments lose their credibility and lose the interest and commitment of the learners and teachers.

REFERENCES

Bindal N., Goodyear H., Bindal T. and Wall D. (2013) DOPS assessment: A study to evaluate the experience and opinions of trainees and assessors. *Medical Teacher*, 35: e1230–e1234.

Bindal T., Wall D. and Goodyear H. (2011) Trainee doctors' views on workplace-based assessments: Are they just a tick box exercise? *Medical Teacher*, 33: 919–927.

Brown N., Hoslgrove G. and Teeluckdharry S. (2011) Case based discussion. *Advances in Psychiatric Treatment*, 17: 85–90.

Bullock A.D., Hassell A., Markham W.A., Wall D.W. and Whitehouse A.B. (2009) How ratings vary by staff group in a multi-source feedback assessment of junior doctors. *Medical Education*, 43: 516–520.

Burford B., Illing J., Kergon C., Morrow G. and Livingston M. (2010) User perceptions of multi-source feedback tools for junior doctors. *Medical Education*, 44: 165–176.

Cheston H., Graham D., Johnson G. and Woodland D. (2021) Changes in UK medical trainees' perceptions of workplace based assessments across 10 years: Results of two cross sectional studies. *Postgraduate Medical Journal*, 98; 1–7. http://dx.doi.org/10.1136/postgradmedj-2020-137907. DOI: 10.7860/JCDR/2019/37913.12594.

COPDEND (2021) A reference guide for postgraduate dental core and specialty training in the UK. Available at www.copdend.org/guidance/dental-gold-guide-2021-edition/ (Accessed 18.5.22).

Happy D., Aditya A., Hadge P., Devkar N. and Vibhute A. (2019) Introduction and comparison of direct observation of procedural skills (DOPS) with conventional method of skill assessment in dental students. *Journal of Clinical and Diagnostic Research*, 13: 13–17. DOI: 10.7860/JCDR/2019/37913.12594.

Hassell A., Bullock A., Whitehouse A., Wood A., Jones P. and Wall D. (2012) Effect of rating scales on scores given to junior doctors in multi-source feedback. *Postgraduate Medical Journal*, 88: 10–14.

Hejri M.S., Jalili M., Masoomi R., Shirazi M., Nedjat S. and Norcini J. (2020) The utility of mini-clinical evaluation exercise in undergraduate and postgraduate medical education: A BEME review: BEME Guide No. 59. *Medical Teacher*, 42(2): 125–142. DOI: 10.1080/0142159X.2019.1652732.

Holmboe E.S. and Hawkins R.E. (2008) *Practical guide to the evaluation of clinical competence*. Philadelphia: Mosby Elsevier.

Holmboe E.S., Hawkins R.E. and Huot S.J. (2004) Effects of direct observation of medical residents' clinical competence training: A randomised control trial. *Annals of Internal Medicine*, 140(11): 874–881.

Holmboe E.S., Huot S., Chung J., Norcini J.J. and Hawkins R.E. (2003) Construct validity of the mini clinical evaluation exercise (MiniCEX). *Academic Medicine*, 78: 826–830.

Jackson D. and Wall D. (2010) An evaluation of the use of the mini-CEX in the foundation programme. *British Journal of Hospital Medicine*, 71: 584–588.

Marriott J.T., Purdie H., Crossley J. and Beard J.D. (2011) Evaluation of procedure based assessment for assessing trainees' skills in the operating theatre. *British Journal of Surgery*, 98: 450–457.

Miller G.E. (1990) The assessment of clinical skills/competence/performance. *Academic Medicine*, 65(9): s63–s67.

Nagurney J.T., Brown D.F., Sane S., Weiner J.B., Wang A.C. and Chang Y. (2005) The accuracy and completeness of data collected by prospective and retrospective methods. *Academic Emergency Medicine*, 12: 884–895.

Norcini J.J., Blank L.L., Arnold G.K. and Kimball H.R. (1995) The mini-CEX (clinical evaluation exercise): A preliminary investigation. *Annals of Internal Medicine*, 123: 795–799. DOI: 10.7326/0003-4819-123-10-199511150-00008.

Norcini J.J. and Burch V. (2007) Workplace-based assessment as an educational tool: AMEE Guide No. 31. *Medical Teacher*, 29: 855–871. DOI 10.1080/01421590701775453.

Nursing and Midwifery Council (2022) Assessment of practice. Available at www.nmc. org.uk/supporting-information-on-standards-for-student-supervision-and-assessment/ practice-assessment/what-do-practice-assessors-do/assessment-of-practice/ (Accessed 17.5.22).

UK Foundation Programme Curriculum (2022) Assessments. https://foundationprogramme. nhs.uk/curriculum/assessments/ (Accessed 17.5.22).

Wall D., Singh D., Whitehouse A., Hassell A. and Howes J. (2012) Self-assessment by trainees using self-TAB as part of the team assessment of behaviour multisource feedback tool. *Medical Teacher*, 34(2): 165–167.

Whitehouse A.B., Hassell A., Bullock A.D., Wood L. and Wall D.W. (2007) 360° assessment (multi-source feedback) of UK trainee doctors: Field testing of TAB (team assessment of behaviour). *Medical Teacher*, 29(2): 171–176.

Whitehouse A.B., Hassell A., Wood L., Wall D., Walzman M. and Campbell I. (2005) Development and reliability testing of a new form for 360° assessment of senior house officers' professional behaviour, as specified by the general medical council. *Medical Teacher*, 27(3): 252–258.

Whitehouse A.B., Higginbotham L., Nathavitharana K., Singh B. and Hassell A. (2015) Team assessment of behaviour: A high stakes assessment with potential for poor implementation and impaired validity. *Clinical Medicine*, 15(1): 7–9.

Whitehouse A.B., Waltzman M. and Wall D. (2002) Pilot study of 360 degree assessment of personal skills to inform record of in-training assessments for senior house officers. *Hospital Medicine*, 63: 172–175.

CHAPTER 18

Appraisal

....

HOW AM I DOING?

This very natural question that we have all asked ourselves is formalised in the appraisal meetings by giving protected time for feedback on a one-to-one basis between appraiser and appraisee. Appraisal builds on all of the support and supervision (Chapter 20) and feedback skills, including multi-source feedback (Chapter 15) covered in other chapters, but is certainly not a substitute for close supervision and feedback on day-to-day work.

Appraisal (sharing some features with and sometimes called, confusingly, formative assessment by educationalists) has been defined as a two-way dialogue focusing on the personal, professional and educational needs of the appraisee which produces agreed outcomes (SCOPME 1996). It is a process of regular, planned reviews between appraiser and appraisee, with support, carried out for the appraisee's benefit. Appraisal, through reflecting on practice, allows both the demonstration of strengths and the revelation of difficulties so that the former may be reinforced and the latter can be put right within the framework of the objectives that were set at the start of the programme. Appraisal should be non-threatening, friendly and supportive and does not result in a judgement or a pass/fail decision. It is sometimes called facilitated self-appraisal.

This chapter covers the concepts involved in appraisal of an appraisee and, more specifically, an appraisee who is junior to you, perhaps a student or trainee. However, you can use the information to prepare for your own appraisals and appraisals of peers.

BACKGROUND TO APPRAISAL

Formative assessment has been extensively applied for healthcare professionals in training for many years. It helps to identify what learners have achieved, might achieve and are now ready to achieve (Torrance 1998). For example, taking part in

DOI: 10.1201/9781003352532-21

a 'mock' objective structured clinical examination or OSCE can familiarise learners with the process of the examination and how it might run, but also gives them feedback on areas they need to develop before the summative OSCE. In the way it offers feedback on performance and identifies areas for development, it takes on the purpose of appraisal.

Many if not all universities have a personal academic tutor system which equally shares many features with an appraisal process (e.g. see University of Worcester 2020). Under this system faculty are expected to:

> monitor the progress of their tutees, discuss and agree developmental objectives and goals with their tutees, support them in making decisions about module choice and employability related plans, maintain a record of meetings, and provide them with an academic reference if required. Personal academic tutors are expected to ensure students who are experiencing personal difficulties that impact on their studies are signposted to the professional student support services available at the University. . . . The personal academic tutor system is intended to provide a stable, holistic and developmental form of support for individual students.
>
> *(UoW 2020, p. 1)*

In the perfect appraisal, appraisees are actively involved in reflecting on their practice, discussing it and sharing ideas about how to develop further towards learning goals. There is a degree of mutuality about the process, and teachers might offer information and insights into the educational opportunities that they can provide.

Appraisal is relevant to and undertaken by healthcare professionals across different disciplines and countries. Appraisal is now a contractual requirement for all UK doctors to maintain their personal and professional development. Frequently in healthcare the relationship is peer-to-peer. Peer appraisal differs slightly from formative assessment, mainly in the nature of the relationship between appraiser and appraisee and the degree to which the appraiser is responsible for the overall progress of the appraisee.

Appraisal for healthcare professionals differs from that in business or industry, as in the latter settings it is often used as a performance management tool and is an uncomfortable mixture of development and judgement.

Appraisals are often undertaken by line managers, tutors, educational supervisors, preceptors or mentors or by colleagues or peers who have been selected, appointed and trained as appraisers (Chambers et al. 2004). This difference will depend upon the discipline in which the appraisee works and the seniority of the appraisee.

CHARACTERISTICS OF APPRAISAL

Table 18.1 lists the general principles of appraisal and shows how it compares with assessment, with which it is often confused.

TABLE 18.1 General Principles of Appraisal and Assessment

Feature	Appraisal	Assessment
Prime purpose	Developmental 'Informing progress'	Judging achievement 'Summing up'
Participants	Appraiser and appraisee	Learner and third party
Methods used	Structured conversation	Varied (see Chapters 16 & 17)
Areas covered	Educational, personal and professional development, career progress, employment (appraisee's agenda)	Learning objectives (third-party agenda)
Process informed by	Appraisee's self-assessment, day-to-day observation by teachers, other work-related inputs, results of assessments and examinations	Outcome of standard, objective tests
Standards of achievement	Internal (personal to the appraisee) and negotiated with the appraiser	Pre-determined by assessing body (cont. . . .)
Output of the process	Record of appraisal having taken place, agreed educational and personal development plan	Pass/fail
Confidential to appraisee?	Yes, in most circumstances	No
Review/appeal	No need, as decisions should always be joint ones	Yes
Outcome	Enhanced education, personal and professional development	Proceed to next stage

THE FOLLET PRINCIPLES

The Follet review looked at appraisal for senior NHS and university staff with both academic and clinical duties (DfES 2001). The recommendations were as follows:

1. The substantive university contract and the honorary NHS contract for clinical academics should be interdependent (Paragraph 41).
2. Universities and NHS bodies should work together to develop a jointly agreed annual appraisal and performance review process based on that for NHS consultants, to meet the needs of both partners (Paragraphs 46–60).

3. The process should:
   - Involve a decision on whether single or joint appraisal is appropriate for every senior NHS and university staff member with academic and clinical duties;
   - Ensure joint appraisal for clinical academics holding honorary consultant contracts and for NHS staff undertaking substantial roles in universities;
   - Define joint appraisal as two appraisers, one from the university and one from the NHS, working with one appraisee on a single occasion;
   - Require a structured input from the other partner where a single appraiser acts;
   - Be based on a single set of documents; and
   - Start with a joint induction for those who will be jointly appraised (Paragraphs 51–60).

The aim of the recommendations was to minimise the need for appraisees to have more than one appraisal. It also facilitates a more easily constructed integrated job plan with line managers or appraisers aware of the commitments and responsibilities of the appraiser across their whole working week. One of the unforeseen benefits of the changes to communications during the COVID-19 pandemic means we are now all more familiar and comfortable with online meetings. This should facilitate these joint appraisals which hitherto have proved difficult at times to set up.

QUESTIONS TO ASK

In the education setting appraisers might help the appraisee, trainee or learner to understand their progress by asking them to consider the following questions (Stuart 2003):

- Am I achieving statutory competences?
- Is there a demonstration of a growing level of skills?
- Is my performance consistent?
- Do I show a growing understanding of the principles underpinning practice?
- Am I demonstrating the development of attitudes and values appropriate to professional practice?
- Is there a demonstration of the ability to engage in reflective practice?

Any feedback on performance must take into account the circumstances under which the appraisee is performing (Phillips et al. 2000).

The appraisal process has links with performance review, as it covers areas of statutory competence and progress, but it is also contextualised to the individual's professional circumstances and needs, rather than making a judgement, and so has some features that overlap with mentoring (see Figure 18.1) (Robinson and Simpson 2003).

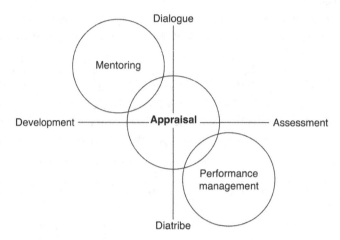

FIGURE 18.1 Relationship between mentoring, appraisal and performance management.

CARRYING OUT APPRAISAL

A good working definition of appraisal is the provision of a structured process by which the appraisee can be helped to define their own learning needs in the light of information they can gather or be given about progress from whatever source. Plans can then be made to meet those needs.

Aims for the appraisal process with appraisees are as follows:

1. To meet regularly. In the best schemes, progress is reviewed frequently (some specify every 2, 3, 4 or 6 months). Annual reviews are generally insufficient in situations whether it is an appraisal between the learner and supervisor, but might be appropriate in a peer to peer process of professional support once in practice.
2. To prevent information coming as a shock during a formal appraisal interview (ongoing feedback should minimise the risk of this).
3. To continue day-to-day supervision, support and feedback on performance.
4. To ensure that the appraisee can achieve the agreed objectives and, where necessary, give or direct them to help.
5. To set the appraisee's objectives within the overall framework of what learners or staff in that grade are expected to achieve, or what appraisees at that stage are expected to be able to demonstrate.
6. To curb the tendencies of unreasonably self-critical appraisees (see also 'imposterism' in Chapter 22).
7. On the whole, appraisal interviews are best conducted on a one-to-one basis. The exception to this is where Follet principles for joint appraisals have been successfully implemented.
8. To respect any promised level of confidentiality. The only exception is where aspects of poor performance come to light when the appraiser has a professional responsibility to protect patients.
9. This proviso should be made explicit at the start of the process.

The following are skills for successful appraisal:

- Listen.
- Reflect back what is being said by the appraisee.
- Support.
- Counsel.
- Treat information in confidence.
- Inform without censuring.
- Judge constructively.
- Identify educational needs.
- Construct and negotiate achievable plans.

Listening is key. Remember what *listening* really means – keep your mouth closed and your ears and brain open, not interrupting, not dominating the conversation, and not going in with pre-judged ideas and conclusions already reached. The balance of talking in an appraisal interview should be roughly 80:20 between the appraisee and the appraiser.

THE APPRAISAL DISCUSSION

Arrange a time when you are both free, and find a quiet room from which your conversation cannot be overheard. Appraisal needs to be prepared ahead and at least an hour set aside. Frequently the material for the appraisal is collated by learners or appraisees in the form of an electronic portfolio throughout the course of the time between meetings. Time will be needed for the appraisee to then go over that material and start the reflection before the meeting, and the appraiser will also need time to become familiar with the contents.

The contents of the portfolio may include any of the examples in the following list. Frequently a professional portfolio will be pre-structured to ensure all the essential elements are covered, including a personal development plan and goal setting for the next period.

1. Collect information from:
   - The appraisee
   - The appraisee's log-book
   - Examination results
   - Courses attended
   - Feedback from other teachers
   - Feedback from other staff, both clinical and administrative
   - Feedback from patients
   - Feedback from students
   - Peer observation and feedback on teaching
2. Some prompts to reflect on for peer appraisal might include:
   - Review of significant event analysis
   - Review of audits and protocol development

- Review of prescribing data, referral data
- Surgical morbidity and mortality
- Measures of external esteem (papers, books, conference presentations)
- Working relationships with colleagues
- Review of teaching management and research activity
- Last year's personal development plan and log of completed learning

3. Agree on an agenda.
4. Structure the discussion. This might be informed by the portfolio.
5. Alternatively, use the competences identified in the core curriculum for their specialty or discipline.
6. Agree the current position. Reinforce strengths and identify problems.
7. Identify ways of resolving problems and other needs.
8. Agree a plan for the future.
9. Agree the date and time of the next appraisal meeting.

USING APPRAISAL TO DEAL WITH PROBLEMS

Sometimes problems concerning a learner are brought to you by others. That trainee may not realise that there is a problem, and when told about it, they may react angrily, deny the problem or accuse those making the comments of bias. This section provides advice on techniques to assist you in such circumstances. However, some appraisees lack insight to such an extent that you may require others to help you (see Chapter 19; see also Chapter 15 on feedback).

Even with peer appraisal you may sometimes need to address difficult areas, and may find it tricky to tackle these. As an appraiser, you have to make a decision. Are patients at risk? Does the appraisee lack insight? If the answer to both questions is yes, you must stop the appraisal and start your local poor performance procedure. If patients are not at direct risk and/or the colleague has insight and is prepared to stop working in that area while seeking some retraining, it may be possible to work on and make note of these issues. If the appraisee becomes angry or defensive, the appraisal should be stopped and referred to the appropriate risk management or clinical governance lead. In peer appraisal there is no obligation, as there would be in an educational supervisory position, to deal with it any further, except for your professional responsibilities in the case of a threat to patient safety.

TIPS FOR DEALING WITH PROBLEMS WITH APPRAISAL

- The whole process must be conducted using description, not judgement. For example: *Description:* 'You have not attended 50% of the training sessions, and there have been three occasions when you were half an hour late for the start of the clinic.' *Judgement:* 'You seem to be lazy and disorganised.'
- A key point: keep it friendly. Being descriptive allows you to assume the role of a concerned friend and adviser rather than an outraged boss. Your role is to nurture the appraisee and not necessarily to like them. Therefore ignore any

verbal or nonverbal anger or aggression that you may feel. Show respect for the appraisee, and it is more likely to be reciprocated.

- Identify and reinforce strengths.
- Problem areas need exact definition, not generalisations. For example: *Definition:* 'Your operations tend to take about 50% longer on average, and your knot tying in the cases I helped you with was insecure and different each time.' *Generalisation:* 'You've got two left hands.'
- Express the problem so as to obtain mutual agreement about how to proceed.
- Such agreement will be much enhanced by objective evidence. For example, this might include witnessing of practical skills, team observation, written tests, case-note review or video.
- Collaborate on constructive solutions. Each specific problem area should have an agreed method of targeted training, the setting of objectives to be achieved and a specified timescale.
- Identify 'carrots' and 'sticks' to promote achievement of objectives. Perhaps this trainee has a course he would like to go on. These must be realistic. If something you promise to aid achievement is not delivered, this will seriously demotivate the appraisee. If threatened sanctions are not applied, future threats will be less effective.
- Troubleshoot subsequent progress. For instance, remove minor obstacles before they become major. Keep tabs on the situation – hoping of course to catch the appraisee doing things right! By taking these actions, when the time comes for review, everyone will be well aware of the expected outcome, and any necessary sanctions can be applied with less confrontation.
- Review regularly until the appraisee is back on course.
- Be unyielding in your minimum expectations. If you have insisted that the trainee should attend 70% of a training programme and they do not comply, you must keep to the prearranged sanction.

Tips from experienced teachers

Appraisal can be a supportive and enjoyable process if done well. If your appraisee is a trainee, it can blur into performance management; aim to keep the two separate.

If your appraisee is a student, the university will likely have a personal tutor system. Ensure you follow the guidelines so that all students get equal and fair support. Don't hesitate to refer/ signpost them to university support structures or advise them to see their GP if you suspect any mental health issues such as anxiety.

If your appraisee is a colleague or peer, it can be a positive process of sharing ideas and best practice. It can also deteriorate into a joint exchange of worries, frustrations and irritations with the day job. Look out for that and don't be drawn in. Look out for and comment on behaviours associated with feelings of imposterism (BAFIs) (see Chapter 22).

> If you are the appraisee, consider what you need and expect from the process, and identify in advance what help you need from the appraiser. You know you would try and help if it was you, so will they!

REFERENCES

Chambers R., Tavabie A. and Mohanna K. (2004) *The good appraisal toolkit for primary care*. Oxford: Radcliffe Publishing.

Department for Education and Skills (DfES 2001) *A review of appraisal, disciplinary and reporting arrangements for senior NHS and university staff with academic and clinical duties*. Follett B. and Paulson-Ellis M. London: DfES.

Phillips T., Schostak J. and Tyler J. (2000) *Practice and assessment in nursing and midwifery: Doing it for real*. London: English National Board for Nursing, Midwifery and Health Visiting.

Robinson P. and Simpson L. (2003) *e-Appraisal: A guide for primary care*. Oxford: Radcliffe Medical Press.

Standing Committee on Postgraduate Medical and Dental Education (1996) *Appraising doctors and dentists in training*. London: SCOPME.

Stuart C. (2003) *Assessment, supervision and support in clinical practice: A guide for nurses, midwives and other health professionals*. Edinburgh: Churchill Livingstone.

Torrance H. and and Pryor J. (1998) *Investigating Formative Assessment*. Buckingham: Open University Press.

University of Worcester (2020) *Personal academic tutoring policy*. Worcester: UoW. Available at https://www2.worc.ac.uk/aqu/documents/Personal_Academic_Tutoring_Policy.pdf (Accessed 4.4.22).

CHAPTER 19

Supporting learners with difficulties and disabilities

···

Duncan Shrewsbury

When exploring the difficulties that learners face, it is helpful to draw on the metaphor of an iceberg: we might only observe the top 10% or so of the iceberg (of what is going on for the learner), but there will be a vast amount going on under the surface of the water that we cannot see.

This chapter focuses on *specific learning difficulties* (SpLD), like dyslexia, and *disabilities*. Definitions for disabilities and SpLD can vary across cultural contexts, but the framework used in practice in the UK is helpful to illustrate the key components (see Box 19.1).

BOX 19.1 DEFINITION OF DISABILITY FROM THE UK EQUALITY ACT (2010), AND OF SPECIFIC LEARNING DIFFICULTIES

A person has a disability if: (a) they have a physical or mental impairment, and (b) the impairment has a substantial and long-term adverse effect on their ability to carry out normal day-to-day activities.

Specific learning difficulties (SpLD) are a constellation of *profiles* of cognitive processing difficulties. These may predominantly affect literacy (e.g. fluency, speed and accuracy of reading and writing) – in which case the particular SpLD may be called dyslexia, or they may predominantly affect numeracy (e.g. handling, manipulation and communication of numerically encoded information). Common examples of SpLD include dyslexia, dyspraxia and attention deficit hyperactivity disorder (ADHD).

Reliable data relating to disabilities and learning difficulties among medical students and doctors is hard to find, but estimates would suggest that around 2% of

DOI: 10.1201/9781003352532-22

medical students (Shrewsbury 2011) and up to 5% of doctors may have specific learning difficulties (Shrewsbury 2016), and maybe around 4% of medical students disclose a disability upon applying to medical school (Shrewsbury 2016). These figures are likely to be under-estimates due to the fear that people may have about disclosure and associated stigma. However, even being generous with these estimates, there is a lower prevalence seen in medical education compared to general population statistics (Shrewsbury et al. 2018).

DOCTORS WITH DISABILITIES

Disabilities are generally thought to consist of a physical, sensory or mental impairment that has an impact on someone's ability to function. People may experience multiple forms of impairment and disability simultaneously. We know that some medical students and doctors will have or experience disabilities. We also know that the representation of people living with disabilities within both higher education and medical training in the UK is disproportionately low, compared to general population data. This is, in part, believed to be due to structural barriers that people with disabilities may face with accessing opportunities and participating equitably (Shrewsbury 2018).

The consideration of how disabilities may be *legally* defined (see Box 19.1) is of relevance to educators, because it provides protection for people living with disabilities against discrimination and also encodes for the provision of reasonable adjustments to facilitate equality of opportunity and participation (UK Equality Act 2010; WHO 2001). This is especially pertinent in the healthcare education context because the environments and organisations in which we teach and learn are generally also employers and public services. This drives a stronger imperative to ensure environments and practices are inclusive.

It is also worth noting the increasingly recognised relationship between working in healthcare and the association with burnout and chronic mental illness, especially among doctors (West and Coia 2019). Chronic mental illness is considered a disability within the majority of legal definitions and frameworks. This means that enduring mental health conditions, and the effects of treatments (e.g. sedative side-effects), must be considered within the definitional framework of disabilities and subsequent duties to provide reasonable adjustments.

Should a learner disclose a disability, or a suspicion of one, they should be supported in accessing formal assessment, drawing on the expertise of a multidisciplinary team (e.g. occupational health physician, occupational therapist and psychologist). In addition to this assessment, it should be noted that there are often government funded initiatives to assist people in accessing the support needed to work. In the UK this would be exemplified by the *access to work scheme*. Some practical considerations and suggestions for supporting learners with disabilities include the following:

- Adopting an individualistic approach with each different learner, drawing on coaching frameworks to ascertain needs and means to meet these. An example of a framework that might be useful is the Egan Skilled Helper Model, broadly summarised in Box 19.2 (Wosket 2006).

- Considering showcasing examples of inclusive practices and how learners with disabilities are supported so that positive outcomes from disclosure can be shared.
- Addressing anxieties relating to stigma and discrimination head-on, through encoding organisational or institutional practice and demonstrating accountability.

BOX 19.2 THE EGAN SKILLED HELPER MODEL (SUMMARISED)

Stage 1: What is going on (here and now)?
- What problems and opportunities are affecting learning and practice?
- What new perspectives can tell us more about these challenges?
- What is of key importance, and what would work best to solve first?

Stage 2: What solutions make sense for me?
- What would you hope to see happen instead?
- What is a helpful goal to work towards, and how should this be worded?
- What will the benefits (or potential consequences) of this be?

Stage 3: How do I secure what I need or want?
- What might help you get to where you need to be? How many different ways can you achieve this?
- What is the best way to achieve your goals for you (e.g. 'Force Field Analysis')?
- What will you do next, and what will your next steps be (e.g. Timeline)?

SPECIFIC LEARNING DIFFICULTIES

The phrase 'specific learning difficulties' (SpLD) is often used as an umbrella term to refer to a range of neurological conditions that impact on people's ability to assimilate, process and handle information. The most prevalent example is dyslexia, which estimates suggest affects about 6% of the general population (Miles 2004) and possibly around 2–5% of medical students and doctors, as noted earlier. Importantly, all of these conditions exist on a spectrum of severity, and co-occurrence is relatively common (Deponio 2004). This means that the way one person may experience their SpLD can be quite different from another, and the way that SpLD may manifest through education, training and practice can also be unique and dynamic.

Many learners with SpLD achieve great successes throughout their lives, but may experience a particular set of difficulties in trying to do so. In response to this, people with SpLD often develop sophisticated coping strategies, which can mean that they progress through certain stages of training successfully. At times, however, these coping strategies can be overwhelmed and the underlying difficulties can manifest and result in unexpected performance issues, or psychological distress. This is why it is not unusual to find that adults with SpLD often get diagnosed later in life, sometimes triggered by an unexpected examination failure (McLaughlin 2015).

Multiple studies have looked at the impact of SpLD like dyslexia on the education, training and practice of doctors. Perhaps unsurprisingly, common difficulties experienced include the following:

- Recall and communication of information from clinical notes or conversations
- Being asked to read clinical notes aloud in front of patients and colleagues
- Poor time management and task prioritisation
- Greater distractibility, and poorer concentration

Whilst these struggles may impact on functioning in the clinical environment, there is nothing to suggest they negatively impact on patient care (Newlands et al. 2015). Experiencing difference and difficulty, however, can have an impact on self-esteem and wellbeing. This is thought to be due to the way in which professional identity (e.g. self-as-doctor) becomes so core to one's global self-concept, that the impact of SpLD on academic self-concept (e.g. arithmetic, literacy, clinical knowledge and clinical skill) can impact on mental health, motivation and openness to talking about and seeking help with their difficulties (Marsh 1990; Shrewsbury 2018). This further highlights the need for educators to be proactive about cultivating a supportive, nurturing and inclusive environment for people to learn and work in, and to foster good relationships and communication with their learners.

REASONABLE ADJUSTMENTS

When considering provision of different forms of support for learners experiencing disabilities or difficulties, it is important for us to consider the imperative to provide 'reasonable adjustments' – both to enable access to and support in education and training and to be taken into account in assessment of performance. In the UK, this imperative is reflected in legislation (UK Equality Act 2010), and as such it is a requirement of organisations to have an open and accountable system in place to proactively assess the need for and provide reasonable adjustments. There are tensions, concerns and misapprehensions about the provision of such adjustments in higher and medical education (Riddell and Weedon 2006).

These are terms that are also frequently misused in debates of widening participation initiatives. To clarify what we mean exactly by reasonable adjustment, it helps to consider how we might also define other measures that are sometimes referred to in relation to supporting learners, especially in the context of assessments (see Table 19.1). From these clarified definitions, it becomes apparent that reasonable adjustments are measures that are intended to 'level the playing field' and support equality of access to an opportunity, rather than to fundamentally alter the construct of what is being taught or assessed.

TABLE 19.1 Applying the UK Equality Act (2010) and Other Definitions to Consider the Terminology of Adjustment, Accommodation, Modification and Compensation

Reasonable adjustment	*A measure employed in order to alleviate or remove the effects of a 'substantial disadvantage'.*
Accommodation	*A measure that differentially affects a student's performance in comparison to a peer group. An accommodation does not alter the nature of the construct being assessed, but does provide differential access so that students with certain characteristics may complete the test with influence from confounding variables minimised (e.g. change in administration of an assessment or response format) (Tindal et al. 1997).*
Modification	*A change in the test, for example, the way it is administered, format of response, that results in a change in the constructs being measured. Modifications affect all students with similar or equal effect (Hollenbeck et al. 1998)*
Compensation	*In the sense of academic performance rather than remuneration in the context of settling a claim or complaint, compensation can be seen as either an* **internal** *or* **external** *process.* **Internal** *compensation: a process by which individuals employ strategies to overcome or minimise the effects of their disability.* **External** *compensation: a process by which those assessing performance make allowances for difficulties associated with the disability (e.g. not deducting marks for poor spelling of dyslexic learner's work). In assessment, compensation is also used to refer to the practice of allowing higher marks in one assessment to compensate for unsatisfactory marks in another.*

In the context of medical education, the most frequently afforded accommodation is an extension to the time in which learners have to sit an assessment, and is usually restricted to written assessments. In childhood, extended time is seen to confer advantage on all students in earlier phases of their education, where both disabled and non-disabled learners improve performance with this accommodation (Elliott and Marquart 2004). However, in adults this effect is not seen, and what is termed the 'accommodation-disability paradigm effect' is seen, where only disabled learners benefit from accommodating conditions, such as extra time (Phillips 1994; Runyan 1991). Retrospective analyses of assessments data for medical student and post-graduate doctors provides no evidence to suggest that the provision of accommodations affords unfair advantage to dyslexic learners, and indeed may suggest that there is still some work to be done to ameliorate disadvantage (Ricketts et al. 2010; Gibson and Leinster 2011; Asghar et al. 2019).

SUPPORTING LEARNERS

When considering how one may support a learner experiencing difficulties or disabilities, it is firstly important to consider how their overall wellbeing and sense of self-esteem has been affected. Some learners may previously have experienced discrimination or fear prejudice. Fostering a culture of positive active bystandership is essential to all inclusivity endeavours, meaning supporting any observer to speak up, and differential confrontation of examples of prejudicial or discriminatory behaviour. These moments of challenge, however, should exist within a wider context of greater cultural change intended to role model and support inclusion of diverse learners. Beyond this, it behoves us to develop a keen curiosity in our learners' approach to learning and work, so that we can ascertain and anticipate learners' needs. Longitudinal studies of adults with learning disabilities concluded that keys to success included the following:

- Self-awareness
- Perseverance
- Appropriate goal setting
- Use of effective support systems

(Goldberg et al. 2003)

Many of these attributes rely on a degree of self-awareness of the experienced disability or difficulty in the context of clinical learning and work. Given the fear of perceived stigma following self-disclosure, it is likely that some learners may be reticent to discuss their diagnosis, disability or difficulty with you as their educator. This must, of course, be respected, but also met with tangible examples of inclusive practice to encourage learners to come forth to discuss their experiences with us. This might also extend, where individuals feel comfortable, to role models sharing their own experiences of success whist living with difference. In other words, we need to cultivate a learning environment that is constantly inclusive and sensitive to difficulties or differences faced by learners so that learners feel less 'at risk' and able to discuss their needs with their educators.

This process also requires an open-mindedness to different ways of learning and working that may not have been typical of historical practices. For example, the consideration of altering working times to accommodate a later start for someone affected by the sedative side effects of their mental health medication. Another example might include being conscious to not ask someone to read aloud or act as a scribe. Indeed, the majority of learners who experience a disability or difficulty tend to have a good idea of what they need in order to cope in specific situations. The key, as an educator, is to foster a relationship where difficulties, limitations and different approaches to learning and coping can continuously be explored, revisited and re-assessed. Seeking support from appropriately qualified individuals (e.g. educational psychologists, specialist tutors or occupational health practitioners) is also vital in establishing a baseline level of understanding for learners' particular difficulties. The report and recommendations from such a specialist can be an incredibly helpful starting point for a longitudinal coaching-like relationship with the learner so that their approaches to learning and working can be optimised.

REFERENCES

Asghar Z., Williams N., Denney M. and Siriwardena A.N. (2019) Performance in candidates declaring vs not declaring dyslexia in a licensing clinical exam. *Medical Education*, 53(12): 1243–1252.

Deponio P. (2004) The co-occurrence of specific learning difficulties: Implications for identification and assessment. In Reid G. and Fawcett A. (eds) *Dyslexia in context: Research, policy and practice*. London: Whurr Publications.

Elliott S.N. and Marquart A.M. (2004) Extended time as a testing accommodation: Its effect and perceived consequences. *Exceptional Children*, 70: 349–367.

Gibson S. and Leinster S. (2011) How do medical students with dyslexia perform in extended matching questions, short answer questions and observed structured clinical examinations? *Advances in Health Science Education*, 16: 395–404.

Goldberg R.J., Higgins E.L., Raskind M.H., et al. (2003) Predictors of success in individuals with learning disabilities: A qualitative analysis of a 20-year longitudinal study. *Learning Disability Research and Practice*, 18: 222–236.

Gov.UK. Equality Act 2010: guidance. https://www.gov.uk/guidance/equality-act-2010-guidance.

Hollenbeck K., Tindal G. and Almond P. (1998) Teachers' knowledge of accommodation as a validity issue in high-stakes testing. *Journal of Special Education*, 32: 175–183.

Marsh H. (1990) The structure of academic self-concept: The Marsh/Shavelson model. *Journal of Educational Psychology*, 82(4): 623–636.

McLaughlin D. (2015) Career development and individuals with dyslexia. *Career Planning and Adult Development Journal*, 31: 151–161.

Miles T.R. (2004) Some problems in determining the prevalence of dyslexia. *Electronic Journal of Research in Educational Psychology*, 2: 5–12.

Newlands F., Shrewsbury D. and Robson J. (2015) Foundation doctors and dyslexia: A qualitative study of their experiences and coping strategies. *Postgraduate Medical Journal*, 91: 121–126.

Phillips S.E. (1994) High-stakes testing accommodations: Validity versus disabled rights. *Applied Measurement in Education*, 7: 93–120.

Ricketts C., Brice J. and Coombes L. (2010) Are multiple choice tests fair to medical students with specific learning disabilities? *Advances in Health Science Education*, 45: 176–182.

Riddell S. and Weedon E. (2006) What counts as a reasonable adjustment? Dyslexic students and the concept of fair assessment. *International Studies in Sociology of Education*, 16: 57–73.

Runyan M.K. (1991) The effect of extra time on reading comprehension scores for university students with and without learning disabilities. *Journal of Learning Disabilities*, 24: 104–108.

Shrewsbury D. (2011) State of play: Supporting students with learning difficulties. *Medical Teacher*, 33: 254–255.

Shrewsbury D. (2016) Dyslexia in general practice education: Considerations for recognition and support. *Education for Primary Care*, 24(4): 267–270.

Shrewsbury D. (2018) *Dyslexia and medicine: The experience and the impact of dyslexia on the education, training and practice of doctors*. Unpublished PhD Thesis, University of Exeter. Available at https://ore.exeter.ac.uk/repository/handle/10871/32896.

Shrewsbury D., Mogensen L. and Hu W. (2018) Problematizing medical students with disabilities: A critical policy analysis. *MedEdPublish*, 7: 45. https://doi.org/10.15694/mep.2018.0000045.1.

Tindal G., Hollenbeck K., Heath W. and Almond P. (1997) *The effect of using computers as an accommodation in a statewide writing test*. Eugene: University of Oregon Press.

West M. and Coia D. (2019) *Caring for doctors, caring for patients: How to transform UK healthcare environments to support doctors and medical students to care for patients.* Manchester: UK General Medical Council.

World Health Organisation (2001) *International classification for functioning, disability and health (ICF).* Geneva: World Health Organisation.

Wosket V. (2006) *Egan's skilled helper model: Developments and implications in counselling.* London: Routledge.

CHAPTER 20

The challenging trainee

....

CHALLENGING TRAINEES: WHERE IS THE PROBLEM?

Sometimes the difficulty lies with the learner, sometimes with the teacher and sometimes with the learner–teacher relationship. There are probably as many causes of this as there are challenging trainees, but there are some recurring themes, which other chapters in this book might also give suggestions for:

- Mismatch between teaching style and stage of self-directedness of the learner (see also Chapters 8 and 9)
- Problems with the learning-group dynamics
- Health-related issues – mental or physical
- Specific learning difficulties (see Chapter 19)
- Problems outside work (e.g. family difficulties, financial problems)
- Disciplinary matters
- Are they in the wrong career?

Multidisciplinary healthcare teachers on a postgraduate certificate in medical education were asked what they found challenging about teaching. Some of their responses are listed in Box 20.1. You will probably recognise things that are true for you.

BOX 20.1 'I FIND IT CHALLENGING WHEN . . .'

- Learners say 'yes' but mean 'no' when I ask whether they understand.
- People sit at the back of the group and talk throughout the session.
- Students relate to me on a surface level and don't incorporate learning into the next scenario.
- Juniors can't get on with other members of the team.

DOI: 10.1201/9781003352532-23

- Students forget what we have covered.
- I have a trainee who is competent clinically, but lazy.
- I have to give advice about moving/changing career.
- Learners know more than me!
- I need to find out what the trainee doesn't know.
- Learners react in an irritated manner or it turns into an argument.
- We can identify the issue but the learner doesn't want to address it.
- People don't listen to reason.
- I need to balance pastoral care/careers counselling with teaching and clinical commitments.
- Trainees say 'teach me something'.
- A trainee is not able to recognise weaknesses or shortcomings.
- I find it difficult to confront trainees with attitude problems.

Is it a communication issue?

One of the keys to preventing or dealing with difficulties lies in the educational rapport between the learner and the teacher. The Johari window (see Figure 20.1) is well established model for thinking about communication (Luft 1970).

The four panes of the window represent how relationships are built up by an accumulation of information from 'self' and 'others' – me and you. As you build relationships with your learners to increase the effectiveness of your teaching, this model might help to explain why some people are considered to have communication difficulties, or are labelled poor communicators, or worse still, why relationships become dysfunctional. Up to a point, the larger the area called the arena in the top left-hand 'pane' of the window, the more productive the relationship will be.

Consider the crossed lines that separate the panes in the 'window' in Figure 20.1 as if they can be moved in the direction of the arrows to vary 'pane' size. The horizontal line represents exposure (disclosure). Here you open up the self, share ideas and information, admit mistakes, and talk about feelings and opinions. As you increase exposure, your facade decreases, but the blind spot may increase due to less time being given to feedback.

The vertical line in Figure 20.1 represents feedback seeking. Here you ask for and encourage feedback, and the 'self' gives 'others' the opportunity to express their feelings in an open and supportive way. If used alone it may increase the facade, as it allows less time for exposure.

You can use either of these behaviours equally, but most people have a preference for one or the other. To enhance relationships you need not change, but alter the balance of these two basic behaviours.

- *Type A:* little exposure, little feedback seeking. These individuals are often perceived as withdrawn, aloof or impersonal, where the unknown square

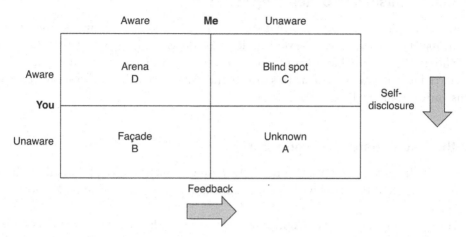

FIGURE 20.1 The Johari window.

(in Figure 20.1) is the largest. This may induce resentment in others, who may take the behaviour personally. It can be common in large bureaucratic organisations.

- *Type B:* increased feedback seeking, little exposure. These individuals decrease the information about themselves that is available to others, while requiring more from others, due to either fear or a wish for power or control. Others may react by withdrawing trust or becoming hostile.
- *Type C:* increased exposure, neglect of feedback. These individuals are oblivious to the effect that they have on others. They have a large blind spot, as the opportunity for feedback is rare. They may be confident of their own opinions, and insensitive, with little concern for the feelings of others. Listeners may become angry and reluctant to tell them anything.
- *Type D:* balanced. These individuals have a large arena, as feedback seeking and exposure are well used. They are open and candid. Initially others may be put on the defensive, but when they are seen as genuine, productive relationships can follow. They induce an open, balanced response in others.

Teachers and learners need to be sensitive about the covert content of the blind spot, the facade and the hidden area, and respect privacy concerning information that is kept hidden for reasons of social training or custom.

Is it a problem with the learner's stage of self-direction?

Although teachers of adult learners appreciate that there is a process involved in developing higher levels of self-direction, it does not always occur to them that their teaching level may be out of step with, or be mismatched to, their learner's current stage (see Chapters 8 and 9).

Is there a mismatch of 'learning styles'?

You will recall from Chapter 7 that there is much discussion about the concept of 'learning styles'. It is true however that learners differ in their expectations of what teaching is 'for' and what it should look like. It helps to have insight into your own preferred learning activities, as this affects the way you teach, and to be aware that this varies from one learner to the next.

Is the issue related to group work?

Probably the commonest clinical teaching setting is a small group, and all teachers will experience difficulties with the reactions and interactions of some members of the group.

A useful summary of behaviours within a group divides actions into talkers, quiet and hesitant or negative (Allery 1998).

Talkers

The Monopoliser: enthusiastic, and often knowledgeable, this learner could be preventing others from contributing. Limit their domination of the discussion by summarising contributions and moving on, interjecting with yes or no answers and inviting others to contribute. Ask them to make written summaries of the group discussion. Split the group into smaller cells.

The Rambler: restrain contributions that cause diversions by asking direct questions of others. Address the problem head on (e.g. say 'That is interesting, but our point is . . .'). Defer until later (e.g. coffee time).

The Eager Beaver: some learners try to answer every question. Acknowledge this help, but suggest that others should be asked for their views, or direct questions to others by name.

The Conferrer: ask yourself why this is happening. Do you need to change something you are doing? Stop talking and listen until they realise. Call them by name and draw them in with a direct question. Ask them whether they have anything to add to the discussion. Brief a co-facilitator to sit next to them to prevent a participant from being distracted.

Quiet and hesitant

The Shy and Timid: allow time for their responses and value their contributions. Boost their confidence through social events. Protect them from mockery within the group.

The Reticent: do they feel indifferent to the group or the task, or do they have something else on their mind? A non-participant may be unsure of the relevance of the task, or may be a reflector, or may be tired after being on call.

The Superior: ensure that you do not have a false stage 4 (S4) learner (see Chapter 8). This is easier said than done and will most likely need a careful one-to-one discussion. Encourage them to share their experience/expertise with the group. Use them to lead on tasks.

Negative

The Complainer: control their fault finding by asking for specifics. Ask others in the group if they agree.

The Clown: humour can be useful, but what is the constant joker really doing? Repeated irritating one-liners might be an attempt to upstage the teacher or to lighten a subject they find difficult. Compliment any serious contribution, and ask for the point behind the comment.

The Arguer: antagonistic combatants like to score points. Avoid lengthy debate ('I think we will have to disagree'). Ask the group to comment – they will often criticise outlandish suggestions. Alternatively, take the person to one side and offer to 'help' if they have a problem.

Other participants can learn a lot from the varieties of opinions expressed in group work and the ways in which they are discussed, and they will also learn from how you deal with the situation. Only if one person's behaviour is seriously preventing others from learning, and after exhausting all other avenues, should you ask a group member to leave.

There are some general principles for dealing with resistance in a group that are devised from the five beliefs of neurolinguistic programming (NLP), known as presuppositions of NLP (Walker 2002).

Perhaps bear these ideas in mind when a learner is frustrating you!

1. The map is not the territory. Everyone has a different world view, and there is no one right model of the world.
2. Knowing other people's maps is useful in order to communicate with them effectively.
3. People make the best choices available to them at the time, given the possibilities and capabilities that they perceive are accessible to them.
4. Separate a person's behaviour from the intention behind it, and respond to the intention.
5. Resistance and objections are often communications about positive intentions that are not being met.

It is useful to presuppose that all behaviour in a group is positively intended and that negative behaviours are separate from the positive intent. Therefore, consider trying to identify the positive intent of the resistant person, and offer them other choices of behaviour to achieve the same positive intention.

Is it an issue of time management?

If your learner persistently arrives after everyone else and can't seem to fit all the work into the day, first check that this is not due to a misunderstanding. Do they genuinely think the 8.30am ward round starts at 9.00am, or do they have conflicting commitments, such as a child to be dropped off at the nursery? This situation might be remedied by a simple renegotiation of working hours. However, some learners never seem to cope well with meeting deadlines. They request extensions for project work, are late for meetings, their clinics over-run and their paperwork is left undone. This might be a time management problem. Discuss it and come to a joint understanding about why this issue has arisen. Sometimes learners have full, difficult lives, and the best you can be is supportive. Offer advice about priority setting, delegation, planning, organisation and not taking on too much.

Are they simply in the wrong career?

People become healthcare professionals for a variety of reasons, parental expectations being just one. Many sources of career advice are now available through education and training organisations and their websites. If a learner really does not like healthcare and is in the wrong career, the only solution may be to change direction.

WHY HEALTH PROFESSIONALS RUN INTO DIFFICULTIES: WIDER ISSUES

Apart from problems with educational processes, there are a number of other reasons why your learners may run into difficulties. We can categorise the various problems into five main areas:

1. Personal conduct
2. Professional conduct
3. Competence and performance issues
4. Health and disability
5. Adverse life events

Personal conduct issues that are not related to being a health professional

Examples of personal conduct issues that have provoked disciplinary procedures for trainees include theft, fraud, assault, vandalism, rudeness, bullying, racial and sexual harassment, child pornography, drunkenness and serious traffic offences. Sometimes the police will be involved.

The normal procedure for doctors in training in the UK is that the three responsible bodies – the lead employer, Health Education England and the training site (Trust, or practice) – must all be involved. So, whoever first becomes aware of an issue will inform the other two. A clear disciplinary process is available for doctors in training, and human resources functions are organised and implemented by the lead employer. Advice on representation and pastoral support will be given.

Professional conduct issues that are related to being a health professional

Examples of professional misconduct include inappropriate behaviour during clinical examinations, falsely claiming qualifications, plagiarism, research misconduct, failure to take consent properly, prescribing issues, improper relationships with patients, improper certification issues (e.g. the signing of cremation forms, sickness certification, passport forms) and breaches of confidentiality.

Again, the lead employer will take the lead under its approved disciplinary procedures. For issues in either of these two first lists, it is very likely the regulatory body such as the General Medical Council will be informed.

Any decision to involve the regulatory body is a very serious one for the professional involved, and this will be a joint decision. Regulatory bodies generally recommend that approved procedures should be followed first at the local level, rather than everything being reported to national regulatory bodies at the earliest stage.

Competence and performance issues

Examples include a single serious clinical mistake, excessively slow surgical operating, poor clinical results (possibly found as a result of audit), persistent poor time-keeping, poor communication or English language skills, and repeated failure to attend educational events. Very basic problems can occur, including inability to take a history or examine a patient, and unsafe use of basic equipment. Most of these can be dealt with through the educational framework. An isolated serious mistake may happen to any practising healthcare professional and usually does not reflect the overall competence of the individual.

Health and sickness issues

Depressive illness is common and sadly under-diagnosed. A few healthcare professionals will have a psychotic illness, and when this is uncontrolled it can be very serious and difficult to manage in the workplace. Alcohol- and drug-related problems occur. Healthcare professionals have physical illnesses just as others do, including multiple sclerosis, diabetes, arthritis and chronic respiratory diseases. Most of these problems can be successfully managed and the individual concerned restored to the workplace.

Adverse life event

Adverse life events may be a contributing factor to any of the previous categories. People may experience horrendous adverse events which occurred outside of the workplace and will often not volunteer such information. An effective educational supervisor, noticing some change in behaviour, might ask 'is everything alright at home?' and discover bereavements, severe illness, accidents, change of job, moving house, lack of family support, and so on. Sometimes healthcare professionals who work in one country have close family living in another and may travel back and forth. This undoubtedly has an effect on the individual's personal and professional life.

Stress is cumulative. Sometimes it may be a small event that tips the balance following a series of major life events – 'the straw that broke the camel's back'.

RISK FACTORS THAT TRIGGER DIFFICULTIES FOR LEARNERS

Certain traits and situations will place your learners at risk of running into problems. Knowing these risk factors will alert you to when you need to be more vigilant with your learners, hopefully either pre-empting and thereby avoiding problems, or detecting them in their early stages.

Personality, behaviour and performance

Several personality characteristics can result in problems with behaviour and performance. For example, perfectionist tendencies can lead to poor time management, and arrogant behaviour may be associated with individuals being unable to recognise their limitations or when they are heading for problems. Although we will not be able to change people's personalities, it is often possible to detect and quantify unacceptable behaviours with multi-source feedback and to help to modify these behaviours with coaching, constructive feedback and, on occasion, sanctions.

Education and training

Healthcare education in different settings can put different emphasis on aspects such as communication skills (both with patients and with colleagues), on multidisciplinary teamworking and on appropriate attitudes and behaviours. This might be governed by cultural and societal norms. Healthcare professionals who are moving from one setting to another might experience challenges of expectations and experiences.

Teamworking

Most of us work in teams, but we don't all work in supportive and effective teams. Working in a multidisciplinary team can be demanding, but good teams are rewarding to work in, result in less stress among their members and provide a good and important sense of support. The dysfunctional team is the opposite of this. People become stressed and hate working. Different understanding of the models of the societal or healthcare hierarchy, for example, might lead one member to ignore the wishes of others and behave in an authoritarian and condescending way to other members.

Leadership (or lack of it)

Trainee healthcare professionals need opportunities to develop leadership skills (see Chapter 22). Leaders should be able to recognise limitations, delegate, predict and plan accordingly, and create a sense of justice. They should have good communication skills and integrity, and give people a sense of control. Unfortunately, some healthcare professionals in senior positions have developed few of these qualities, either through lack of training or opportunity.

Cognitive impairment

This term encompasses concerns about a person's memory, reasoning or decision making. It is uncommon, but some senior healthcare professionals have run into problems of underperformance, when further investigations have revealed loss of short-term memory and dementia. Cognitive impairment may result from long-standing alcohol-related problems, certain neurological disorders, electroconvulsive therapy (ECT), severe head injury, stroke and coronary heart disease. It can be very difficult to diagnose cognitive impairment and to differentiate it from depression. Expert referral and assessment are necessary.

Organisational culture and climate

Organisational climate relates to staff perceptions of what it is like to work in the organisation, and organisational culture is also about expected behaviours, leadership style and values. Ideally, we would all like to work in an open, fair, friendly, sensitive and supportive culture where we feel appreciated and valued. Working in a culture of institutional bullying and intimidation, scapegoating and poor leadership is stressful and can lead to unhelpful behaviours in return. It should not be tolerated. Leaders who are ignorant, arrogant, dictatorial, hostile or boastful can cause many problems – for example, less efficient working and high rates of staff absence and turnover, as people get fed up and look for opportunities to leave for other jobs where they feel more appreciated.

Heavy workload

Although the number of hours worked per week has slowly declined for healthcare professionals generally, the intensity and complexity of practice have greatly increased, and there are still some pockets of heavy workload and a 'long-hours' culture. Lack of sleep and shift working can result in poor performance and can make existing mental and physical health problems worse. A heavy workload may cause burnout. Shift working is especially risky at times when levels of sleepiness are high, such as between 1 am and 6 am, but in general can have adverse physiological effects on the individual. Ensuring that there are proper timetabled breaks will help.

WAYS IN WHICH A PROBLEM MAY PRESENT

We can identify several early signs of trainees (and colleagues) being in difficulty:

- The disappearing act: not answering bleeps, frequent sick leave, not attending teaching sessions, failure to turn up for work or learning events
- Low work rate: slow in performing procedures, clerking patients and dictating letters, non-participation in group work, destructive group behaviour, not keeping up to date, failing to prepare for teaching, failure in exams
- Ward rage: problems working in the team, shouting at colleagues, inability to give instructions to or take instructions from staff
- Rigidity: low tolerance of uncertainty, difficulty in making priority decisions
- Bypass syndrome: nurses and other colleagues avoid asking the doctor to do anything
- Career problems: examination difficulty, disillusionment with medicine
- Insight failure: rejection of constructive feedback, defensiveness, counter challenge
- Unkempt: poor personal hygiene or inappropriate dress

WHAT SHOULD WE DO IN PRACTICE?

When learners are in difficulty, the training organisation should follow a set procedure. An example for doctors in difficulty is provided in Figure 20.2. The process and elements to think about if setting up such a service, are described here.

Phase 1: the referral

Highlighting the concern must be done confidentially and, ideally, with the learner's knowledge.

Phase 2: meeting the individual

An introduction is essential, including an explanation that this process is intended to help the person and is not a telling off or disciplinary meeting. Ask the individual to tell their story. Rather than have an unstructured and often rambling conversation, structure the conversation. Frame the meeting, and say that after the introductions you will be asking about the situation in four areas as follows:

1. The career history from undergraduate to the present time, including the person's career aims
2. The present problem as the person perceives it
3. Health issues and any adverse life events
4. The plan of action proposed – this may be to offer a diagnosis and a plan of actions to help, or more frequently you will need to obtain further information and meet again

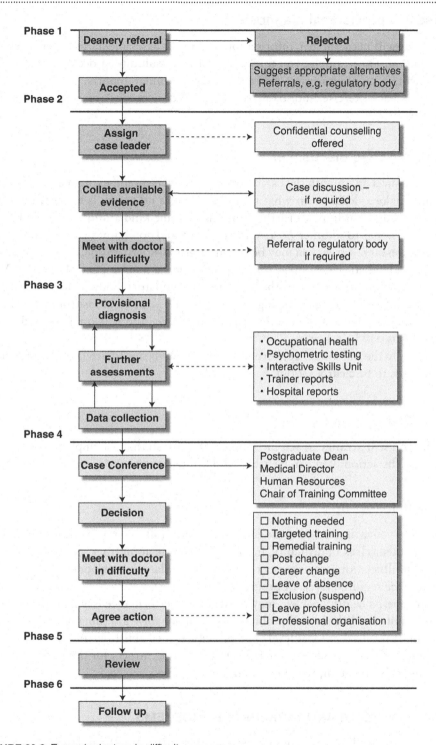

FIGURE 20.2 Example doctors in difficulty process.

Phase 3: a provisional diagnosis

Often you will need further information and other assessments in order to clarify the situation. For example, you might ask for a consultant-led occupational health assessment, a communication skills assessment, trainer reports, a further multi-source feedback exercise, and so on. You should then arrange to meet again to review all of this.

Phase 4: a case discussion

When you meet again with the extra information, you should explain all of the findings and make a decision on what to do. Sometimes no action is needed, but often you will need to put in place further training of some kind and/or move the healthcare professional to another post. Career advice and sometimes career counselling may be necessary. Rarely you may be required to advise suspension, or even to advise that the individual leaves their training programme and/or post altogether. Very rarely you will need to refer to the professional regulatory body. Before doing this, you must discuss the case at the highest level within your local institution/organisation. Once the referral has gone in, it is unstoppable, and it is often unpredictable what actions will be taken.

Hopefully the individual concerned will agree with the advised course of action, which needs to be clearly set out.

Phase 5: the review

Usually you will arrange to see the individual again so that the implementation and success of the action plan can be assessed. Has improvement occurred?

Phase 6: follow-up

Sometimes you will need to arrange a longer-term follow-up of certain individuals who find themselves in difficulty, in order to keep them on track. Sometimes this is because of illness, or a requirement from their regulatory body, or because they do not make the required levels of progress.

Remember, a health problem may present as a performance issue, and vice versa. If you do not establish the real problem, you will not solve anything, but many problems can be resolved at local level. The principles of establishing and using the facts (and not opinions), constructive feedback and setting targets for improvement, and following these through, will work well in most cases.

EARLY DIAGNOSIS AND TACKLING OF PROBLEMS

If you are involved in managing an individual in difficulty, the following principles will be helpful.

1. *Do it now:* Tackle the problem when it occurs, not at the end of the placement or not at all.
2. *Find out the facts:* Don't jump to conclusions. Obtain information from all sides.
3. *Share the problem:* Don't do it all on your own.
4. *Explain the problem:* Discuss the problem constructively with the individual concerned, and plan how to get back on course. Sometimes no one has sat down with the individual and explained what the difficulty is, and how this may be put right. Sometimes people will say that this was the first time that anyone had mentioned to them that they have a communication skills or teamworking problem.
5. *Give support:* Appropriate encouragement and positive feedback do work.

GETTING BACK ON TRACK: GUIDING PRINCIPLES

The National Clinical Assessment Service (NCAS) has described 11 key principles for handling performance concerns (NCAS 2006a). These are as follows.

1. Patient safety must be the primary consideration.
2. Healthcare organisations are responsible for developing policies and procedures to recognise performance concerns early and act swiftly to address those concerns.
3. Policies for handling performance concerns should be circulated to all healthcare practitioners.
4. Avoid unnecessary or inappropriate exclusions of practitioners.
5. Separate investigation from decision making.
6. Staff and managers should understand the factors that may contribute to performance concerns.
7. Performance procedures should contribute to the organisational programme for clinical governance.
8. Good human resources practice will help to prevent performance problems.
9. Healthcare practitioners who work in isolated settings may require additional support.
10. Individual healthcare practitioners are responsible for maintaining a good standard of practice.
11. There must be commitment to equality and diversity.

Back-on-track framework

In addition, NCAS has also outlined seven guiding principles for helping healthcare professionals who are in difficulty (NCAS 2006b).

1. *Clinical governance and patient safety:* Patient safety must come first.
2. *A single framework guiding individual programmes:* Use of a framework must encompass common principles, which are applicable in different specialties and for different grades.

3. *A comprehensive approach:* Identify and deal with problems comprehensively, identifying all of the issues, dealing with the needs of the individual and the organisation, and keeping the need to protect patient safety as a primary concern. Communication skills are often a problem, so work closely with communication skills teachers to help to identify and improve communication.

4. *Fairness, transparency, confidentiality and consent:* You must be fair and open about what you do. The confidentiality of the person in difficulty needs to be protected. Copy letters to the organisations involved, to occupational health (where applicable), and to the person in difficulty so that they know exactly what has been said and why. However, there is a guiding principle here about the need to know, so such information should only be given to those helping in the process. Patients need to be properly informed if they are being seen by an individual who is on a return-to-work programme. Fairness also involves being aware of and practising fairness in terms of the legislation on equality of opportunity with regard to age, gender, ethnicity, religion, sexual orientation and disability.

5. *Ongoing and constant support:* This is essential. Support for some individuals in difficulty may be necessary for several years, sticking with it despite setbacks. In certain cases, individuals may continue to need support for over ten years. Good progress can still occur even after this time, but it can be a long hard journey with considerable setbacks on the way. In such cases the remedial training team and the healthcare organisation can be under considerable load. Often such teams need breaks from training after dealing with an individual in difficulty, as remedial training can put considerable stress on the whole team. You may need to be aware of and recognise this as a significant issue.

6. *Success and failure:* Although you hope that dealing with the problems of individuals in difficulty will help them to succeed and get back on track, this is not always the case. Think of what to do if a programme of return to work does not succeed, and how to spell out what is to happen if objectives are not achieved. Sometimes, for those individuals with severe physical or mental illness, despite all measures to cope, the only solution may be an early retirement on medical grounds. Here obviously the continuing involvement and close collaboration of a senior consultant in occupational medicine is essential. On rare occasions, in other situations, where the individual is felt to pose a danger to patients, a referral to the appropriate regulatory body will be appropriate. If you are dealing with individuals in difficulty, you must acknowledge that you cannot succeed in every case. You also need support from your professional organisation.

7. *Local resolution drawing on local and national expertise:* Use local procedures first. Sharing your experiences is also very valuable at the local and/or regional level. People need to be trained at the local level in managing poor performance so that they know what to look out for, what to do, and when and where to refer on for help if necessary.

FUNDING

Who pays for the person to be re-trained? This can be a very difficult issue. For those who are trainees and who are already in approved training programmes, it is easier, as the postgraduate training organisation will keep some posts for such eventualities. For healthcare professionals who are employed or contracted in career posts, some healthcare organisations are willing to fund or part-fund a return-to-work programme, including help with courses, for a specific period of time according to a programme of training and assessment. For certain professionals there can be a considerable problem of locum costs for backfilling the work of the individual while they are away re-training.

The situation can be dire for individuals who are unemployed, who are not trainees, or who have been suspended or erased from the professional register for several years. However, they may expect to be given a job immediately after remediation. Often such individuals are in considerable difficulty in many areas, have a chaotic life situation, are in debt, and are unable to fund their re-training. The suggestion that such individuals should take out a loan, when they may already be in considerable debt and have no creditworthiness at all, is not viable. A clear policy and ring-fenced funding are required to help to rehabilitate such desperate individuals. Remember that not everyone is remediable (see Section 20.9).

REMEDIABILITY WITH REGARD TO CLINICIANS IN DIFFICULTY

Remediability refers to whether an individual's problems may be successfully addressed and their career put back on track, or whether the prognosis is so poor that other measures need to be considered. In the area of remediation, we need to know what we may take on with the hope of successful remediation back into practice, or whether we need to consider other measures such as referral to the regulatory organisation or advice on resignation or retirement from the post. Can we predict how well a person in difficulty will respond? To some extent the answer is yes. Here is a classification that you might find useful, which is partly derived from discussions at the Network of Expertise Group at the NCAS, and which is summarised in Table 20.1.

Capacity to learn

Some individuals may have lost the capacity to learn, perhaps due to brain injury, various neurological disorders or the development of cognitive impairment. Some of these cases represent really sad situations. Without capacity to learn, the prognosis is poor.

Knowledge or skill deficit

If a specific area of knowledge or skill deficit has been identified, and the healthcare professional recognises this fact, has insight and is willing to learn, focused training

TABLE 20.1 Remediability

Capacity to learn	May have reached limitations	Prognosis poor
Learning deficit	More training will often help	Prognosis good
Arousal and motivation	Too bored or too overwhelmed	Prognosis good
Distraction	Problems elsewhere (e.g. health)	Prognosis good
Alienation	Deep-rooted feeling of injustice	Prognosis very poor
Lack of insight	No acceptance of a problem	Prognosis very poor

in that area will help. Such a deficit may respond well to specific training. Obviously it is essential to monitor progress in order to demonstrate that improvement has occurred. Here the prognosis is good.

Arousal and motivation

Some individuals may be too bored or too overwhelmed to work and learn effectively. These are problems with workload. This may be due to an overwhelming clinical workload and sleep deprivation sapping any motivation to work. However, in some cases healthcare professionals seem to have a lot of time off, appear bored and uninterested in their work, and take a lot of motivating to do anything. A change of post, inspirational trainers and role models, and regular meetings with the supervisor may help. The prognosis here is good.

Distraction

Many individuals are distracted – sometimes by health issues, but more often by adverse life events outside of work. These include bereavement, family illness, financial problems, break-up of relationships, and so on. Many people have multiple problems. Such difficulties often present as problems in workplace performance. If you can sort out what are the real problems underlying this, you stand a really good chance of helping the individual to get back on track. If you can do this, the prognosis is good.

Alienation

Once the individual is alienated, angry, has a feeling of injustice and lacks belief that they have a problem which can be helped, the prognosis is very poor indeed. Anger and hostility significantly obstruct help offered to the individual. For example, an individual who feels that they have been incorrectly singled out and victimised by their regulatory body may find it very difficult to recognise areas for improvement and to construct a personal development plan. Time and energy may be spent pursuing senior or government involvement for support, when this time might be better spent trying to improve clinical activities. Here the prognosis is very poor.

Lack of insight

In some ways, lack of insight may have features of alienation (see previous section), but not always. However, lack of insight is the most serious problem of the lot. An individual who lacks insight into their problematic behaviours or attitudes or their knowledge or skill deficits has a very poor prognosis.

BEHAVIOURS AND THEIR PROGNOSIS: ARE THEY TREATABLE?

It is almost impossible to change personality. However, we may be able to change behaviours – but not in all cases. Feedback on performance, with good evidence to back it up (e.g. from Multisource Feedback (MSF)) is the key to achieving behaviour change. For example, individuals have been helped to work better within a team, and understand how to relate to other team members through the use of evidence from an MSF exercise, role-play sessions with experts on clinical communication, and constructive feedback on such behaviours. Continued monitoring of the individual's performance, using MSF in many cases, produces an acceptable level of performance which is sustained in the longer term.

There are pre-conditions for changing behaviours. The individual needs to be sufficiently intelligent, stable and perceptive, and have insight into their problems. As noted earlier, lack of insight is a considerable problem in this area, as is a history of previous unsuccessful attempts to change and not being motivated to change. Unless the individual sees a reason to change and really wants to do so, it will be very difficult to achieve success.

Trainees challenge us in many ways, daily. Some trainees have support, education and training issues that once identified, we can address. Some will have pervasive difficulties, and for those we need to seek further help. The principles in this chapter should help make a plan and successfully return learners to practice or be able to identify when they need to be advised to seek a different future path. As educators and mentors, we need to be aware of our limitations in some of these difficult situations we will find ourselves in.

REFERENCES

Allery L. (1998) *Dealing with challenging group members.* Two sides of A4. Number 4. Cardiff: School of Postgraduate Studies, University of Wales College of Medicine.

Luft J. (1970) *Group processes: An introduction to group dynamics.* Palo Alto, CA: National Press Books.

National Clinical Assessment Service (2006a) *Handling concerns about the performance of healthcare professionals: Principles of good practice.* London: National Clinical Assessment Service.

National Clinical Assessment Service (2006b) *Back on track: Restoring doctors and dentists to safe professional practice.* Framework document. London: National Clinical Assessment Service.

Walker L. (2002) *Consulting with NLP.* Oxford: Radcliffe Medical Press.

For healthcare educators in relation to medical education research and scholarship

....

CHAPTER 21

Research and scholarship in medical education

Definitions in health professions education research

···

The terminology and vocabulary in research can be confusing and perhaps off-putting to new researchers. In this section we have included some definitions or explanations of the commonest terms.

It is important to know whether your project is research, service evaluation or audit (HRA 2017) not least because possibly only if it is research will you need to apply for the all-important, yet time consuming, ethics committee approval. We will return to the subject of ethics approval later.

Research is a careful study of a subject, especially in order to discover new facts or information.

Evaluation looks at the value or impact of a policy, programme, practice or service with a view to making recommendations for change. Evaluation research is part of research, and this is about assessing the worth of something that is already in place (Lovato and Wall 2014).

Audit looks at actual practice and compares it to pre-determined standards and/or expectations of practice.

A useful checklist for your project, if you are not sure can be found here: www. hra-decisiontools.org.uk/research

The Philosophy of research: The theoretical basis of research includes the philosophical foundations which underline the research construction and methodology. Such concepts influence the research assumptions, how the research is done, the role of the researcher and the types of knowledge which will be produced (Illing 2014). Elements include the following:

Ontology, the study of being. It is concerned with the nature of existence and the structure of reality ('What is there to know?')

Epistemology, the theory of knowledge, its origins and nature, and the limits of knowledge (What sort of 'knowing' are we looking for?)

DOI: 10.1201/9781003352532-25

Methodology, the research design and plan (How can we find out?)
Methods, the techniques used for data collection (Will these enable us to find out?)

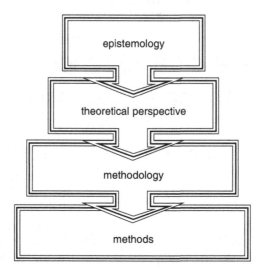

FIGURE 21.1 A Crotty diagram.

Constructing a Crotty diagram as you ask yourself these philosophical questions can help ensure you have aligned these elements to your research question and will lead to appropriate data that can address your research question (Crotty 1998; see Figure 21.1).

A paradigm is a particular world view or set of theories. These include positivism, post positivism, critical theory with feminist and Marxist perspectives, and the constructivist or naturalistic perspectives.

Positivism is based on the belief that all knowledge is based on what we can measure, and can be advanced only by observation and carefully controlled experiments (the 'scientific method'). This uses a hypothesis testing framework (e.g. drug A works better in type 2 diabetes than drug B). This has been the dominant perspective in the sciences going back to the 17th century. Part of this belief is that science is accurate and certain; there is a 'knowable truth' if we look hard enough.

Post positivism developed as a response to the growing understanding that the scientific method cannot be applied to all questions. Post positivism questions the objectivity and certainty of the scientific method. This leads to an understanding that probability has replaced absolute certainty, and approximate truth replace absolute truth.

In both positivism and post positivism, the map of a research process is as follows:

- The aim of the study
- Testing the hypothesis

- Cause and effect
- Generalisability
- Adding to the sum of existing knowledge
- Rigour – especially emphasis on validity and reliability

Interpretivist research rejects the idea that human behaviour is governed by general universal laws. Instead the starting point is that the social world can only be understood through the frame of reference of individuals, their understanding of the world around them, and their interpretations and meanings. Because the values and beliefs of researchers cannot fully be removed from their inquiry, those using an interpretivist paradigm believe research *on* human beings *by* human beings cannot yield objective results. Thus, rather than seeking an objective perspective, interpretivists look for meaning in the subjective experiences of individuals engaging in social interaction. Many interpretivist researchers immerse themselves in the social context they are studying, seeking to understand and formulate theories about a community or group of individuals by observing them from the 'inside'.

Constructivism is the view that knowledge and then following on from this, all meaning, is not discovered but is socially constructed. So meaning is not brought new but is constructed out of existing ideas, objects and concepts.

Critical theory: This looks at positivism and interpretivism as both being somewhat incomplete accounts of social behaviour, as both neglect the political and ideological contexts which may influence much of human behaviour. Critical theorists' intentions are to transform society – and to bring about a more just and equal democratic society.

Feminist research: this looks at and challenges several types of research that do not empower otherwise invisible groups within society; it looks at sexism and power issues in research. It is not just about women, but can include disadvantaged groups such as benefit claimants, asylum seekers or victims of sexual violence. (One example of feminist research is the initiative some years ago to get more girls into scientific and technological careers – e.g. the *Girls into Science and Technology Project*, see www.gist.foundation)

The research process (sometimes called a research protocol) may be considered as a series of logical steps:

- The purpose of the research
- The scope
- Expected outcomes
- The research idea
- Literature search
- The research question
- Design of the study
- Collecting the data
- Analysis of the data
- Writing it up

- Timeline
- Staff involved
- Costs involved
- Publicising the research

THE RESEARCH QUESTION

What is the question which you are trying to answer? This is the basis of your research and should be the very first thing you define and clarify in your mind. It should be:

- **Clear:** it provides enough specifics that the purpose is clear without needing additional explanation.
- **Focused:** it is narrow enough that it can be answered thoroughly in the time, or with the resources, available.
- **Concise:** it is expressed in the fewest possible words.
- **Complex:** it is not answerable with a simple 'yes' or 'no', but rather requires synthesis and analysis of ideas and sources prior to composition of an answer.
- **Arguable:** its potential answers are open to debate rather than accepted facts.

If you are going to succeed, especially if you are embarking on a whole PhD programme of research, it must be a question about a subject about which you are genuinely interested and enthusiastic (Writing Centre 2022). Even a student project needs to engage you, otherwise your commitment might flag!

Once you are clear about your question, what sort of data will you be collecting?

Quantitative research is about numbers, measurements, statistical testing to accept or reject a research hypothesis.

Qualitative research is about exploring the social aspects. It looks at relationships and experiences of people and groups in their natural settings and how that has been shaped by the complexity of human behaviours and the cultural environments in which they live and work.

Mixed methods research uses methods from both quantitative and qualitative research to build a picture, maybe using data from interviews and text analyses, and then survey data analysed with various statistical methods. The specific element that makes it 'mixed' and not just 'multiple' methods is that both forms of data are used to interrogate each other to give a rich picture.

AN INTRODUCTION TO QUANTITATIVE RESEARCH

Some may say this uses a 'scientific' theoretical framework, with hypothesis testing, collections of numerical data and using various statistical methods to describe the data. Often there are comparisons of one set of data with another, using p values and tests of significance.

However, health education research is very much more than just randomised controlled trials! Nevertheless, knowledge of the null hypothesis, sampling, surveys, experimental methods, consensus methods, psychometrics (looking at assessment scores) and meta-analysis will be helpful to the health education researcher (Norman and Eva 2014).

The null hypothesis

A type of hypothesis that proposes at the start that no statistical significance exists in a set of given observations. If there are differences in sets of observations, then statistical testing will tell us the probability that these have occurred by chance.

- P value of 0.05 means a 1 in 20 probability by chance
- P value of 0.01 means a 1 in 100 probability by chance
- P value of 0.001 means a 1 in 1000 probability by chance

Sampling and populations

A population survey looks at everyone in that population (e.g. all anaesthetics registrars in West Midlands). A sample looks at a part of the whole population (e.g. all anaesthetics registrars in the West Midlands with more than four years' experience in the specialty).

These are various types of sampling, which might be random or non-random.

With random sampling, each person in the population has an equal chance of being selected. Each in the population to be studied is given a number, and selection made by published tales of random numbers or random number generators. With systematic random sampling, perhaps a one in ten sampling is then done. With stratified random sampling, stratified into layers such as doctors, nurses, physiotherapists and then random sampling is applied. With cluster sampling, areas would be chosen at random and then include all in these areas.

Non-random sampling includes convenience sampling, with subjects near at hand and easy to recruit, or purposive sampling, which samples a group with a certain characteristic, such as all patients in the practice with type 2 diabetes. Snowballing is when the researcher asks an initial group of people to participate and asks these to recruit others.

Statistical power calculations

Power is an estimate of how likely the study is to produce a statistically significant result for a difference between groups of a given size. Put another way, how big a study population will be needed to detect a true difference between groups? A p value of 0.05 is usually taken to indicate a significant difference. Power should be greater than 0.8, and computer packages will calculate this for you. This is rarely needed in education research – as randomised experimental studies are rare.

Surveys

The use of surveys is common in health education research. They aim to measure certain events, behaviours and attitudes. A survey may use a questionnaire (postal or email), interviews, face-to-face, by Zoom meeting or by telephone. A cross-sectional survey looks at one point in time. In contrast, longitudinal surveys look at more than one point in time (e.g. repeating the survey to show whether changes have taken place or not).

Questionnaire design

A questionnaire can give a broad picture of a research topic. It can reach a lot of people, and collect much information in a relatively short period. This enables comparisons of groups within the study and can be repeated over time to give longitudinal picture. A questionnaire is cheaper in terms of effort than interviews and focus groups, but beware asking questions, that you have seen other people include perhaps, that do not address your research question. You will end up with a large and potentially unwieldy data set.

Many validated questionnaires already exist, so look around first. If you do decide to design and use a questionnaire of your own design, then following some basic principles will help (Oppenheim 1992; Berk 2006). It is, as always with any research, paramount to have a clear research question. Then decide on what you are going to measure. Choose the right questions to ask and design the response options (called the anchors). Pilot testing to check e.g. readability and any difficult to understand questions is an essential step, and this includes analysis. Field testing may also be needed, before the main study is ready to go. Think out how you are going to analyse these questions before you send out the questionnaire.

Before you start, think about and write down what exactly you need to measure. What do you wish to compare with what? Do younger people differ from older people in their responses for example? If so, then put in a question about age or date of birth. It is not unusual for expert researchers to be approached for help with the analysis of questionnaire results who come with a spreadsheet of data they have collected. They wish (for example) to compare UK, EU and international graduates' responses – but have not asked about graduate origin.

Here is a basic framework to follow. Start with an introduction – a paragraph of what the study is about, and where it has come from. Begin with some simple questions (tick box format), which are not off putting or too personal. (Some years ago I collected examples of poorly designed questionnaires for teaching purposes. One began with the very first question, 'What is your sexual orientation?') You might choose to include some Likert questions (stem and 1–5 scale format). Leave questions of a personal nature to the end. Finally have a free comments box right at the end, again for responders to comment in their own words. Here you may get some wonderful answers, which you would have never thought of yourself. (I had a comment about 'star performers' which captured exactly what I was looking for as part of my PhD research.)

Say thank you at the end of the questionnaire, and give directions about where to send it. Sometimes a small token of appreciation is given (not large enough to attract claims of bribery) or the offer of inclusion in a prize draw might be made to encourage participation, especially if students are your participants.

Use clear simple language, proof read and proof read again. Check grammar and punctuation and avoid double negatives. Keep to one concept per question – do not ask two questions in one sentence.

Avoid unfamiliar words. Avoid statements that suggest the answer and avoid abbreviations, as these may mean completely different things to different people. For example, some years ago in the UK the Medical Training Application Service was often referred to as 'MTAS'. But it can also mean Massage Therapists Association of Saskatchewan, the Merthyr Tydfil Alzheimer's Society and the Manchester Tram Appreciation Society.

How can you obtain the best possible response rate? (Edwards et al. 2002) looked at 292 randomised trials of 75 interventions. The key strategies are as follows:

- A short simple questionnaire – not too crowded
- A covering letter on headed notepaper from a respected organisation
- A personalised letter (Dear Dr Wall – not Dear Sir)
- Hand signed by the researcher
- A subject interesting and relevant to the responder
- Coloured paper better than white (yellow and pink best – but avoid blue)
- Pre-paid reply envelope or some way of easily returning the questionnaire
- Follow up and repeat questionnaire to non-responders

If you are interested, there is much more to read about design and analysis of questionnaires in Berk (2006) and Oppenheim (1992).

Experiments

The true experiment has a test group and a control group with random allocation, or a pre-test and post-test study on a whole study population. The quasi-experiment is if two groups are compared but not randomised, when randomisation is not possible (e.g. student performance in a medical school with a problem-based curriculum versus another with a traditional curriculum). Occasionally a natural experiment may be studied. For example, when the Quality and Outcomes Framework was introduced into UK general practice, the performance of training and non-training practices was compared (Houghton et al. 2006).

Consensus methods

There are three methods which can attempt to build a consensus of opinion. These are the Delphi technique, the nominal group method and the snowball review.

Delphi technique

Delphi is now an important archaeological site in Greece. In ancient times it housed the Temple of Apollo. The Oracle, a priestess in the Temple, when asked a question whilst in a trance, would utter ecstatic speech. This was interpreted and translated into meanings by the priests. She was considered very wise and consulted over many important Greek decisions of state. She would often give cryptic pronouncements. Hence we have the name the Delphi technique, where wise people were consulted and gave their considered opinions.

The Delphi is a postal/email consensus method. A group of expert volunteers receive written open-ended questions. Responses are then compiled into a questionnaire and sent back out to the expert group. Members are asked to rate levels of agreement. Results are analysed and sent back to experts, who again rank levels of agreement. Statistical testing is used to help ascertain a consensus. Variations, or modified Delphi techniques, also exist.

Nominal group method

In a group situation, instructions and explanation of the problem are given to the group members. To begin, there is silent thinking of ideas by each group member, without consultation with other group members. Then ideas are listed, with each member contributing, but no debate at this stage. The facilitator writes the ideas down on flip chart. This is followed by group discussion. Then there is voting and ranking of ideas by the group.

Snowball review

This is a group-based process aimed at ensuring all views are taken into account. Each group member makes a list of points. Individuals join up in pairs and discuss, negotiate and agree a list as a pair. Each pair then forms a group of four and again discusses and agrees as a foursome. Two groups of four form an eight who discuss until agreement is reached.

The name 'snowball' describes the game of rolling a snowball down a hill. The snowball starts small, but picks up more and more snow on the way down.

Psychometrics

Psychometrics is the field of study concerned with the theory and technique of psychological measurement, which includes the measurement of knowledge, abilities, attitudes, personality traits and educational measurement. In health professions education, psychometrics is primarily concerned with the construction, validation and performance of measurement instruments and assessments such as questionnaires, multiple choice questions or OSCEs, for example.

Such research questions may include the following:

How many stations do we need to make our OSCE reliable?
How many raters do we need for our multi-source feedback to be reliable?
Do different raters give different assessment scores?
How fair and reliable is the multiple mini interview selection process?

(Goodyear et al. 2007)

(See also Chapter 16 on assessment.)

Meta analyses

Meta analysis is the analysis of other analyses. It is the systematic review of previous studies on a defined research question. It involves the collecting and aggregating the results of many studies on a selected topic (e.g. can we teach communication skills?). It will involve much statistical work and qualitative analysis to obtain an answer and usually involves a team of researchers (see later section on Best Evidence Medical Education).

Analysis of the data

You should design the analysis in at the beginning, before you collect any data. Some questionnaires turn out to be impossible to analyse because no thought went into the analysis beforehand. So think first before you send out the questionnaire. Test it out in the pilot phase before you do the main study. Or, as our woodwork teacher used to say at school, *'Measure it twice and cut once!'*

Get expert advice from someone who knows about this.

Statistics

A great book for learning about and doing the statistics for your research is *Discovering Statistics* using IBM SPSS Statistics (Field 2017). The subject is treated with humour and is made easy to understand and to use.

Statistical data analysis

First of all, some basic summary statistics can be very valuable – so explore the data first of all. Obtain numbers, frequencies, mean, median, standard deviation and range. Are there any outliers, and can these be dealt with? Display your information in graphs and diagrams. Do there seem to be any differences? Is your data normally distributed or not? Is it parametric or non-parametric?

Comparing one group with another

Comparative testing, comparing one group with another, together with tests of significance is a common statistical technique. Depending on your type of data these tests may include Chi Square, Mann Whitney and Kruskal Wallis, T tests, ANOVA, Wilcoxon signed rank tests and correlations. Detail of these tests is beyond the scope of this book but will be found in any statistics textbook. Get expert advice on which ones to use when – think of it as being similar to getting expert radiological advice to help you make a diagnosis; we don't all need to know everything!

How reliable is your data?

Does the questionnaire measure in a consistent way? Individual items can be measured separately and the questionnaire as a whole. Cronbach's alpha is often used here – (value 0 to 1). Other tests include Split-half reliability and Kappa. Test-retest reliability is another technique. We list them here to demonstrate the range of analytical processes available but again, most clinician-educator-scholars will not need to be familiar with many, just enough to ensure you make the right selection to analyse your data.

In terms of reliability values, a value of Cronbach's alpha of 0.7 or above is considered reasonable for a research study, and 0.8 or above for an assessment tool.

Reducing your data into a few key themes

Factor analysis is a data reduction method. In a series of responses, it enables the reduction of the numerical data into a small number of variables that are key discriminators or predictors of difference. Questions load into groups if answered in a similar way. The mathematics is very complex! However, using the statistics programme SPSS this is not too difficult to do. In research on a Teaching Styles Questionnaire, data from a 96-item questionnaire was 'collapsed' into six main groupings – leading to a paper and a textbook on six teaching styles (Mohanna et al. 2007).

AN INTRODUCTION TO QUALITATIVE RESEARCH

Qualitative research explores the social aspects, the relationships and the experiences of people and groups in their natural settings. It has been shaped by the complexity of human behaviours and cultural environments. It may be considered to be about theory building, finding explanations about behaviours and understanding what is going on, rather than hypothesis testing and experimentation.

Its origins come from anthropology, sociology, education and history. It explores the objects of study within their natural environment and seeks to understand the complexity of human and social situations. It looks at the role of context – where situations are anchored in time, space, and cultures. It is about the careful understanding of what we do and why.

Methodologies in qualitative research

Ethnography: This arose from anthropology (emersion by living with groups or populations to try and understand their ways and culture) but is now more often used at a more local level to understand the meanings of activities and behaviours of a particular social group (e.g. the study of male student culture in a medical school).

Grounded theory: This explores social phenomena by developing theoretical explanations based on practical experiences and observations on the study participants – grounded and created from the data (e.g. developing a model of feedback in health professions education).

Case study: This is the in-depth analysis of a programme, an event or a group (somewhat like a clinical case report). It often draws on data from several sources to build the understanding from multiple perspectives – called *triangulation* (e.g. what influences medical students to become paediatricians?). The word *triangulation* is originally a navigational technique to fix one's position using compass bearings from usually three fixed points.

Phenomenology: This is about understanding the essence of a social phenomenon from the perspective of those who experience it – often studying a small group of people in a defined activity (e.g. experiences of students interacting with standardised patients).

Hermeneutics: This uses the experiences of individuals to look at meaning making, particularly in developing understanding of their religious, political, historical and socio-cultural contexts.

Narrative research: This uses storytelling as a means of communicating, arranging and interpreting human experiences by finding the inner meanings from the story – the moral of the tale (e.g. means of teaching empathy or professionalism).

Action research: This is a way of producing change through the research process with active engagement by the researcher in the research process (e.g. the design and implementation of a new induction course for students).

Methods used in qualitative research

An excellent account of the tools for collection of data and for its analysis can be found in Coffey and Atkinson (1996). We continue our list of definitions in this section to provide an overview, which you may then need to go on to read more about.

Interview: This is a conversation between a subject and a researcher. Interviews may be of several types:

- The in-depth interview – one research question explored in depth
- The semi-structured interview – several open-ended questions asked and explored
- The structured interview – several questions and fixed responses to each

Interviews are often recorded and transcribed verbatim for analysis. As a rough rule of thumb, it takes at least ten times the length of the interview to listen and type it all up in a document. So a 10-minute interview may take 100 minutes (or longer) to type it up for analysis.

Focus group: This is a group of usually between 4 and 12 people as participants and a facilitator, with a group discussion on a relevant topic of research. The focus group can give multiple perspectives, can draw out diverse experiences and facilitate an interchange of ideas and debate on the topic being considered. Usually the focus group is recorded and the conversation typed up verbatim. In addition, the facilitator will also make field notes on what they thought was going on – and their reflections on it. Disadvantages include the power dynamic between facilitator and participants, and the reluctance of participants to reveal sensitive and personal issues to others in such a group (a one-to-one interview may be better here).

Observation: This is watching a defined activity taking place (e.g. the giving and receiving of feedback on a ward round). The observer makes field notes, and the activity may be audio recorded or video recorded in the ethnographic tradition.

Textual document collection and assembly: This is where the researcher collects a series of documents such as curricula, evaluation reports, assignments, teaching materials and so on, and analyses these.

Analysis of qualitative data

How do we make sense of a set of qualitative data? How do we find the meanings and interpret what is going on? Reading the data is the first step – immersion and deep engagement with the data. Then thinking and reflecting on the data, and reading it again, and questioning the meaning of the data. Sometimes the meanings will seem to come out of the page at you – but not always. It is good to have an experienced colleague who will also look at the text and give their interpretations as well.

Coding – organising the data into categories or themes

One way to start organising the data is to go through the document and attach codes, like labels, to chunks of text for which the researcher has decided there is a meaning. Several codes may be grouped together to create themes. Memos should be written about what it all means – as the ideas become more abstract.

This can be done with a printed document, the interview transcript for example, and a series of coloured highlighter pens, or on the computer in Word using a series of colours to highlight the text to label the codes. Qualitative analysis software programmes exist, such as NVivo™ (QSR International 2020) which can be very useful but take a lot of learning how to use it! Its use may not be necessary for a short project.

Thematic analysis is one of the commonest ways of analysing qualitative data. Here you are looking for themes that you can create from the data. You may develop a branching system of themes, concepts and general ideas by going in and out of your data and building the whole picture up as you look at and think about the data in the interviews you have done and transcribed (see also Braun and Clarke's (2021) book in which they revisit their foundational 2006 '*6 stage mode of thematic analysis*').

Narrative analysis: This is the analysis of stories which people tell – often to illustrate a particular point or theme. A student may tell their pals about the time they turned up an hour late for an operating room session and received a telling-off by the surgeon concerned. So what was the moral of the tale here? Turn up on time!

TABLE 21.1 Analysis of Narrative

Element	Question
Abstract (optional)	*What was this about?*
Orientation	*Who? What? When? Where?*
Complication	*Then what happened?*
Evaluation	*What is the point?*
Result	*What happened in the end?*
Coda (optional)	*Narrative finishes*

Narratives have a rather specific distinct structure with formal and identifiable properties, often in the same and repeatable order (see Table 21.1).

Life history research is another research example where narrative is used widely.

Text and discourse analysis: This is about looking at language in its social situation – with data at the level of language and how we use it. This can be in conversations, and also in documents, novels, reports and so on. It can help us understand the meanings and power relationships in an interaction. Examples include the doctor–patient consultation, compared with doctor to doctor conversations, and adults speaking with children for example.

How do we achieve rigour in qualitative research?

Here is a series of questions to ask of a qualitative study:

- Did the researcher describe a theoretical framework and methods used at all stages of the research?
- Were the research questions clearly stated?
- Was the context clearly described?
- Was sampling clearly described and justified?
- Was the sampling comprehensive so as to ensure generalizability of the conceptual analysis (diverse range of individuals and settings for example)?
- How was the field work undertaken?
- Could the evidence of interviews transcripts, analysis etc. be inspected by others?
- Were the data analysis clearly described and theoretically justified?
- Did the data analysis relate to the original research questions?
- Was the analysis repeated by another researcher to ensure reliability?
- Did the researchers make use of any quantitative data to test qualitative conclusions if appropriate?
- Did the researchers give any confounding or contradictory findings?
- Was sufficient original evidence presented (quotations numbered and sources given) to illustrate and justify conclusions made?

Ethical aspects of health professions education research

Ethical aspects of health professions education research are about rules of conduct and principles relating to moral behaviour (Illing 2014). These are discussed next.

Consent

Remember that there are differences between informed consent and implied consent.

Implied consent

A major difference exists between implied consent and informed consent. With implied consent, the way a patient behaves indicates whether they give permission to do something. There is no formal agreement. For example, a patient who calls to make an appointment, or rolls up their sleeve for a blood pressure to be taken, is giving implied consent to treatment.

Informed consent

Informed consent is a legal term, with a series of principles to be satisfied. These are as follows:

- The individual is competent and can understand to what they are consenting to.
- The individual is making the decision voluntarily – without coercion.
- The individual has received sufficient information to decide.
- A plan of the research has been explained to the individual.
- The individual understands the terms being used in the above.
- The individual has decided to take part.
- The research has been authorised.

Informed consent includes the question of what does taking part involve on behalf of the subjects of research. This needs to be explained to participants in advance. Agreement to take part needs to be voluntary. Gaining consent may be by giving full information as to what is involved, signing a consent form, or by returning a questionnaire.

There are very specific aspects of consent regarding video and audio recordings, see Box 21.1.

BOX 21.1 VIDEO AND AUDIO RECORDINGS

When making or using recordings, you must respect patients' privacy and dignity, and their right to make or participate in decisions that affect them. This means that you must:

Give patients the information they want, or need, about the purpose of the recording.

Make recordings only where you have appropriate consent or other valid authority for doing so.

Ensure that patients are under no pressure to give their consent for the recording to be made.

Where practicable, stop the recording if the patient asks you to, or if it is having an adverse effect on the consultation or treatment.

Anonymise or code recordings before using or disclosing them for a secondary purpose, if this is practicable and will serve the purpose.

Disclose or use recordings from which patients may be identifiable only with consent or other valid authority for doing so.

Make appropriate secure arrangements for storing recordings.

Be familiar with, and follow, the law and local guidance and procedures that apply where you work.

Source: Taken from General Medical Council (GMC 2022).

Confidentiality

Professional confidentiality is about privacy, protecting the identity of participants and their details so that no discovery of identity can be made on the basis of certain characteristics. This is very familiar to healthcare professionals in their clinical practice and is no different in research. Data must not be published or made publicly available in a form which identifies individuals, and no-one outside the research team should have access to the raw data which will be kept safe and eventually destroyed.

Anonymity

Anonymity is assured if names are not requested. For example, a questionnaire sent once to all registrars in paediatrics in England, with no identifiers on the questionnaire and no names requested, is anonymous. However, it will be impossible to send reminders to non-responders.

ETHICAL APPROVAL

The role of ethics regulation in research is a vital principle, to prevent both local, personal breaches of professional ethics but also minimise the risk of ever seeing institutional recurrences such as the Nazi atrocities and the Tuskegee syphilis experiments in the name of scientific research (Petrova and Barclay 2019). The process for ethics approval varies from country to country, and from discipline to discipline. Universities have their own ethical committees and generally students working for degrees are expected to submit a research protocol to the ethics committee for approval. If the project involves patients, healthcare staff or healthcare premises, it will also need to be considered by an NHS ethics committee. If and when research is submitted for publication, editors will ask about ethics approval, and this will need to be stated in the manuscript submitted.

Clinical research is clearly defined as we saw earlier (HRA 2017). Only research needs research ethics committee review. Service evaluation, clinical/non-financial audit and usual practice in the UK do not.

Within the National Health Service the situation is more complex for educational research. Health Education England (HEE) has given guidance to health professions trainees doing educational research projects:

> Virtually all potential projects in education fall into the scope of a 'service evaluation' rather than research per se. As such their governance is simple and straightforward. These do **not** normally require research ethics approval.
> *(Health Education England 2022, emphasis in original)*

This document also recommends two further potential sources of help for small projects. These are the Local Research Ethics Committee (LREC) chairperson and a University Ethics Committee lead.

However, in the UK the Integrated Research Application System (IRAS 2021) is the body for ethical approvals for all health, social and community care research in the UK. IRAS is a single system for applying for the permissions and approvals for health and social/community care research in the UK. It shares information with the following organisations:

- Administration of Radioactive Substances Advisory Committee (ARSAC)
- Confidentiality Advisory Group (CAG)
- Gene Therapy Advisory Committee (GTAC)
- Health Research Authority (HRA) for projects seeking HRA Approval
- Medicines and Healthcare products Regulatory Agency (MHRA)
- NHS/HSC R&D offices
- NHS/HSC Research Ethics Committees
- National Offender Management Service (NOMS)
- Social Care Research Ethics Committee

This can be a system of complexity, red tape and delays. For example, one paper reported a low-key study by interview and questionnaire which resulted in 491 exchanges with 89 individuals involved in research ethics and governance, and generated 193 pages of email text – excluding attachments (Petrova and Barclay 2019)!

BEST EVIDENCE MEDICAL EDUCATION

Just as with clinical practice, teaching should be based on evidence of what works best. The Best Evidence Medical Education (BEME) movement has defined this as: 'The implementation by teachers and educational bodies in their practice, of methods and approaches to education based on the best evidence available'. Five steps have been recognised in the practice of BEME. These are framing the question, developing a search strategy, evaluating the evidence, implementing change and evaluating that change (Masoomi 2012; see also the BEME Collaboration www.bemecollaboration.org).

Healthcare professionals are trained to make clinical decisions that are based on evidence. However, when it comes to teaching, many abandon this approach and base everything on tradition and intuition. Healthcare teachers sometimes believe that evidence to support or reject educational approaches is not available. Students of health professions education often argue against principles of educational theory on the grounds that 'there is no evidence that they work'.

This is sometimes true, but in other circumstances evidence is not found because it is sought in the wrong place, using inappropriate databases (e.g. Medline). In 1999 the Association for Medical Education in Europe (AMEE) published the first developments of the Best Evidence Medical Education (BEME) Collaboration (Harden et al. 1999). As of February 2022, there are now 70 such reviews listed on the BEME website (BEME 2022).

The Best Evidence Medical Education Collaboration is an international group of individuals, universities and professional organisations committed to the development of evidence informed education in the health professions through the following statements:

- The dissemination of information which allows teachers and stakeholders in health professions to make decisions on the basis of the best evidence available.
- The production of reviews which present the best available evidence and meet the needs of the user.
- The creation of a culture of best evidence education amongst individuals, institutions and national bodies.

The goal of BEME is to provide and to make available the latest findings from scientifically-grounded educational research. This will enable teachers and administrators to make informed decisions about the kinds of evidence-based education initiatives that boost learner performance on cognitive and clinical measures.

BEME rejects the legacy of health professions education in which decisions have been made based on pseudoscience, anecdotes and flawed comparison groups rather than empirical evidence. The BEME approach contends that in no other scientific field are personal experiences relied on to make policy choices, and in no other field is the research base so limited (BEME 2022).

The first BEME review was on the teaching of communication skills (Aspegren 1999). This is still one of the very best, with many valuable learning messages. These include the following valuable messages:

- Communication skills can be taught.
- They are learned.

- Communication skills are best maintained by practice.
- Teaching should be experiential, not instructional.
- Content should be problem defining.
- The least competent students improve the most.
- Men take longer to learn than women do.

Therefore good-quality evidence can inform our practice on how best to teach using experiential methods (patients, role players, video recording and constructive feedback on performance).

However, educationalists are still being requested to come and 'give a lecture on communication skills'.

Some examples among the many examples of BEME reviews now published include the following:

- BEME Guide 27 – on doctor role modelling in medical education (Passi et al. 2013)
- BEME Guide 62 – a systematic review of teaching interventions to equip medical students and residents in early recognition and prompt escalation of acute clinical deteriorations (Balakrishnan et al. 2020)

CONCLUSION

Try not to let the complexities of ethics review or logistics put you off! There are many questions unanswered in educational research, and your idea might just represent a breakthrough!

This chapter has only been able to outline some of the key areas in the research process, and you will need to consult specialist literature for the detail of how to apply some of these principles. You can also get help and advice from senior experienced researchers in your organisation, or your local university or local, national or regional professional body, before starting your work. Remember that ASME (the Association for the Study of Medical Education) and AMEE (the Association for Medical Education in Europe) run courses on research methods in health professions educational research. Royal Colleges are another valuable source of information, help and advice.

REFERENCES

Aspegren K. (1999) BEME guide 2 teaching and learning communication skills in medicine – a review with quality grading of articles. *Medical Teacher*, 21(6): 563–570.

Balakrishnan A., Dong C., Law L.S-C., Liaw S.Y., Chen F.G. and Samarasekera D.D. (2020) BEME guide 22 a BEME systematic review of teaching interventions to equip medical students and residents in early recognition and prompt escalation of acute clinical deteriorations. *Medical Teacher*. DOI: 10.1080/0142159X.2020.1763286.

BEME – best evidence medical education collaboration (2022) Available at www.bemecollaboration.org/Published+Reviews/ (Accessed 20.2.22).

Berk R.A. (2006) *Thirteen strategies to measure college teaching*. Sterling, VA: Stylus Publishing, LLC.

Braun V. and Clarke V. (2021) *Thematic analysis: A practical guide.* Thousand Oaks, CA: SAGE.

Coffey A. and Atkinson P. (1996) *Making sense of qualitative data.* Thousand Oaks, CA: Sage Publications Inc.

Crotty M. (1998) *The foundations of social research.* Thousand Oaks, CA: Sage Publications.

Edwards P., Roberts I., Clarke M., DiGuiseppi C., Pratap S., Wentz R. and Kwan I. (2002) Increasing the response rate to postal questionnaires: Systematic review. *British Medical Journal*, 324: 1183–5. DOI: 10.1136/bmj.324.7347.1183.

Field A. (2017) *Discovering statistics using IBM SPSS statistics.* 5th edn. London: Sage Publications Limited.

GMC (2022) Available at www.gmc-uk.org/ethical-guidance/ethical-guidance-for-doctors/making-and-using-visual-and-audio-recordings-of-patients/principles (Accessed 3.4.22).

Goodyear H.M., Jyothish D., Diwakar V. and Wall D. (2007) Reliability of a regional junior doctor recruitment process. *Medical Teacher*, 29: 504–506.

Harden R.M., Grant J., Buckley G. and Hart I.R. (1999) BEME guide no. 1: Best evidence medical education. *Medical Teacher*, 21(6): 553–562. DOI: 10.1080/01421599978960.

Health Education England (2022) Educational research – guidance for HEE fellows. Available at www.hee.nhs.uk/sites/default/files/documents/Educational%20Research-%20Guidance%20for%20HEE%20Fellows.pdf (Accessed 23.2.22).

Health Research Authority (2017) What is research? Research, evaluation or clinical audit. Available at www.hra-decisiontools.org.uk/research/docs/DefiningResearchTable_Oct2017-1.pdf (Accessed 1.4.22).

Houghton G., Wall D., Norton B. and Wyatt S. (2006) Do GP training practices achieve higher QOF points? A study of the quality and outcomes framework in Birmingham and the black country. *Education for Primary Care*, 17: 557–571.

Illing J. (2014) Thinking about research, theoretical perspectives, ethics and scholarship. In Swanwick T. (ed) *Understanding medical education – evidence, theory and practice.* 2nd edn. Oxford: Wiley Blackwell, pp. 331–347.

IRAS (2021) The integrated research application system (last updated 27th July 2021). Available at www.hra.nhs.uk/about-us/committees-and-services/integrated-research-application-system/ (Accessed 23.2.22).

Lovato C. and Wall D. (2014) Programme evaluation: Improving practice. Influencing policy and decision making. In *Understanding medical education – evidence, theory and practice.* 2nd edn. Oxford: Wiley Blackwell, pp. 385–399.

Masoomi R. (2012) What is the best evidence medical education? *Research and Development in Medical Education*, 1(1): 3–5.

Mohanna K., Chambers R. and Wall D. (2007) Developing your teaching style: Increasing effectiveness in healthcare teaching. *Postgraduate Medical Journal*, 83: 145–147.

Norman G. and Eva K.W. (2014) Quantitative research methods in medical education. In *Understanding medical education – evidence, theory and practice.* 2nd edn. Oxford: Wiley Blackwell, pp. 349–369.

Oppenheim A.N. (1992) *Questionnaire design, interviewing and attitude measurement.* New edn. London: Continuum.

Passi V., Johnson S., Peile E., Wright S., Hafferty F. and Johnson N. (2013) BEME guide 27 doctor role modelling in medical education. *Medical Teacher*, 35(9): e1422–e1436.

Petrova M. and Barclay S. (2019) Research approvals iceberg. *BMC Medical Ethics.* Available at https://doi.org/10.1186/s12910-018-0339-5 (Accessed 23.2.22).

QSR International (2020) Nvivo™. Available at www.qsrinternational.com/nvivo-qualitative-data-analysis-software/home (Accessed 4.1.23).

Writing Centre (2022) How to write a research question. Available at https://writingcenter.gmu.edu/guides/how-to-write-a-research-question (Accessed 20.2.22).

For healthcare educators in relation to the management, leadership and governance of healthcare education

....

CHAPTER 22

Educational leadership

....

BACKGROUND

What does a good leader look like? In the UK there has been a recognition in the recent past of a need for greater engagement of doctors as leaders both in developing education and training and in healthcare service development. Although there is now considerable overlap in roles and responsibilities in healthcare, a need for greater clinical and especially medical engagement was identified in two major reviews of UK healthcare organisation and provision (Darzi 2008; Tooke 2008).

> The doctor's frequent role as head of the healthcare team and commander of considerable clinical resource requires that greater attention is paid to management and leadership skills regardless of specialism. An acknowledgement of the leadership role of medicine is increasingly evident.
>
> *(Tooke 2008)*

Tooke had been asked to lead an inquiry into the implementation of a controversial reform of UK postgraduate medical education and training under the policy initiative, Modernising Medical Careers. This was aimed at speeding up the production of fully trained specialists. The speed with which these changes were introduced (coupled with an inadequate online application process supporting the first phase of change) resulted in widespread system deficiencies and countless tales of personal difficulties in career progression. The subsequent inquiry attributed fault to a policy of healthcare training and education that aspired to 'good enough' rather than 'excellence' (Tooke 2008).

The same inquiry identified confused or deficient professional engagement, particularly with regard to matters of education and training. As a result, a call was made for a national lead for medical education, and stronger collaborations, within

DOI: 10.1201/9781003352532-27

the health education sector. The medical profession was urged to develop a mechanism for providing leadership of education and training across the whole profession. Aspiring to excellence would require doctors in particular, but also all others engaged in education and training, to step up as leaders in their profession.

These recommendations required expansion of the number of healthcare professionals involved in aspects of leadership, and new training initiatives to equip them for this task. Modifications were also required for the structure of postgraduate training to provide training in leadership.

The second influential review (Darzi 2008) placed emphasis more broadly on enabling all the health professions to lead and manage the organisations in which they work:

> Greater freedom, enhanced accountability and empowering staff are necessary but not sufficient in the pursuit of high quality care. Making change actually happen takes leadership. It is central to our expectations of the healthcare professionals of tomorrow.
>
> *(Darzi 2008)*

In a move designed to encourage leadership, suggestions were made for investment in programme of clinical and board leadership with all clinicians encouraged to be 'practitioners, partners and leaders in the healthcare system' and placing a new emphasis on 'enabling NHS staff to lead and manage the organisations in which they work' (Darzi 2008, p. 13).

In the UK, a National Leadership Council (NLC) was suggested to create a step change in the development of leadership, 'responsible for overseeing all matters of leadership across healthcare' (Darzi 2008). The consultation process that informed the NLC development emphasised that the drive for leadership should permeate all levels and grades of the healthcare organisation: 'Leadership at all the levels'. There was a strong emphasis on clinical leadership, but a similar drive for the NLC, which went on to become the NHS Leadership Academy, to work with people and professional groups from all backgrounds.

As a consequence of these reviews, the Department of Health released *Inspiring leaders: leadership for quality* (DoH 2009) which suggested identification and development of leadership potential had four underpinning principles (see Box 22.1 and Figure 22.1).

BOX 22.1 TALENT AND LEADERSHIP FRAMEWORK

1. Co-production – the engagement of people across 'the system' to work together to make change happen
2. Subsidiarity – ensuring that decisions are made at the right level, and as close to the user as possible

3. Clinical ownership and leadership – building on the concept of staff as 'practitioners, partners and leaders'

4. System alignment – aligning different parts of the system towards the same goals as a way of achieving complex cultural change

Source: DoH (2009).

DEVELOPING LEADERSHIP POTENTIAL IN OTHERS

Interview research has suggested that leadership training is regarded as important, and overall, senior leaders recognised the need to develop personal qualities, the ability to lead and work in teams, how to manage and improve services and how to set direction for change (Nicol et al. 2014; Wilkie and Mohanna 2017). The difficulties of organising this however and fitting it in with the needs of service delivery and existing curricula has been highlighted.

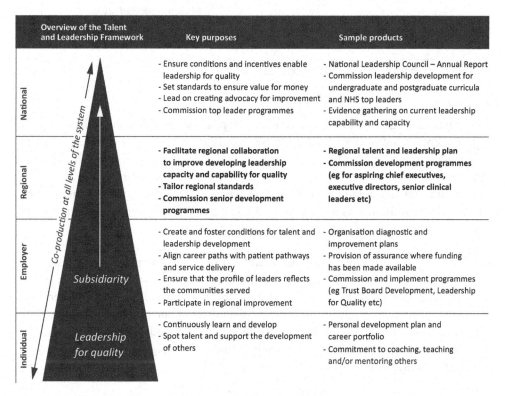

FIGURE 22.1 Talent and leadership framework. *Source:* DoH (2009).

TABLE 22.1 Leadership 'Eras'

Era	Period	Theory	Description
Trait	1840s	Great Man	Focus on natural born leaders
	1930s–1940s	Trait	Focus on identifying traits and characteristics of effective leaders
Behavioural	1940s–1950s	Behavioural	Focus on the actions and skills of leaders
Situational	1960s	Contingent and Situational	Focus on leaders adapting their style, taking into account the environment
New leadership	1990s	Transactional	Focus on leadership as a cost-benefit exchange
	1990s	Transformational	Focus on an inspirational style pushing followers to higher and higher levels of achievement
	2000s	Shared	
	2000s	Collaborative	Focus on followers leading each other
	2000s	Collective Servant Inclusive Complexity	Focus on engaging followers. Person-centred style Focus on the whole system of an organisation

Source: Taken from Benmira and Agboola (2021).

So, the challenge for those involved in health professions education is: how can you help to identify and develop leadership potential in others? Many different and varied theories of leadership (and management) make even an overview of the required characteristics confusing (Chambers et al. 2007; Wilkie and Spurgeon 2009).

Benmira and Agboola have recently reviewed the 'evolution of leadership theory' and suggest four main eras in leadership thinking: trait, behavioural, situational and new leadership (see Table 22.1; Benmira and Agboola 2021).

- *Trait theory:* This emphasises personal qualities. Developing from an idea of the inspirational leader with innate qualities, this evolved into an understanding that what counts is the characteristics or traits that leaders possess (either from personality or through training). A consistent set of such traits has been hard to identify, however. The implication of this theory for leadership teachers is that it seems to suggest leaders are 'born not made' which might mean limited impact from training opportunities.

- *Behavioural theory:* This focusses on largely learned behaviours and suggests that a person's 'leadership style' or collection of behaviours is what matters and that this can be taught and trained for. It does not emphasise the context the leader works in however or the impact of environment on their leadership abilities.
- *Situational leadership:* This suggests that different tasks call for different leaders with a varying skill mix. This recognises the mutuality of leadership interactions that depend on the characteristics of the followers and the environment as much as the leader. This theory speaks to the reported difficulties some trainee-leaders have found in implementing new ideas.
- *'New Leadership':* This category includes transactional leadership which utilises incentives and exchanges to engender followership, and transformational leadership depending more on the empowering of individuals. Other models in the 'new era' have tended to recognise the potential for learners to emerge as leaders depending on context and support. This suggests the importance of whole team awareness of change management.

THE NHS LEADERSHIP ACADEMY

Following a system-wide change in thinking about healthcare leadership, courses, programmes, books and guidance have proliferated. Some of these will suit some learners more than others. The resources section identifies a range of health professions development opportunities.

What we have seen since those early days however is that authentic leadership roles, embedded in practice, are needed to create sustainable change in services and individuals. On the job development opportunities allow potential leaders to develop in a supportive environment and spread their ideas and thinking to other members of the multidisciplinary team. New leaders report that 'going away' on a course does not necessarily help them when they come back to the workplace brimming full of new ideas and expectations. If they don't also have the change management or team leadership tools to manage the team they left behind, they can find it hard to implement system change, even at a ward, practice or departmental level.

The NHS Leadership framework (see Figure 22.2) can be a useful tool to facilitate thinking about the multi-faceted experience of healthcare leadership (NHS Leadership Academy 2013). An associated self-assessment questionnaire can be used to form the basis of an interactive workshop with students or trainees in any discipline.

The model describes nine-dimensions of leadership (note, not leaders), and the questionnaire is free to access; however you will need to register for a free NHS Leadership Academy ID on Profile, and register for 'Healthcare Leadership Model' under Available programmes.

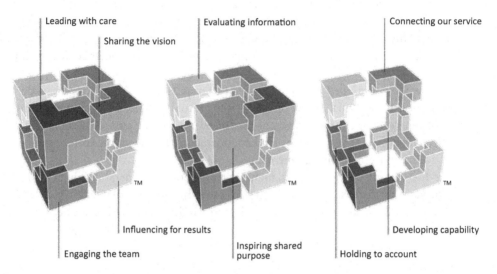

FIGURE 22.2 Healthcare leadership model. *Source:* https://www.leadershipacademy.nhs.uk/resources/healthcare-leadership-model/

LEADERSHIP DEVELOPMENT ACTIVITIES

Quality improvement projects (QIPs)

Skills *for* leading projects are best developed *by* leading projects. Often trainees are full of ideas for service improvement that they rarely get a chance to experiment with or implement. An effective form of educational supervision can be to engineer time and opportunity for learners to plan, carry out and evaluate small scale quality improvement projects. The skills to organise, negotiate, delegate, encourage others, implement and evaluate are leadership skills. Resources to help support QIPs in the form of e-modules be found here: www.rcgp.org.uk/qi-ready (you will need to register, but it is a free resource and you do not need to be an RCGP member).

Multi-source feedback (MSF, or 360-degree assessment)

An effective conduit for development as professionals, team members and leaders is through eliciting and responding to feedback. A 360-degree assessment tool, developed by the NHS Institute for Innovation and Improvement, is available from the Leadership Academy website. This enables a trainee to elicit views on how team members view the behaviours of them as a potential leader. Thus it identifies areas to be developed or particular strengths of an individual.

Shadowing

Buddying potential leaders with colleagues in positions of influence in other organisations can allow 'cross-fertilisation' of ideas, close observation at first hand and the development of transferable qualities. By occasionally spending time in another's workplace, you can compare and contrast the qualities and behaviours that are required for success.

Experimentation or simulation

Leadership development programmes often include simulation exercises. This provides a safe environment in which variables can be adjusted to test out actions and reactions in a team arena, with different individuals taking the position of leader. Both on courses and in the workplace, exercises can be developed for departments and teams to practise acting under pressure.

ADDIE (analyse, design, develop, implement, evaluate)

ADDIE refers to a system that was originally developed for instructional media design (primarily in e-learning), which can be adapted to become a form of project development exercise (Allen 2006). This can be used as the basis of an effective game for thinking about leadership activity (see Box 22.2).

BOX 22.2 THE ADDIE GAME (ANALYSE, DESIGN, DEVELOP, IMPLEMENT, EVALUATE)

This is an exercise for two small mixed-professional groups.

Preamble: The COVID-19 pandemic has hit the hospital, and 20 temporary staff at all levels have been brought in to help cover staff illness and increased healthcare demand. They have never worked in your Trust before.

Task: Design a short activity that will allow the permanent employees to meet and introduce themselves to the temporary staff and decide who will do what during the emergency season.

ADDIE:

- **Analyse** the problem: Perform a short task analysis. How do people usually get to know each other?
- **Design** the activity: Develop objectives, sequence.
- **Develop** the activity: Outline how they will perform the activity and trial it.
- **Implement** the activity: Describe the activity to the other group.
- **Evaluate** the activity: Groups vote on both schemes.

THE IMPORTANCE OF ORGANISATIONAL SUPPORT

Leaders do not emerge overnight. Leadership capacity must be proactively developed within an organisation to encourage new leaders. Some organisations are better at this than others. Effective organisations encourage mentoring in the workplace (see Chapter 17). Box 22.3 shows how effective organisations support and encourage new leadership.

BOX 22.3 ORGANISATIONAL SUPPORT FOR DEVELOPING LEADERS

- Mentoring: An effective mentor should ensure that inexperienced leaders set realistic and challenging objectives while enabling effective use of the fresh perspective and energy that they bring.
- Achievable goals: with a degree of responsibility and influence promote personal development and motivation.
- Effective interim evaluation: during as well as after the project, should assess the success of developmental opportunities and give essential feedback to the learner.
- Ensure that you develop training and development opportunities for those in existing positions of leadership, as well as for inexperienced newcomers.

Source: Modified from Cragg, in Chambers et al. (2007).

WORKPLACE-BASED LEARNING

With a supportive organisation, aspiring leaders can experiment in the higher-stakes setting of a practice-based project. Leaders must have innovative ideas and the ability to implement change. A project that is under their control but effectively supervised will unearth hidden abilities. To minimise the risk that funding will disappear part of the way through, as priorities change, you should ensure that there is active engagement by the organisation so that projects can be discussed and developed together with the aspiring leader, and that activities are as congruent with the development plan of the organisation as they are with that of the project lead.

IMPOSTERISM

One significant area an educational supervisor or mentor can help with for aspiring new leaders is the so called 'imposter phenomenon'. Described as 'a creeping sense of professional inadequacy' (Morgenstern and Dallaghan 2020), it has been suggested that imposterism is an almost universal finding at some time in the career trajectory from student to senior healthcare professional. Despite external evidence to the contrary, when suffering a bout of imposterism, our learner (or we?) might feel they are out of their depth and about to be 'found out'. Achievements are minimised or put down to 'luck'.

It appears to arise in high-achievers, perfectionists and hyper self-critical individuals and might be pervasive in all their interactions with others. If left unchecked it can lead to anxiety, depression and burn-out. The challenge in recognising it is that it exists along a spectrum with factors for success such as conscientiousness and attention to detail. Despite their success, affected individuals never seem to achieve an inner sense of satisfaction; they may resort to working ever harder to the point of exhaustion. It seems to occur at times of transition, perhaps when a person moves from the safety of an area in which they did well to one that is more challenging e.g. high school into university, university into health professions training, training to fully fledged autonomous healthcare professional. Being surrounded by new colleagues who appear to be succeeding effortlessly, when they might be struggling with the transition, reinforces their belief in their own inadequacy.

Morgenstern and Dallaghan use the term *Behaviors Associated with Feelings of Imposterism* (BAFI) to describe one way we might recognise when it is happening and when we might be able to step in to help. Colleagues with BAFI might exhibit avoidance behaviours, they might not put themselves forward for projects or jobs, because they 'know' they will fail; or because they fear that people don't really like them and might be jealous of their success. This can result in 'hiding out'. The corollary of that of course is you cannot get a job you do not apply for, so the resulting lack of success further fuels the sense of inadequacy. (See Box 22.4 for a suggested self-assessment quiz.)

BOX 22.4 YOUNG IMPOSTER SYNDROME QUIZ

1. Do you secretly worry that others will find out you're not as bright and capable as they think you are?
2. Do you sometimes shy away from challenges because of a nagging self-doubt?
3. Do you tend to chalk your accomplishments up to being a 'fluke', 'no big deal' or the fact that people just 'like' you?
4. Do you hate making a mistake, being less than fully prepared, or not doing things perfectly?
5. Do you tend to feel crushed even by constructive criticism, seeing it as evidence of your 'ineptness'?
6. When you do succeed, do you think 'Phew, I fooled them this time, but I may not be so lucky next time'?
7. Do you believe that other people (students, colleagues, competitors) are smarter and more capable than you?
8. Do you live in fear of being found out, discovered, or unmasked?

Responding 'Yes' to five or more of these questions is considered a positive finding of imposter syndrome.

Source: Adapted from Villwock et al. (2016).

How can we, as educators, help? These suggestions are adapted from Morgenstern and Dallaghan (2020):

1. Start early in training to let learners (and faculty) know that having feelings of imposterism is a nearly ubiquitous occurrence. Consider sharing your own experiences.

2. At points of transition in the education continuum, including stepping up to a leadership role, remind learners what they are likely to sense in the next few months and reassure them that the perceptions are common, real and often situationally appropriate.
3. When faculty are undergoing development for mentoring/advising/coaching roles, address imposterism to raise awareness and also to allow them to express any feelings they might have.
4. Consider running sessions that address:
    *   The value of some sense of discomfort to avoiding complacency and driving lifelong learning.
    *   The importance of forgiveness of failure in self and others.
    *   The risks and benefits of setting perfection as one's personal standard of performance.

CONCLUSION: LEADERSHIP AND CREATIVITY

There is much interest in the way in which 'creativity' might apply to healthcare service development. Effective leaders frequently provide new direction, inspiration and ideas, which implies imagination and creativity. However, if their function is to be catalysts, their main roles may be to recognise or enable creativity in others.

Perhaps creative leaders are those who can find better ways of doing things, either themselves or through others. However, if such inspiration is associated with inadequate communication skills (or feelings of imposterism?), this situated leadership (leadership demonstrated at the point where it is needed) might go unnoticed and untapped. To ensure implementation, creative leadership must be associated with effective support and 'followership'.

We might all need to adopt the oscillating position, sometimes be leaders and at other times be followers. Mutual respect, open-mindedness and the ability to speak up and to listen are essential leadership qualities.

Aspiring leaders might become disillusioned about the ability of the healthcare system to react and respond to challenge. You can protect learners from the risks of cynicism by helping them to develop as 'imaginative professionals' (Power 2008; Barnett 2008). This model links the inner world of values with the external world of public policy, and predicts that some protection can be obtained against the corrosive effects of 'performativity'. Performativity results when tasks are organised (or required) that seek to raise standards by looking directly at outcomes, rather than inputs or processes. It can infuriate healthcare professionals who characterise it as a 'tick-box' exercise. Healthcare leadership needs to find a new voice. By engaging with the process of change in healthcare through leadership and speaking out about the shared values of healthcare workers, you can cultivate an environment in which 'creative professionalism', a new inclusive discourse, can flourish (Barnett 2008).

RESOURCES

The Healthcare Leadership self-assessment tool is free to access and available here:

www.leadershipacademy.nhs.uk/resources/healthcare-leadership-model/
supporting-tools-resources/healthcare-leadership-model-self-assessment-tool
Other resources can be found here: www.leadershipacademy.nhs.uk/resources

Examples of established UK training programmes

The King's Fund: For 'Support at every stage of your leadership journey' www.kingsfund.org.uk/courses
National Health Service: 'Programmes to help you grow as a leader' www.leadershipacademy.nhs.uk/programmes
- The Edward Jenner programme to build foundation-level leadership skills
- Mary Seacole programme for those in their first leadership role
- Rosalind Franklin programme for mid-level leaders aspiring to lead large and complex programmes departments, services or systems
- Elizabeth Garrett Anderson programme for middle to senior leaders, to help challenge the status quo, drive lasting change and prepare for senior roles (leads to an MSc in Healthcare Leadership)
- Nye Bevan programme for senior leaders who want to move into a board role
- Stepping Up programme for tailored support for Black, Asian and minority ethnic (BAME) leaders
- Ready Now programme to support senior BAME leaders to move into board level positions and significantly more senior roles

Royal College of Nursing (RCN) Clinical Leadership programmes: www.rcn.org.uk/professional-development/professional-services/leadership-programmes
- Introduction to Leadership programme, designed for levels 2–4; 'to help you grow in confidence as a leader'
- The Developing Leadership programme, designed for nursing staff level 5 or equivalent
- Clinical Leadership programme for future clinical leaders working at levels 6 and 7; to 'help you to create a culture of innovation and give you the confidence to lead a team through organisational change'
- System Leadership programme to 'Guide you through the complex political structures to help implement changes to policy and practice', designed for level 8 and above
- Demonstrating Value 'to equip frontline staff with the skills, tools, and techniques for change'

- **Royal College of General Practitioners:** Offers training in 'Compassionate, collaborative and inclusive leadership approaches' www.rcgp.org.uk/training-exams/discover-general-practice/leadership-and-management.aspx
- **Royal College of Physicians** www.rcplondon.ac.uk/education-practice/courses/topic/leadership
- **Royal College of Surgeons** www.rcseng.ac.uk/careers-in-surgery/careers-support/leadership

REFERENCES

Allen M. (2006) *Creating successful e-learning: A rapid system for getting it right first time, every time.* San Francisco, CA: Pfeiffer.

Barnett R. (2008) Critical professionalism in an age of supercomplexity. In Cunningham B. (ed) *Exploring professionalism.* London: Institute of Education.

Benmira S. and Agboola M. (2021) *BMJ Leader,* 5: 3–5. DOI: 10.1136/leader-2020-000296. Available at https://bmjleader.bmj.com/content/leader/5/1/3.full.pdf (Accessed 3.4.22).

Chambers R., Mohanna K. and Spurgeon P. (2007) *How to succeed as a leader.* Oxford: Radcliffe Publishing.

Darzi A. (2008) *High quality care for all. NHS next stage review.* London: Department of Health. Available at https://assets.publishing.service.gov.uk/government/uploads/system/uploads/attachment_data/file/228836/7432.pdf (Accessed 3.4.22).

Department of Health (2009) Available at www.aemh.org/images/AEMH_documents/2018/16_Inspiring_leaders_Dept-of-health.pdf (Accessed 3.4.22).

Morgenstern B. and Dallaghan G.B. (2021) Should medical educators help learners reframe imposterism? *Teaching and Learning in Medicine,* 33(4): 445–452. DOI: 10.1080/10401334.2020.1856112.

NHS Leadership Academy (2013) *Healthcare leadership model.* Leeds: The Leadership Academy. Available at www.leadershipacademy.nhs.uk/resources/healthcare-leadership-model/structure-healthcare-leadership-model (Accessed 3.4.22).

Nicol E., Mohanna K. and Cowpe J. (2014) Perspectives on clinical leadership: A qualitative study of the views of senior healthcare leaders in the UK. *Journal of the Royal Society of Medicine,* 107(7): 277–286.

Power S. (2008) The imaginative professional. In Cunningham B. (ed) *Exploring professionalism.* London: Institute of Education.

Tooke J. (2008) *Aspiring to excellence: Findings and final recommendations of the independent inquiry into modernising medical careers.* London: MMC Inquiry. Available at www.asit.org/assets/documents/MMC_FINAL_REPORT_REVD_4jan.pdf (Accessed 3.4.22).

Villwock J.A., Sobin L.B., Koester L.A. and Harris T.M. (2106) Impostor syndrome and burnout among medical students: A pilot study. *International Journal of Medical Education,* 7: 364–369.

Wilkie V. and Mohanna K. (2017) View from the top: A thematic analysis of interviews with top healthcare leaders in the UK about leadership and how UK GPs should prepare for it. *BMJ Leader,* 2018(2): 136–139.

Wilkie V. and Spurgeon P. (2009) *Management for new GPs.* London: Royal College of General Practitioners.

CHAPTER 23

Applying education and training to the requirements of the healthcare system

This chapter looks at several challenging areas of practice including:

- Clinical governance
- Involving the public and patients in the planning and delivery of healthcare
- Involving patients in teaching
- Putting changes into practice

Many of these skills require the development of the organisation as well as helping individual professionals to develop specific skills. Leaders of clinical governance must learn how to motivate others while taking a wider perspective that encompasses the work of other management and clinical professionals. Individual practitioners should link their clinical practice closely with research evidence, and must listen to the views of patients and the public with regard to healthcare system priorities.

TEACHING ABOUT CLINICAL GOVERNANCE

Clinical governance is about implementing care within an environment in which clinical effectiveness can flourish, by establishing a facilitatory culture. Implementation of clinical governance is only possible if practitioners know what it is (see Box 23.1), what the organisation requires, and how to apply appropriate knowledge, skills and attitudes in practice. Education in isolation from active practice or without the necessary resources (e.g. skills, access to information technology, and the time available to professionals and non-clinical staff to undertake the associated work) cannot achieve the successful implementation of clinical governance.

DOI: 10.1201/9781003352532-28

BOX 23.1 COMPONENTS OF CLINICAL GOVERNANCE

- Clinical audit
- Risk management
- Evidence-based clinical practice
- Development of clinical leadership skills
- Managing the clinical performance of colleagues
- Continuing education/professional development for all staff
- Health needs assessment
- Learning from mistakes
- Effective management of poorly performing colleagues

Source: Adapted from the National Centre for Clinical Audit (NCCA 1998).

TEACHING ABOUT THE MEANING OF CLINICAL GOVERNANCE

Clinical governance cannot be taught effectively from the perspective of a single discipline in a classroom, because establishing clinical governance necessitates a change in culture. Teaching should include learning about negotiation, political awareness and finding out others' opinions, roles and responsibilities. Effective implementation of clinical governance requires the whole organisation to be flexible to change in response to individuals' learning and application of clinical governance in their workplaces. A combination of activities is likely to be needed, such as paper-based and electronic newsletters, workshops, lectures, seminars and tutorials and involvement of learners in practice-based quality improvement projects (QIPs) to try out and test ideas. Projects should be reviewed both in departmental or practice meeting to disseminate good practice and also in the individual's appraisal, and learners could compile a portfolio describing their contribution to their practice's or unit's programme of developments or overall clinical governance effort. Many organisations publish guidance on how to initiate and complete a QIP (e.g. the RCGP learning network at www.rcgp.org.uk/qi-ready; you will need to register to access the learning materials).

The components of clinical governance were originally set out in a UK government White Paper (NHS 1997). Since then, different organisations (NCCA 1998; RCGP 1998; RCN 1998) have applied the meaning of clinical governance to their special areas of interest (see Boxes 23.1–23.3).

BOX 23.2 APPROACH ADOPTED BY THE ROYAL COLLEGE OF GENERAL PRACTITIONERS TO CLINICAL GOVERNANCE

Protecting patients
- Registration/revalidation of professional qualifications
- Identifying unacceptable variations in care and areas in need of improvement

- Managing and minimising poor performance of colleagues
- Risk management

Developing people
- Continuing professional development or lifelong learning
- Development and implementation of guidelines and protocols for 'best practice'
- Personal accreditation
- Recognising and celebrating success

Developing teams and systems
- Learning from what other teams do well
- Clinical audit
- Development and implementation of guidelines and protocols for 'best practice'
- Recognising and celebrating success
- Evidence-based clinical practice
- Improving cost-effectiveness
- Listening to the views of patients and carers
- Practice accreditation
- Through all of the above, promoting accountability and transparency

A baseline for individual learners might be as follows:
- To identify their own learning needs and plan an appropriate educational programme
- To know something of their organisation's strategic or business plan
- To have basic skills in critical appraisal and searching for evidence relevant to best practice in their field
- To know the government's clinical priorities relating to them
- To be able to undertake clinical audit
- To know what constitutes clinical and non-clinical risks in the course of their work or in the workplace
- To understand accountability and its relationship to the healthcare system
- To be engaged in risk minimisation and know how to act if a significant event occurs
- To know how to involve consumers and act on their feedback as an integral part of day-to-day work

Source: RCGP (1999).

BOX 23.3 PROCESSES FOR CLINICAL GOVERNANCE ADOPTED BY THE ROYAL COLLEGE OF NURSING

- Patient- or client-focused approach
- Integrated approach to managing and improving quality

- Effective multi-professional teamwork
- Information sharing and networking
- Open culture: learning from mistakes

Source: RCN (1998).

When teaching learners about the implementation of clinical governance, you are likely to encounter the following challenges:

- Teaching the theory when the infrastructure and resources (information technology and software, data collection, support and accountability systems) to practise in this way are inadequate.
- The managers and chief executives of healthcare organisations possibly having little understanding of the topic and how to facilitate its application.
- Teaching evidence-based practice to individuals whose colleagues do little to follow suit.
- Encouraging professionals to own standards or guidelines of good practice, or to set their own.
- Running multi-professional CPD when professionals from single disciplines cling to their territorial traditions (SCOPME 1997).
- Teaching about national priorities and establishing the extent and nature of their local adoption where there may be conflicting guidelines.
- Limited knowledge of the evidence for and constraints on best practice in prescribing.
- Teaching professionals to view 'health' as a broad concept that encompasses physical, mental, social and environmental well-being.
- Teaching the benefits of a learning, non-blaming culture when professionals operate in a competitive environment, and mistakes and complaints are viewed as serious failures.
- Teaching the theory of cost-effectiveness when there are few systems for fair and responsible prioritisation of resources at local or national levels.
- Learning how to establish meaningful user/non-user involvement in policy, planning and monitoring of care.
- Understanding the legal implications of containment of demand and maintenance of performance standards.
- Motivating learners to want to make change work when multiple ongoing amendments to healthcare system policies and priorities have left them 'change fatigued'.
- Finding protected time to do the work involved in undertaking clinical governance effectively.

Promoting understanding about what the organisation requires will focus on making sure that the principles of good practice in the application of clinical governance are fulfilled in a coordinated way across the patch. These will include the following:

- Delivering local priorities such as those in the healthcare organisation's local delivery plan
- Addressing national healthcare priorities
- Clinical and management practices being based on best evidence as far as possible
- Setting up structures and systems for delivering the components of clinical governance

Teaching the application of clinical governance in practice will require education about how to do the following:

- Establish and maintain a quality improvement culture
- Motivate others to integrate the core components into their everyday work
- Evaluate changes in practice
- Specify and measure health gains
- Use the most appropriate type of consumer involvement for particular settings or situations
- Obtain and apply information about populations or clinical matters

Your clinical governance educational programme might have a multi-pronged approach, as follows:

- Teaching practitioners different ways to find out about patients' concerns and what they would like to see changed (the term 'patient' is used here to include user, non-user, carer and the general public) (McIver 1993).
- Teaching managers how to organise a coherent plan for clinical governance across their practice, unit or organisation. This will involve knowing what the priorities are in relation to the organisation's strategic goals and may include any and every aspect of organisational development, mapping out baseline resources, undertaking a needs assessment, improving information systems and establishing a learning, non-blaming culture.
- Teaching clinicians how to identify and agree several priorities on which to focus their clinical governance development in accordance with both the organisation's priorities and their own professional priorities.
- Teaching non-clinical staff to identify and agree several priorities for clinical governance in line with the priorities of both the organisation and their clinical colleagues. Ensuring that those in supportive posts realise that their contribution is vital for healthcare professionals to be able to provide effective face-to-face care.

- Encouraging each set of staff as uni-disciplinary or multi-professional groups to develop action plans in those agreed priority areas that either incorporate the core components or justify why core components are not relevant. Their action plans should make the purpose, process, expected outcomes and people's roles and responsibilities clear.
- Encouraging interaction between managers and healthcare professions should ensure that the 'bottom-up' priorities are consistent with 'top-down' priorities. This should help managers to see that healthcare professionals have the resources necessary to implement clinical governance, and healthcare professionals to view managers in a positive light with regard to improvement in the quality of care and services.
- Teaching those involved in implementing clinical governance the importance of monitoring progress and outcomes and revising associated action programmes as necessary.
- Developing a learning culture within the organisation, and developing new ways of working and problem solving (Garcarz et al. 2003).

TEACHING HOW TO INVOLVE PUBLIC AND PATIENTS IN THE PLANNING AND DELIVERY OF HEALTHCARE

It is difficult to teach the theory of involving the public and patients in the planning or delivery of healthcare without learners also obtaining first-hand practical experience. When required to establish what people think, many health professionals turn to a questionnaire survey. This has many disadvantages – for example, the great potential for exclusion of elderly, visually impaired, mentally ill and homeless people, depending on how participants are identified and the actual method that is chosen. Teachers must therefore have considerable practical knowledge and understanding of ways in which biases in sampling and processing surveys can be minimised (see also Chapter 21).

Such teaching requires a combination of knowledge and application of research methodology, information gathering, management, health policy, needs assessments, health economics and communication (see Box 23.4). Some teaching may be delivered through traditional methods such as lectures, seminars and workshops describing others' experiences. However, you must also provide opportunities for facilitated hands-on experience, perhaps by:

- Linking a less experienced practice, ward or department with ones that have undertaken successful consultation exercises previously
- Inviting an expert facilitator to lead a group of professionals through the planning and execution of real examples
- Arranging 'shadowing' to allow less experienced professionals to observe more expert professionals
- Undertaking a planned consultation

BOX 23.4 CRITERIA THAT SHOULD BE TAUGHT AS GOOD PRACTICE IN ANY EXERCISE THAT INVOLVES AND ENGAGES THE PUBLIC OR PATIENTS IN THE PLANNING OR DELIVERY OF HEALTHCARE

- Specify the purpose of the consultation.
- Create a timetabled programme at the planning stage. Include details of the aim, method, expected outcomes, feedback and review.
- Ensure that the method of obtaining the views of users, carers and the public is appropriate for the question posed and the information required.
- The exercise should be necessary. Is the information already available elsewhere?
- Select an appropriate method and be able to justify this choice.
- There should be sufficient resources to carry out a well-constructed consultation process.
- Lay involvement should be sought and achieved at an early stage in the process of planning or providing care.
- Seek statistical advice early on to find out how many people to survey and check the design.
- Feed back the results to those who contributed to the exercise.
- Decisions or changes should be made as a result of the exercise. If they were not, this lack of change should be justified.
- The consultation process should involve a representative group of people central to the purpose of the consultation. The extent to which the target population groups were included, the processes by which the citizens were involved, the response rates and whether the consultation process favoured representatives with particular skills should all be stated.
- The learner should be aware of the impacts, benefits and drawbacks of involvement of the public.
- The learner should be aware of how conflicts of interest (e.g. competing priorities) were resolved.

Source: From Chambers et al. (2003).

INVOLVING PATIENTS IN TEACHING

Consider training patients to become effective teachers, including involving them in teaching healthcare teachers about utilising patients as teachers. Patients can be trained to become standardised patients – that is, patients who have a specific condition and are taught to present themselves consistently to allow healthcare students or professionals to practise, or be assessed on, communication, diagnostic or examination skills. Standardised patients are not to be confused with simulated patients. The latter are actors who are trained to present themselves as having a particular condition. The consistency fostered by using either standardised or simulated patients is beneficial for the purposes of assessment. Learners are able to test different management approaches in a 'safe' environment, and to obtain feedback about the effectiveness of each – a unique and invaluable opportunity that cannot be provided in the clinical setting (see more on this in Chapter 19).

In order to develop patients as effective teachers, you must teach them to succeed when faced with presentations, meetings, focus groups, surveys, role playing and facilitation. When considering utilising patients as teachers, you should address the following issues:

- Commitment, building trust, and engaging with, empowering and promoting the inclusion of patients as teachers
- Practical issues (e.g. travel, parking, accessibility, communication)
- Respecting patients and taking their diverse and individual needs into account
- Prompt and appropriate payment and non-monetary rewards
- Power differentials and empowering patients

BOX 23.5 KEY COMPONENTS OF PATIENT-CENTRED CARE FOR WHICH IT COULD BE PARTICULARLY BENEFICIAL TO INVOLVE PATIENTS AS TEACHERS

- Partnership: help for someone with a problem, achieved through partnership between that person and health professionals.
- Empowerment: help for patients with problems to find the best ways of helping themselves.
- Judgement: the person with the problem is the only one who really understands their experience and problem.
- Values: people's values and priorities change with time. They may be quite different from the health professional's values, but no less valid.
- Autonomy: a fundamental right of every individual. Illness, disability, low income, unemployment and other forms of social exclusion mean a loss of some aspects of autonomy in society.
- Listening: active non-judgemental listening is core to helping people, and crucial to gaining an understanding of people's problems.
- Shared decision making: people with ongoing problems need to be able to take their own decisions about the care of their clinical condition, based on expert information communicated to them by health professionals. Patients do value shared decision making, but not as much as other key attributes of consultations, such as having a doctor or nurse who listens, and being provided with easily understood information. Shared decision making leads to concordance, which should be the goal of all shared decision-making encounters between health professional and patient.

Effective teaching in this domain will focus on helping learners to appreciate what patient-centred healthcare delivery means (see Box 23.5) and the balance to be achieved between patients' needs and preferences. Patients in a teaching role will have more impact on learners than a professional teacher when discussing the feelings of vulnerability, isolation and loss of control that accompany illness.

Patient-teachers can help learners to appreciate the potential power imbalance that is created by the superior knowledge of the healthcare professional. They can promote shared decision making as the middle ground between informed choice, where decisions are left entirely to the patient, and traditional, paternalistic medical decision making. This means two-way information giving (medical and personal) between the clinician and the patient concerning all of the options available, with the final decision being made jointly.

Tips from experienced teachers

- If you do recruit patients as teachers of health professionals and/or managers, prepare them well and look after them.
- Be clear about the purpose.
- Target the patient contribution for maximum gain. Don't exhaust them or keep them hanging around.
- Enable your patient-teacher to be well prepared and confident. Describe the nature of the learners and what sort of things will be most useful for them to hear about.
- Protect the patient from the 'audience'. Don't allow the patient-teacher to be hassled or to be expected to answer questions that are too challenging or personal.
- Encourage learners to realise the benefits of hearing the patient's perspective at first hand.

TEACHING ABOUT CHANGE

Much is known about the effects of change on an organisation and workforce. However, the gaps between theory and practice and the general lack of application of research into clinical practice are well recognised. This is the focus of translational medicine. Effective ways of teaching about changing practice, such that those changes are widely put into place, continue to be elusive.

People underestimate the barriers and hurdles to be overcome before change will be made and sustained. These barriers include the following (from Dunning et al. 1998):

- Lack of perception of relevance
- Lack of resources
- Short-term outlook
- Conflicting priorities

- Difficulty in measuring outcomes
- Lack of necessary skills
- No history of multidisciplinary working
- Limitations of the research evidence on effectiveness
- Perverse incentives
- Intensity of contribution required

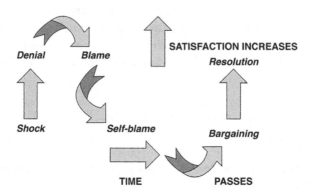

FIGURE 23.1 Stages of change.

Any teaching programme that is intended to involve and motivate learners to effect changes in practice must address those barriers that the individual learner can influence. It should also provide the necessary additional knowledge and skills for learners to be able to understand the need for change and the practical means to put change into practice. Even then, change will not be possible unless healthcare service managers are committed to it and are prepared to alter the environment to make it happen.

You must help learners to understand how people react to change (see Figure 23.1). Initially they are surprised, even if change is anticipated. Then they move from surprise/shock to denying that it will happen. After the denial phase they look for somebody to blame for what has happened – often the individual(s) who announce the change. After general blame comes self-blame.

Part of the next stage, the bargaining, involves negotiating that if they do it *this* way they are going to be able to do *that*. Eventually they arrive at the resolution phase, where they have accepted the organisational change.

Different people pass through the stages of change differently according to individual and situational factors. When change is imposed, people are generally much more resistant and move more slowly. If the effect of the change is serious, feelings about it will be stronger and longer will be spent in the denial, blame and self-blame stages.

PLANNING FOR CHANGE

The effective teacher will help learners to address change by clarifying where they are heading and identifying the causes of dissatisfaction. Learners should plan how to reach their target and find their way in staged steps to measure their progress.

Learners should be taught to recognise the roles that people play in response to change. For example:

- The rebel – 'I don't see why I should'.
- The victim – 'I suppose you will make me, but I will drag my feet'.
- The oppressor – 'You all have to do it'.
- The rescuer – 'I will save you all from this terrible change'.

TIPS FOR MAKING CHANGES

Give learners a checklist for planning change that they can adapt to their particular situation.

- Have realistic time scales and be flexible.
- Provide clear communication about what is happening.
- Consult with all staff, identifying all problems as they occur.
- Plan for more resources and time than you expect to use.
- Fix interval markers of progress.
- Feed information back to everyone about what is happening.
- Identify anxieties and try to resolve them.
- Consider the effects of this change on other services and people.
- Beware of too many changes taking place at once.
- Recognise that change can be hijacked by vested interests, and the direction altered.
- Be prepared to change direction if necessary.
- Beware of a lack of commitment from others.

MOTIVATING PEOPLE TO CHANGE, TO DO A BETTER JOB

The best way to discover what motivates people is to ask them. People are motivated by different things. Some of the best motivators for fulfilling health professionals' needs are:

- Interesting and/or useful work
- A sense of achievement
- Responsibility
- Opportunities for career progression or professional development
- Gaining new skills or competences
- A sense of belonging to a healthcare organisation or practice team
- Personal or written congratulations from a respected colleague or immediate superior
- Public recognition
- Announcement of success at team meetings
- Recognising that the last job was well done and asking for an opinion on the next one

- Providing specific and frequent feedback (positive feedback first)
- Providing information on how the task has affected the performance of the organisation or the management of a patient
- Encouragement to increase their knowledge and skills to do even better
- Making time to listen to ideas, complaints or difficulties
- Learning from mistakes and making visible changes

Human nature makes people respond better to praise than to punishment. So when you teach others about motivation, emphasise the importance of praise and celebrating people's achievements.

As with any feedback, start with the positive things (see Chapter 15). Praise should come:

- Immediately after the successful completion of part or all of a particular task
- From someone who knows what the task involved (not a remote committee)
- From an understanding of what the task involved

REFERENCES

Chambers R., Drinkwater C. and Boath E. (2003) *Involving patients and the public.* 2nd edn. Oxford: Radcliffe Medical Press.

Dunning M., Abi-Aad G., Gilbert D., et al. (1998) *Turning evidence into everyday practice.* London: King's Fund.

Garcarz W., Chambers R. and Ellis S. (2003) *Make your healthcare organisation a learning organisation.* Oxford: Radcliffe Medical Press.

McIver S. (1993) *Obtaining the views of health service users about quality of information.* London: King's Fund.

National Centre for Clinical Audit (NCAA) (1998) *Autumn newsletter.* London: National Centre for Clinical Audit.

National Health Service Executive (1997) *The new NHS: Modern, dependable.* London: Department of Health.

Royal College of General Practitioners (RCGP) (1999) *Practical advice on the implementation of clinical governance in primary care in England and Wales.* London: Royal College of General Practitioners.

Royal College of Nursing (RCN) (1998) *Guidance for nurses on clinical governance.* London: Royal College of Nursing.

Standing Committee on Postgraduate Medical and Dental Education (SCOPME) (1997) *Multi-professional working and learning: Sharing the educational challenge.* London: Standing Committee on Postgraduate Medical and Dental Education.

Further resources

Association of Standardized Patient Educators. Available at www.aspeducators.org/.

CHAPTER 24

Values based education and training[1]

··

THE CHALLENGE OF DEFINING PROFESSIONALISM

In all health systems, all around the world, it would be difficult to find one that did not place central emphasis on 'professionalism', both in codes of conduct for healthcare practitioners and as a key element of curriculum design. If you were to ask patients, most likely they would not find professionalism hard to define; it would include elements of 'doing the right thing', 'being trustworthy' and 'being good at their job'. However, an international definition has proven hard to pin down despite a wealth of literature (O'Sullivan et al. 2021). It is not surprising therefore, that a consensus on how to ensure healthcare graduates achieve the high standards expected of them, and how to teach and assess professionalism, has not developed.

In addition, in some regions of the world we are seeing a change in the way the healthcare professions are seen by regulators, patients and the public. We see perhaps less emphasis on self-regulation and more focus on managerial control to ensure 'professionalism'; plus what has been called a 'democratisation of knowledge' so that information is not just in the hand of a privileged few but available to be consulted by all, via the internet and other sources. Definitions that hinge on possession of expert knowledge are perhaps becoming less relevant.

In the UK, in a 2005 report on healthcare professionalism, the Royal College of Physicians (RCP) defined medical professionalism as 'a set of values, behaviours and relationships that underpin the trust the public has in doctors' (RCP 2005). In their most recent attempt at a definition in 2018 the RCP concludes: 'There is increasingly

---

[1] Some of the content of this chapter, by the same authors, also appears in Wass V. (ed) (2023) *WONCA family medicine series: Family medicine in the undergraduate curriculum: Preparing medical students to work in evolving health care systems*. Taylor & Francis/CRC Press. (In press). With kind permission of the publisher and the authors and editors of both publications.

DOI: 10.1201/9781003352532-29

a gap between what doctors are trained to do and the realities of modern practice'. They abandoned the search for a revised definition of professionalism and instead aimed to: 'explain, expand and interpret' their earlier definition (Tweedie et al. 2018).

DEFINING VALUES

One of the clues to why trying to define professionalism and use it to inform education and training is difficult lies in the important inclusion in the RCP definition of 'values'. Values are those principles which tend to determine a person's behaviour; principles which are 'action-guiding' but which can mean different things to different people. Even the word 'values' itself is hard to define. Sacket and colleagues defined it as the 'preferences, concerns and expectations' of individual patients and, we might add, of practitioners (Sacket et al. 2000).

A crucial feature of both healthcare and healthcare education is that they are values-laden activities. This can sometimes lead to differences of opinion in what 'doing the right thing' means. For example, situational judgement tests are widely used for selection or assessment in many industries and require candidates to imagine themselves into a scenario and decide how they might act. In order to be marked there needs to be some alignment with a panel of experts, model answer or 'ideal responses' (e.g. UCAT 2022). Model answers will be context specific and may not transfer well from one setting to another. Since healthcare deals with often difficult and frequently emotional decision-making, those values will be both complex (e.g. what do we mean by 'best interests'?) and sometimes conflicting (such as, at times, the two values of 'person-centred care' and 'public health'). Citizens, healthcare professionals and patients will hold a range of values as drivers for behaviours, arising from professional and personal codes and belief systems, from their experience and from their preferences. Values-based practice has been defined as 'a process that supports balanced decision making within a framework of shared values where complex and conflicting values are in play' (Fulford et al. 2012).

Consider the Academy of Medical Educators standards for medical educators, which includes the following 'core values' expected of healthcare teachers. How would you align yourself with these values? How might you demonstrate them in your annual appraisal as an educator?

AoME (2021) core values

Core value 1: Demonstrates professional identity and integrity

1. Works within a professional framework relevant to medical education.
2. Complies with relevant standards of professional practice.
3. Is an advocate for medical education.
4. Demonstrates a commitment to equality, diversity and inclusion.

5. Demonstrates an ethical educational philosophy.
6. Supports inter-, trans- and multi-professional education, learning with, from and about other professionals to improve collaborative care.

Core value 2: Is committed to scholarship and reflection in medical education

1. Is active in their own professional development as an educator.
2. Enhances the practice of medical education through analysis and a commitment to personal reflection.
3. Responds appropriately to feedback from colleagues, learners, patients and carers.
4. Advances medical education through scholarly endeavours of creation, application, synthesis and dissemination.

Core value 3: Demonstrates respect for others

1. Equality and diversity
   a. Ensures equality of opportunity for patients, students, trainees, staff and colleagues.
   b. Actively promotes and respects diversity in discharging their educational responsibilities.
2. Respect for wider society
   a. Balances the needs of high-quality service delivery with the needs of high-quality medical education.
   b. Is committed to providing safe and effective learning at all times.
3. Respect for patients
   a. Acts with due consideration for the emotional, physical and psychological well-being of patients, including maintaining the dignity and safety of patients at all times when discharging educational duties.
   b. Enhances the care of patients through medical education.
4. Respect for learners
   a. Acts with due consideration for the emotional, physical and psychological well-being of learners and identifies and signposts well-being support for learners.
   b. Supports learners in their personal and professional development.
5. Respect for colleagues
   a. Acts with due consideration for the emotional, physical and psychological well-being of colleagues within the interprofessional team.
   b. Supports all colleagues in their personal and professional development.

Core value 4: Promotes quality and safety of care

1. Ensures the safety of patients at all times.
2. Promotes high-quality clinical care.
3. Works within appropriate clinical governance and risk management frameworks, and maintains professional registration where appropriate.
4. Appropriately supports and manages learners in the clinical environment.

PROFESSIONALISM AND FITNESS TO PRACTISE: A COMPLEX RELATIONSHIP

In an attempt to 'professionalise' the behaviour of physicians, one response has sometimes been to increase regulatory measures of control such as revalidation and performance management. For example, the Indian Medical Council (Professional Conduct, Etiquette and Ethics) Regulations are currently being considered for revision. There is a risk however that such a rules-based approach to healthcare decision making in fact risks doing just the opposite, to 'de-professionalise and erode trust' (Shrewsbury and Mohanna 2010).

Kane, commenting on the proposed Indian revisions, calls for the medical profession to redefine professionalism for itself since a:

> purely control-based regulatory response to this [crisis of trust in the medical profession], as is being currently envisaged by the Parliament and the Supreme Court of India, runs the risk of undermining the trusting, interpersonal relations between doctors and their patients.
>
> *(Kane and Calnan 2017)*

This view is echoed by authors who see a risk that a punitive or regulatory approach, focussing on fitness to practise in the undergraduate curriculum, also fosters a negative view of professionalism which students and trainees may then perceive as a drive to avoid poor performance rather than develop good practice (O'Sullivan et al. 2021). Is there a risk that this sends a message to healthcare students that professionalism means 'staying out of trouble' or, worse still, 'not getting caught'? Innovations in undergraduate curricula such as elements of reward or commendation for excellence, perhaps in activities that extend outside the taught components and beyond the assessed components, attempt to redress this.

The impact of the null curriculum – negative, unintended learning experiences – particularly in the clinical setting, shows the importance of ensuring an alignment between our espoused values and the behaviours that are rewarded if we are to avoid negative role models for our students in the workplace (see Chapter 9). We can also see however that teaching about, and for, professionalism includes a need to help our students develop the tools to continue to monitor and develop professionalism both in themselves and others. We need to give our students the skills to reflect on what they see in practice, notice and respond to situations where behaviours are falling below expected standards and empower students to speak up on behalf of patients if they observe actions raising patient safety concerns. This might include reflective writing after clinical encounters, encouragement to document learning events and the skill and confidence to open 'courageous conversations' (NHSLA 2021).

VALUES-BASED PRACTICE (VBP)

Consider the role of the named nurse or therapist, or that of the GP or family physician, who takes pride in the role of advocate for her patient. Advocacy is perhaps considered one of the guiding principles (or values) that generalists will use, helping to signpost a patient through the mass of healthcare uncertainty. The enactment of professionalism in this context requires not a list of preferred (or 'right') outcomes, or adherence to rules, but fluidity with a process through which the expert family physician helps the patient make decisions that 'fit' with the way they see the world. However, it is also clear that some patients rely on what they perceive as expert-decision making from the healthcare professional to guide their choices and actions. In such a situation therefore, it is always important to make sure we explore the values of the patient as well as our own. We can think of healthcare professionalism as the competence of being able to explore and balance the three domains of the values of the patient, scientific healthcare values and our own personal values. An important element of the model of values-based practice is that of *dissensus*: that difference in values are explored and acknowledged, but are not necessarily 'merged' or agreed upon, as they would be in a consensus-building model. Differences of values remain differences, equally valid and readily available to enable decisions to be made sometimes one way and sometimes another depending on specific circumstances (Fulford et al. 2012, p. 179).

In May 2021 a straw-poll of around 50 colleagues across South Asia and the UK was carried out by the authors. Our respondents were experienced trainers, workplace-based assessors and examiners, and they were all in active clinical practice as GPs. It was not a scientific survey, more the email equivalent of a chat over coffee. Box 24.1 summarises their comments on aspects of professionalism, where there was agreement:

BOX 24.1 CORE ELEMENTS OF PROFESSIONALISM SHARED BY A GROUP OF GPS ACROSS SOUTH ASIA AND THE UK

Aspects of professionalism that graduates:

Should know:

- That community epidemiology of disease is different from hospitals
- The limits of their knowledge and skills,
- How to coordinate and oversee care within a team
- How generalist and specialist care fit together
- The importance of advocacy
- The importance of data management
- Financial and managerial aspects of healthcare provision

Should be able to do:

- Act in the best interests of the patient in front of them
- Solve problems
- Implement and apply policies and evidence
- Balance 'today's conversation' with future decision making with the patient
- Listen to the patient using 'ears, eyes and heart'
- Engage in population-based health systems development

Should be:

- Curious and interested in the patient
- Able to change – themselves, their approach, their systems
- Creative, imaginative leaders and owners of decisions
- Aware of the importance of creating a collaborative culture

Whilst these core aspects of professionalism were similar, Box 24.2 shows that some differences were seen that perhaps arise from differences in social context. Some of the GPs we asked seemed to be saying that there are some elements of professionalism that are expressed differently in their communities. There was a recognition that some of these elements are in a state of flux as healthcare systems develop which illustrates the importance of a focus on dissensus for critical thinking in decision making. The VBP model requires us to keep such differences in values visible and unsilenced, so they can be taken into account.

It seems likely that the positions represented by the two columns in Box 24.2 are expressions of values that should be considered to exist to a greater or lesser extent in all doctors and all citizens; both doctors and patients will sit somewhere on a spectrum between the two positions in terms of the importance of an aspect to them. It also seems likely that individual doctor–patient relationships will negotiate a way between the two positions depending on the individual values in play in that particular doctor–patient dyad, for any specific decision being considered. Perhaps there is in fact only one element of professionalism, the ability to recognise and respond creatively and imaginatively to such differences of values.

BOX 24.2: AREA OF VALUES-BASED DISSENSUS

UK GP trainers	South Asian GP trainers
The importance of work-life balance and knowing when to say no	*Being the best or 'never fail' approach*
Person-centered decision making	*Rules-based decision making*
Equality between patient and doctor	*Hierarchical culture, doctor expected to 'know'*

UK GP trainers	South Asian GP trainers
Primacy of patient in decision making	*Tendency towards doctors leading decisions*
Individualism in decision making	*Collectivism in decision making eg family involvement*

TEACHING VALUES-BASED PROFESSIONALISM IN PRACTICE

Consider the case outlined in Box 24.3. GPs around the world are likely to recognise similar scenarios. Try to put yourself in the shoes of the teacher in Box 24.3 and work through the exercise beneath.

BOX 24.3 CASE STUDY FOR TEACHING PROFESSIONALISM AND VALUES-BASED DECISION MAKING

Imagine you are in clinic when the student you are supervising knocks on your door.

'Is it ok if I quickly ask your advice?' they say. You look at the paper they have brought and see the name of a long-standing, elderly patient of yours. Your heart sinks as you notice the result showing a Prostate Specific Antigen (PSA) result of 12ng/ml. (The normal age adjusted upper limit in your local lab is 6.5.)

'The patient is not here' says your trainee, 'but his daughter is coming in later to get the result. She says she wants to talk about what the options are before deciding what the best thing will be to do for her Dad. Can I tell her the result?'

You think back to when you last saw your patient, when his dementia had started to significantly progress. You remember the close relationship this daughter has with her father and how he trusted and depended on her.

'Come in and sit down', you say to your student, 'this is not going to be a quick conversation.'

---

1. What options are open to you as the supervisor to manage this 'teachable moment'?
2. What would your first step be?
3. What are the complex and competing values at play in this scenario?
4. What is the range of possible outcomes?

Suggested responses:

1. What options are open to you as the trainer to manage this 'teachable moment'?
   You could say no: the daughter needs to make an appointment to bring her father along and, if the patient agrees, a joint consultation can be held. This draws on a principles-based model of healthcare ethics, where a patient's autonomy

is paramount and from this flows the principle of confidentiality. Your patient must consent to their information being shared, and all conversations about them should take place with them present.

You could say yes: its fine to disclose the information to the daughter. On a best-interests basis, the patient is no longer able to understand and retain some elements of the information given. His dementia (not the fact of the diagnosis but the impact of the condition) prevents him expressing an informed decision, so his daughter as the person who has some insight into what sort of decisions he has made in the past about his health is best placed to act on this behalf.

Either option could be right, depending on the patient and the context. In addition you might feel that if there is bad news to be broken, it is better to discuss this with the family before the patient or even that a referral straight to a consultant urologist is needed.

A values-based approach to professionalism means being open to the possibility of dissensus or difference in views. A good teacher uses this case as a way to demonstrate the importance of further exploration rather than jumping to a conclusion.

In addition, this might be a time to remind your student about the place of legal interventions such as the UK Lasting Power of Attorney for patients who lack capacity (Gov.uk 2007). Clinically you might need to check that your student knows what treatment options should be discussed and explained for a raised PSA and the pros and cons of the treatment options, including no further treatment.

2. What would your first step be?

A good teacher displays elements of professionalism by role modelling. An appropriate first step here might be to acknowledge that this is a difficult decision to be made and that there might be more than one 'right' course of action. You could congratulate your student for bringing it to you for discussion. This demonstrates the importance of 'knowing what to do when you don't know what to do', and appropriately seeking help from others, rather than following a potentially inappropriate course of action. By showing that we don't always know, we make it possible for students to feel that is also safe for them to say they don't know – a starting point for learning.

Whatever the decision, the consultation skills for such conversations with the patient or his daughter might be challenging. You could role play the imagined scenario and encourage the student to practise with phrases that might be useful and try to anticipate and prepare for different responses. You will want to ensure your student can manage the consultation and their approach to the patient and his family in a 'balanced' way without undue influence. (Your challenge is that here and now you are both in clinic, and there will be lots of other pressures on your mind, time being foremost perhaps.)

3. What are the complex and competing values at play in this scenario?

We might not know this patient, or his daughter, but we do know that since this is a healthcare scenario, there will be a range of values in play, some of which have been identified (best interests, respect for autonomy, importance of seeking help if you are not sure what the best course of action is). There will be others which will occur to you as you reflect on the case, such as first do no harm.

4. What is the range of possible outcomes?

Either the daughter, the father, or both might get angry or upset about the situation. The learner might also be upset at having to break bad news or manage their own uncertainty in the face of questions from the family. The possibility of cancer, the additional burden of further illness in a family living with dementia, the complexity of interpreting such blood test results (there may be a question for later about why the test was done; does the patient have distressing symptoms?) and the decision making about further tests or treatment are all areas of potential difficulty. But an effective consultation will guide this patient through these, and a good teacher will be able to use this case as a way of helping this student develop elements of professionalism for future practice.

FIVE TIPS FOR TEACHING PROFESSIONALISM

From our discussions with colleagues, trainees and trainers around the world we have developed five tips for teaching values-based professionalism in health professions education (see Box 24.4).

BOX 24.4 TEACHING VALUES BASED PROFESSIONALISM

1. Health professions educators and supervisors have a responsibility to create a climate that fosters debate about differences in values, to encourage discussion and exchange of ideas and develop an understanding that there may be more than one appropriate course of action.

2. Time, space and emotional support from tutors might be needed to encourage learners to reflect on personal motivating values as this might be a new activity for students used to 'finding out the right answer'.

3. The emphasis on seeking and rewarding individual high-achievers 'doing the right thing' in training should shift to a focus on developing 'imaginative professionals' with the ability to explore complex and conflicting values.

4. Critical reflection, such as in learning logs or diaries, should be encouraged as a 'safe space' to explore personal views and reactions to clinical challenges.

5. Values based practice should be considered an ongoing approach to developing professionalism and professional practice as an undergraduate and beyond.

REFERENCES

Academy of Medical Educators (2021) *Professional standards.* Cardiff: AoME. Available at www.medicaleducators.org/write/MediaManager/Documents/AoME_Professional_Standards_4th_edition_1.0_(web_full_single_page_spreads).pdf (Accessed 10.4.21).

Fulford K.W.M., Peile E. and Carroll H. (2012) *Essential values-based practice.* Cambridge: Cambridge University Press.

Gov.uk (2007) Lasting power of attorney. Available at www.gov.uk/power-of-attorney (Accessed 25.5.22).

Kane S. and Calnan M. (2017) Erosion of trust in the healthcare profession in India: Time for doctors to act. *International Journal of Health Policy and Management,* 6(1): 5–8.

NHS Leadership Academy (2021) Courageous conversations. Available at https://people.nhs.uk/guides/courageous-conversations (Accessed 27.8.21).

O'Sullivan H., van Mook W., Fewtrell R. and Wass V. (2021) Integrating professionalism into the curriculum: AMEE Guide No. 6. *Medical Teacher,* 34: e64–e77.

Royal College of Physicians (RCP) (2005) *Doctors in society: Medical professionalism in a changing world.* London: RCP.

Sacket D.L., Straus S.E., Scott Richardson W., Rosenberg W. and Haynes R.B. (2000) *How to practice and teach EBM.* 2nd edn. Edinburgh and London: Churchill Livingstone.

Shrewsbury D. and Mohanna K. (2010) Influencing medical professionalism: Innate, caught or taught? *Education for Primary Care,* 21(3): 199–202.

Tweedie J., Hordern J. and Dacre J. (2018) *Advancing medical professionalism.* London: Royal College of Physicians.

University Clinical Aptitude Test (UCAT) (2022) Available at www.ucat.ac.uk/about-ucat/ucat-scoring (Accessed 7.4.22).

Index

Note: Page locators in **bold** indicate a table. Page locators in *italics* indicate a figure.

Printed in the United States
by Baker & Taylor Publisher Services